ENDOCRINOLOGY RESEARCH AND CLINICAL DEVELOPMENTS

RENIN-ANGIOTENSIN SYSTEM

PHYSIOLOGY, ROLE IN DISEASE AND HEALTH IMPLICATIONS

ENDOCRINOLOGY RESEARCH AND CLINICAL DEVELOPMENTS

Additional books in this series can be found on Nova's website under the Series tab.

Additional e-books in this series can be found on Nova's website under the e-book tab.

PHYSIOLOGY – LABORATORY AND CLINICAL RESEARCH

Additional books in this series can be found on Nova's website under the Series tab.

Additional e-books in this series can be found on Nova's website under the e-book tab.

ENDOCRINOLOGY RESEARCH AND CLINICAL DEVELOPMENTS

RENIN-ANGIOTENSIN SYSTEM

PHYSIOLOGY, ROLE IN DISEASE AND HEALTH IMPLICATIONS

AYAKO HIMURA
AND
TAKESHI SATO
EDITORS

Nova Biomedical
New York

Library of Congress Cataloging-in-Publication Data

ISBN: 978-1-62417-788-0

Library of Congress Control Number: 2012955909

Published by Nova Science Publishers, Inc. † New York

Contents

Preface

The renin-angiotensin system (RAS) is a major hormonal system that plays an essential role in regulating salt-water balance and blood pressure. In this book, the authors discuss the physiology, role in disease and health implications of RAS. Topics include the function of the renin-angiotension-aldosterone system in ISIAH rats with stress-sensitive arterial hypertension; RAS implications for eye diseases, obesity and diabetes, and cardiovascular disease; intensive blockade of renin-angiotensin systems; glomerular renin-angiotensin system activation; the role of vitamin D in RAS; the renin-angiotensin system in the pathogenesis of intracranial aneurysms; and a discussion on whether angiotensin-converting enzyme inhibitors are a contradiction for contrast-induced nephropathy prophylaxis?

Chapter I - Expression of genes of the renin-angiotensin system (RAS) was studied in ISIAH rats with a stress-sensitive form of arterial hypertension in comparison with normotensive WAG strain. Renin (*Ren*), angiotensinogen (*Agt*), angiotensin converting enzyme (*Ace*), and AT1A and AT2 receptors (*Agtr1a* and *Agtr2*) mRNA levels in the renal, myocardial, adrenal, and some brain (hypothalamus and medulla oblongata) tissues was measured by the Real-time PCR. In the 4-month-old ISIAH rats, expression of *Ren*, *Ace,* and *Agtr1a* in the renal tissue was significantly lower than in the WAG counterparts. However, in the younger 1.5-month-old ISIAH rats, the low level of *Ace* and *Agtr1a* expression was combined with two time enhanced expression of the *Ren* gene.

In the young ISIAH rats no changes in myocardial genes expression were found. In myocardium of the adult ISIAHs, *Agtr1a* expression was slightly decreased, but the *Ace* mRNA was increased up to 80% as compared to WAG rats. This enhancement is proposed to be associated with myocardial hypertrophy.

Significant increase of *Agt* mRNA in the both hypothalamic and brainstem tissues of the young ISIAH rats may play a crucial role in enhancement of Ang II. Such increase in brain Ang II synthesis along with enhanced AT1A expression in medulla oblongata may lead to activation of the central sympathetic tone. The increase of *Agtr2* mRNA in hypothalamus may be considered as compensatory mechanism. All changes in brain genes expression were found only in the young, not adult ISIAH rats.

The adrenal function in the adult ISIAH rats is altered to a large extent. Hormonal response of the ISIAHs to acute stress disclosed an elevated aldosterone response. As for adrenal RAS gene expression, only *Agtr2* mRNA level in the young, not adult, ISIAHs was decreased by one third as compared to WAG controls.

It may be concluded that the development of the stress-sensitive arterial hypertension is associated with changes in the activity of the RAS. At the first step of the development of stress-dependent hypertension in the ISIAHs the activation of RAS is related to the conversion of Agt in the brain and kidneys, also imbalance in the brain and adrenal expression of the Ang II receptors. The hypertensive status at the second step pathology is stable and corresponds to the low-renin hypertension with enhanced sympathetic and HPAS responsiveness to stress.

Chapter II - The goal of this chapter is to review the most relevant scientific evidence supporting the role of the renin-angiotensin system (RAS) activation, in the pathogenesis of age-related macular degeneration (AMD) and diabetic retinopathy (DR), two leading causes of blindness in elderly and people of working age respectively, and highlight the importance of Angiotensin II (Ang II), prorenin, and prorenin receptor in the etiology of these diseases. Early AMD, include the presence of waste material in the form of focal deposits named drusen below the retinal pigment epithelium (RPE) and within Bruch's membrane, a stratified extracellular matrix situated between the choriocapillaris and RPE. Late (wet) AMD is characterized by inflammation and the growth of leaky new abnormal blood vessels under the RPE from the subjacent choroid known as choroidal neovascularization. The early stage of DR, non-proliferative diabetic retinopathy is identified by deposits forming in the retina. Proliferative diabetic retinopathy is characterized by neovascularization on or adjacent to the optic nerve and vitreous, pre-retinal hemorrhage, which occurs in the vitreous humor or front of the retina and ischemia. Extracellular matrix turnover (ECM), inflammation, and neovascularization are key cellular processes that play a central role in the pathogenesis of these deaseases. The scientific evidence to support the proposed role of Ang II, prorenin, and prorenin receptor-mediated cellular effects on subretinal deposits formation, inflammation and neovascularization is reviewed in depth.

Chapter III - For a few decades now, the renin-angiotensin system (RAS) has been well known for its implication in the regulation of blood pressure and fluid homeostasis. Furthermore, dysregulation of the RAS has been implicated in many pathological states including obesity, hypertension, diabetes and chronic kidney disease. Due to the elevated consumption of foods that are rich in fat, salt and glucose, typical of a Western diet, obesity and diabetes are two of the greatest causes of morbidity and consumption of health care resources in North America. Interestingly, inhibition of the RAS has been shown to induce weight loss, and increased activation of the RAS in obesity suggests a potential link between the RAS and obesity-related hypertension. Indeed, increased adipose tissue cell size has been associated with a stimulation of the local RAS activity in this tissue which then spills over into the circulation. This in turn contributes to an increase in the circulating levels of angiotensin II and may thus produce a vasoconstrictive state. Moreover, constant fat accumulation eventually causes adipose tissue inflammation, oxidative and nitritive stress which can promote the development of insulin resistance and, with time, type 2 diabetes which are also consequences of local RAS overactivation in the pancreas. Clinically, RAS inhibitors are by far the preferred anti-hypertensive treatment in patients at risk of developing diabetes as they do not impact negatively glucose homeostasis regulation. This chapter will detail the implication of the RAS in the pathology of obesity and diabetes.

Chapter IV - The renin-angiotensin system (RAS) is a major hormonal system that plays an essential role in regulating salt-water balance and blood pressure. Angiotensin II (Ang II) is the major active mediator of RAS. Ang II exerts its effects by activating a number of receptors, primarily type 1 (AT1R) and type 2 (AT2R). The role of both of these receptors in cardiovascular physiology and pathology has been widely studied. Besides stimulating salt and water retention via aldosterone, AT1R activation is thought to promote vasoconstriction, inflammation, oxidant stress and smooth muscle cell hypertrophy, whereas AT2R is believed to oppose the actions of AT1R. Lectin-like oxidized low density lipoprotein scavenger receptor-1 (LOX-1) is one of the major receptors responsible for binding, internalizing and degrading oxidized low density lipoprotein (ox-LDL). The activation of LOX-1 is also known to be related to the pathogenesis of several cardiovascular diseases. Recent findings, including those from our laboratory, have indicated that LOX-1 and Ang II receptors, especially AT1R, have a mutually facilitative interaction in the genesis of atherosclerosis, hypertension, myocardial ischemia, and cardiac remodeling. This chapter summarizes the interplay between LOX-1 and AT1R or AT2R in the pathogenesis of several cardiovascular diseases.

Chapter V - Intensive blockade of renin-angiotensin system has been tested in the treatment of renal disease associated to micro or macroalbuminuria, in congestive heart failure and also after myocardial infarction. Several authors have reported a superior effect of the combination of ACE inhibition and ARBs on microalbuminuria and on clinical proteinuria in patients with primary nephropathies as well as in type 1 and type 2 diabetic patients. A systematic review and meta-analysis has addressed this issue suggesting that concomitant therapy with an ARBs and an ACE inhibitor leads to greater reductions in proteinuria than monotherapy.

Nevertheless, there are no evidences that this kind of therapy can reduce renal disease progression to end stage renal failure. The ONTARGET trial cast some shadows on the use of dual blockade of renin-angiotensin system in ischemic cardiopathy. The combination of the ACE inhibitor and ARBs was associated with more adverse events without an increase in benefit in terms of cardiovascular mortality and morbidity reduction. On December, 20th 2011 Novartis announced that following the interim review of data from the ALTITUDE study a decision to terminate the trial has been taken on the recommendation of the independent Data Monitoring Committee overseeing the trial. Is this the end for dual blockade as therapeutic resource? Some could reasonable think that this is the safer position. But, are there alternative treatments for proteinuria? The answer unfortunately is not. In most patients there is not ethiological treatment for proteinuric renal disease, at least in this moment. It could be plead that ARBs megadosage could be the alternative to dual blockade. There are some reports on the use of very high dosage of ARBs for treatment of proteinuria; nevertheless we have not adequate head to head comparison which shown wether this option is more or less effective than dual blockade and, most important, wether it is safer.

Chapter VI - Sustained pathological glomerular remodeling accompanied by prominent cell proliferation and aberrant extracellular matrix (ECM) formation is the central biological feature of progressive glomerulonephritis (GN) leading to glomerular dysfunction and sclerosis. Accumulating evidence from clinical and basic research indicates that multiple mediators participate in the structural alterations of nephritic glomeruli. In particular, angiotensin II (Ang II), the principal bioactive peptide of the renin-angiotensin system (RAS), mediates glomerular hypertension, cell proliferation and pathological ECM remodeling in various types of progressive glomerular diseases. Recently, apart from the systemic Ang II-generating system (systemic RAS), the local (tissue) Ang II-generating system (local RAS) has been recognized and emphasized to be critically involved in Ang II-mediated pathological tissue remodeling (fibrosis). It is now evident that the kidney expresses all elements (renin, angiotensinogen, angiotensins, and angiotensin converting enzymes as well as their receptors) of the RAS, and locally produced Ang II contributes to not only kidney ontogeny but also to regulation of blood pressure (BP) and progression of chronic kidney disease (CKD). The purpose of this chapter is to review the role of kidney RAS, with particular focus on the role of glomerular RAS in the pathological glomerular remodeling observed in progressive GN.

Chapter VII - The primary function of the renin-angiotensin system (RAS) is to maintain fluid homeostasis and regulate blood pressure. It has been noted that vitamin D and RAS share many of the same risk factors, including both indirect - environment (seasonal and air pollution) and direct - genetics risk factors (human leukocyte antigen, vitamin D receptor, angiotensin-converting enzyme variants, microRNA, and apolipoprotein E).

Vitamin D has been known as a regulator of bone and mineral metabolism by regulating of calcium absorption in the gut and reabsorption by the kidney. The vitamin D receptor (VDR) is present in many tissues. Vitamin D and VDR may effect on the endothelial cells, blood pressure, cardiopathy, renal functions, and keratinocytes via modulating RAS.

The combination of vitamin D and RAS blockade has been proved to be effective synergistically in medicine.

Chapter VIII - "In recent years, the pathophysiology of intracranial (cerebral) aneurysms has been explored by several studies and multiple factors involved in the formation and rupture of intracranial aneurysms have been identified. Currently, researches indicate that the renin-angiotensin system (RAS) is one of the many factors potentially involved in the pathogenesis of intracranial aneurysms. This chapter discusses the pathogenesis of intracranial aneurysms, the nature and pathophysiology of the RAS, and how the RAS, specifically the brain RAS, plays a role in the pathogenesis of intracranial aneurysms."

Chapter IX - Contrast-induced nephropathy (CIN) is reported to be the third leading cause of acute renal failure.The role of angiotensin-converting enzyme (ACE) inhibitors in CIN is controversial. Some studies pointed out that it was effective in the prevention of CIN, while some concluded that it was a risk for CIN, especially for patients with pre-existing renal impairment. Nevertheless, it is a common practice in many centers to prescribe ACE inhibitors before coronary angiography. The most likely mechanisms leading to CIN are medullary hypoxia due to decreased renal blood flow (RBF) secondary to renal artery vasoconstriction and direct tubular toxicity by contrast media. Furthermore, experimental data suggest that an activated renin-angiotensin-aldosterone system, increased endothelin-1, and reactive oxygen species play a role in the pathogenesis of CIN and these can be inhibited by using ACE inhibitors.

In this context, the Authors review the medical literatures and discuss the pathogenesis, the role of renin-angiotensin-aldosterone system on the development of CIN and ACEI's effect on CIN.

In: Renin-Angiotensin System
Editors: Ayako Himura and Takeshi Sato
ISBN: 978-1-62417-788-0

Chapter I

Function of the Renin-Angiotensin-Aldosterone System in the ISIAH Rats with Stress-Sensitive Arterial Hypertension

***L. A. Fedoseeva*[1,*], *E. V. Antonov*[1,3], *L. O. Klimov*[1], *G. M. Dymshits*[1,2] *and A. L. Markel*[1,2]**
[1]Institute of Cytology and Genetics, Siberian Branch of the Russian Academy of Sciences, Novosibirsk, Russia
[2]Novosibirsk State University, Novosibirsk, Russia
[3]Institute of Physiology, Siberian Branch of the Russian Academy of Medical Sciences, Novosibirsk, Russia

Abstract

Expression of genes of the renin-angiotensin system (RAS) was studied in ISIAH rats with a stress-sensitive form of arterial hypertension in comparison with normotensive WAG strain. Renin (*Ren*), angiotensinogen (*Agt*), angiotensin converting enzyme (*Ace*), and AT1A and AT2 receptors (*Agtr1a* and *Agtr2*) mRNA levels in the renal, myocardial, adrenal, and some brain (hypothalamus and medulla oblongata) tissues was measured by the Real-time PCR. In the 4-month-old ISIAH rats, expression of *Ren*, *Ace,* and *Agtr1a* in the renal tissue was significantly lower than in the WAG counterparts. However, in the younger 1.5-month-old ISIAH rats, the low level of *Ace* and *Agtr1a* expression was combined with two time enhanced expression of the *Ren* gene.

In the young ISIAH rats no changes in myocardial genes expression were found. In myocardium of the adult ISIAHs, *Agtr1a* expression was slightly decreased, but the *Ace* mRNA was increased up to 80% as compared to WAG rats. This enhancement is proposed to be associated with myocardial hypertrophy.

[*] E-mail: frumgarts@ngs.ru or fedoseeva@bionet.nsc.ru.

Significant increase of *Agt* mRNA in the both hypothalamic and brainstem tissues of the young ISIAH rats may play a crucial role in enhancement of Ang II. Such increase in brain Ang II synthesis along with enhanced AT1A expression in medulla oblongata may lead to activation of the central sympathetic tone. The increase of *Agtr2* mRNA in hypothalamus may be considered as compensatory mechanism. All changes in brain genes expression were found only in the young, not adult ISIAH rats.

The adrenal function in the adult ISIAH rats is altered to a large extent. Hormonal response of the ISIAHs to acute stress disclosed an elevated aldosterone response. As for adrenal RAS gene expression, only *Agtr2* mRNA level in the young, not adult, ISIAHs was decreased by one third as compared to WAG controls.

It may be concluded that the development of the stress-sensitive arterial hypertension is associated with changes in the activity of the RAS. At the first step of the development of stress-dependent hypertension in the ISIAHs the activation of RAS is related to the conversion of Agt in the brain and kidneys, also imbalance in the brain and adrenal expression of the Ang II receptors. The hypertensive status at the second step pathology is stable and corresponds to the low-renin hypertension with enhanced sympathetic and HPAS responsiveness to stress.

The Abbreviations

BP	blood pressure
RAS	renin-angiotensin system
Ren	renin
Ren	gene encoding Ren
Agt	angiotensinogen
Agt	its gene
ACE	angiotensin converting enzyme
Ace	its gene
ACE2	angiotensin converting enzyme type2
Ace2	its gene
Ang II	angiotensin II
AT1A	Ang II receptor type 1A
Agtr1a	gene encoding AT1A
AT2	Ang II receptor type 2
Agtr2	gene for AT2
PRR	renin/prorenin receptor
PRR	or *Atp6ap2,* gene for PRR
Rpl30	ribosomal protein L30 gene
dNTPs	deoxyribonucleoside triphosphates
ACTH	adrenocorticotropic hormone
PCC	plasma corticosterone concentration
PAC	plasma aldosterone concentration

Introduction

Essential Hypertension

The hypertensive disease is a pathological condition whose major symptom is sustained increase in arterial blood pressure (BP) leading to damage of the organs of the cardiovascular system, of the other target organs as well, predominantly the kidneys. It is a major cause of cerebral insult, myocardial infarction, and renal failure [1].

These complications are, in turn, the main causes of morbidity and mortality in the developed countries. Thus, in 2008, cardiac and cerebrovascular diseases ranked, respectively, first (24.6 %) and fourth (5.4 %) as causes of death in the USA [2]. According to the WHO estimates, roughly 7.3 millions of deaths were related to high BP in 2008 and 23.6 million would presumably be in 2030 [3]. The hypertensive disease may be well defined as an alarming worldwide health problem.

There prevails the notion that BP is a finely regulated physiological parameter affected by a multitude of controls whose actions are integrated at the level of the whole organism, thereby providing an adequate blood supply of all the tissues and organs despite varying metabolic demands [4].

Genetic factors contribute largely to BP regulation. There is a correlation between the BP estimates for parents and offspring, it has been documented for familial aggregation that the BP values are more similar within than between families [5]. Environmental and nutritional agents, life style are also contributors to the pathogenesis of hypertensive disease, being recognized as modifiable risk factors. The observed variations in BP are thought to be genetically determined by 30 – 60 % [6], and, importantly, result from the combined action of numerous genes, when the contribution of each gene alone being is small. A half of the rest of variation in BP is due to environmental impacts, which include alcohol, smoking, diet, stress, and low physical activity [4]. Hence, one is dealing here with a mosaic of environmental-genetic interplay defining a mean level around which the BP fluctuates in each individual.

Essential hypertension (EH) constitutes about 90 – 95 % of all the hypertensive states in humans [7]. In contrast to the rare cases when a single gene mutation underlies hypertension, EH is determined by polygenic mechanisms, a true mosaic made up of neural, hormonal, and cellular deviations, all under the influence of life style and environmental agents. In the monogenically controlled forms of arterial hypertension, most genetic deviations are related to the system involved in regulation of the salt and water metabolism. This justifies assignment of a key role to genetic deviations in water-salt metabolism with reference to EH.

The results obtained with animal models furthered understanding of the pathogenesis of the hypertensive disease. Although animals cannot reproduce the entire clinical pattern of human hypertension, they are informative concerning specific events and features in hypertensive disease allowing control over changes occurring during experimental interventions. For reviews of animal models of arterial hypertension, see [8, 9]. The relevant literature is abundant. Regrettably, no animal strain developed to this day can incorporate all pathogenic hypertensive mechanisms operative in humans, because the EH in humans looks as heterogeneous in the underlying mechanisms and etiology. As a result, every genetic animal model corresponds to one of specific form of human hypertension.

ISIAH Rat Strain

The rat strain with inherited stress-induced arterial hypertension (ISIAH) is the result of many years of selection at the Institute of Cytology and Genetics in Novosibirsk [10]. The ISIAH rats are advantageous models for studying the progression of the hypertensive disease under the influence of psychoemotional stress, a significant provocative agent of arterial hypertension formation in humans, in the view of many researchers. To develop the experimental model of stress-sensitive arterial hypertension, rats were selectively bred for many generations for enhanced responsiveness to emotional stress, manifested as an exaggerated increase in BP, [11]. Importantly, the selection was aimed at raising BP under stress; its other concomitant effect was a rise in basal BP, which reached 160-170 mm Hg. Emotional stress produced in the strain under selection an additional rise of 35-40 mm Hg, so that the high value of 200 mm Hg was attained. In this way, a state was simulated where genetic predisposition to arterial hypertension development was exaggerated under the effect of mild emotional stress.

Numerous physiological and biochemical characteristics of the ISIAH rats have been analyzed through the years. It has been demonstrated that changes in the brain noradrenergic regulatory system in this strain may be responsible for both the increase in BP and alteration in stress reactivity. The functional features of the noradrenergic brain system are probably related to the increased activity of the sympathetic nervous system. This is observed as an increase in adrenaline concentration in the adrenal medulla and in activity of the major enzymes of its biosynthesis [12, 13]. The most pronounced structural changes in the ISIAH adrenals have been described for the cortex glomerular zone producing aldosterone [14, 15]. Amstislavsky et al. [16] have also indicated that the adrenal cortex is enlarged in the ISIAH rats. These hypertrophic changes could be partly prevented by administration of enalapril, an inhibitor of the angiotensin converting enzyme (ACE) [17], or losartan, a blocker of the angiotensin II (Ang II) receptors [18], during the prepubertal period. This preventive effect provided evidence indicating that the renin-angiotensin system (RAS) plays a significant role in the development of hypertrophy in the glomerular zone of the adrenal cortex in the ISIAH rats. Subsequently, the secretory activity of the adrenal cortex was compared in the ISIAH hypertensive and WAG normotensive rats. Comparisons provided direct support for increased secretion in the ISIAH strain, which was mainly due to enhanced biosynthesis of glucocorticoid hormones [19].

Changes in the function of the hypothalamic-pituitary-adrenocortical axis in the ISIAH rats concern both its central and peripheral components.

The basal expression of the gene encoding the key regulatory peptide proopiomelanocortin in the pituitary is increased [20]. This system can be rapidly mobilized by certain stressful stimuli.

This mobilization manifests as an elevation in the corticotropin releasing hormone (CRH) mRNA in the hypothalamus and adrenocorticotropic hormone (ACTH) content in pituitary tissue and plasma [21]. The hormonal response of the adrenal cortex to stress can be much higher in the ISIAH rats than in WAG controls. The plasma corticosterone level is significantly higher in the ISIAH rats after 5 min emotional stress exposure [21, 22].

Renin-Angiotensin-Aldosterone System and Hypertension

Taking into account the key role of the RAS in long-term regulation of fluid volume and blood pressure (BP), also as a target in hypertension treatment, the RAS genes were traditionally regarded as candidates for the hypertensive disease. In conditions of reduced renal perfusion pressure, salt loss or decreased fluid volume, or sympathetic activation, renin is released from the juxtaglomerular cells in the kidneys. It cleaves the inactive synthesized in the liver peptide angiotensinogen (Agt). As a result, angiotensin I (Ang I) is formed. It is converted to angiotensin II (Ang II) by the angiotensin converting enzyme (ACE). Ang II binds to its receptors in the cells of the vascular smooth muscle causing vasoconstriction and in the adrenal glomerular zone inducing aldosterone secretion. Vasoconstriction of the peripheral arteries and the aldosterone-mediated sodium and water reabsorption in the kidneys lead to an increase in systemic BP and counteract the decrease in renal perfusion pressure dependent on arterial narrowing. In the last decade, additional links of the RAS, the novel system members and their biosynthetic pathways have been identified. Besides Ang II, a broad spectrum of bioactive angiotensin peptides, including angiotensin (1 – 7), has been established [23, 24]. Ang (1–7) is synthesized by ACE2, an ACE homolog insensitive to ACE inhibitors (ACEi) [25, 26]. At least four receptors interact with these angiotensin peptides: AT1, AT2, AT4 and Mas [27, 28]. Renin, earlier considered as an enzyme only, can act as a direct cellular mediator with its own receptor PRR (prorenin/renin receptor) [24]. In this chapter, we analyze the expression of both the classical RAS genes and the novel ones, such as *Ace2* (the gene coding ACE2), the angiotensin receptor AT2 gene *Agtr2* and the PRR gene *Atp6ap2* (*PRR*).

Within the last years, there has been a resurgence of the idea that aldosterone plays an important role in the pathogenesis of EH. The titles of the relevant papers were thought-provoking and eloquent: "Aldosterone and arterial hypertension" [29], "Mechanisms of hypertension: the expanding role of aldosterone" [30], or "Aldosterone: A forgotten mediator of the relationship between psychological stress and heart disease" [31]. The "auld acquaintance" mediator of hypertension and heart disease quite obviously could not be undeservedly forgotten. With reference to chronic stress as an acknowledged risk factor of the development of hypertension and cardiovascular diseases, Kubzansky and Adler [31] wrote that adrenaline and to a certain extent cortisol are the main culprits of cardiovascular complications under stress, although the production of aldosterone is greatly enhanced, and ACTH is known as one of the stimulators of aldosterone synthesis. As Kubzansky and Adler [31] have aptly noted, the possible increase in the aldosterone secretion was disregarded, when examining the mechanisms of the stress effects on the heart and blood vessels.

The unique model of stress-sensitive arterial hypertension, ISIAH rats, offered us opportunities for examining the problem in a new light and to estimate the possible contribution of aldosterone to the pathogenesis of the stress-dependent form of arterial hypertension.

Antonov et al. [32] have analyzed the content of aldosterone and glucocorticoids in experimental myocardial infarction (EMI). In the acute phase of EMI, aldosterone sharply increases in the ISIAH rats. We suggest that extracardiac compensation of cardiac failure is stronger in the hypertensive rats. When cardiac necrosis is pronounced, steroidogenesis shifts towards precisely aldosterone, not glucocorticoids, due to the renal blood flow restriction and activation of the renin-angiotensin-aldosterone system.

However, the basal functional activity of the RAS in the ISIAH rats was considered to be reduced. For example, renin activity in the plasma and renal tissue tends to be lower in ISIAH as compared to WAG rats [16]. During repeated measurements, plasma aldosterone concentration in the ISIAH rats was reduced or did not differ significant from that in normotensive WAG and Wistar rats. The ISIAH strain did not differ from the normotensive controls in ACE activity in lung tissue and blood plasma [33]. However, under stress conditions, the ISIAH rats were characterized by a greater increase in lung ACE activity (restriction stress) and plasma aldosterone concentration (mild stress of blood loss or emotional stress) [34]. These data indicate that the potential ability to respond of the RAS to certain stimulatory factors including emotional stress is enhanced in the ISIAH rats, and this system was probably involved in the formation of the stress-induced arterial hypertension.

In recent years, the paradigm shifted from emphasis on the role of systemic RAS in regulation of fluid volume and electrolyte balance, BP and pathophysiology of cardiovascular and renal diseases to that on the local tissue RAS. Numerous studies have demonstrated the importance of the local RAS in the brain, heart, peripheral vessels, adrenals, and kidneys [35–39]. Against this background, we analyze the expression of the RAS genes in organs most significant in terms of BP regulation: the kidneys, myocardium, adrenals, lungs (only *Ace*) and brain structures such as the hypothalamus and medulla oblongata.

A unifying pathway for EH has been hypothesized [40]. The development of secretory EH is thought to occur via two phases. The first phase which is known as “hyperkinetic” is characterized by increase in cardiac output and by episodes of vasoconstriction presumably due to hyperactivity of the sympathetic adrenal system related to changes in the central regulatory mechanisms.

The second phase is defined by morphological and functional changes shifting hypertension to the salt- and renal-dependent form in which peripheral organs, the kidneys in particular, are more significant players [40]. With this in mind, we studied the expression of the RAS in young (1.5 months of age) and mature (4 – 7 months) rats with the hypertension presumably at different developmental stages of the disease.

Methods

Experimental Animals

Young (1.5 months of age) and adult (4 – 7 months of age) rats of two inbred strains, hypertensive ISIAH and control normotensive WAG, from the Center for Genetic Resources of Laboratory Animals of the Institute of Cytology and Genetics (Siberian Branch of the Russian Academy of Sciences) were used in the experiments. All animal procedures were approved by the Animal Resources Committee at this Institute.

All the procedures were carried out in accordance with the International Guidelines for Animal Experimentation (the UFAW Handbook on the Care and Management of Laboratory and Other Research Animals).

RNA Isolation

Animals were decapitated under light ether anesthesia. Organs and tissues (hearts, kidneys, adrenal glands, lungs and such brain structures as hypothalamus and medulla oblongata) were immediately extracted, snap-frozen in liquid nitrogen and stored at -70°C.Total RNA was isolated by the method of phenol-chloroform extraction [41]. After RNA isolation, an additional deproteinization was done by phenol-chloroform (1:1) extraction followed by chloroform extraction to remove the residual phenol. Remaining genomic DNA traces were removed by treatment with DNase I (Promega, USA) according to the manufacturer's instructions. Purified RNA was quantified spectrophotometrically.

Reverse Transcription

Reverse transcription was performed in 50 μl of solution containing 1 – 3 μg of the isolated RNA, 0.25 nmol primers (N_9 – random nonanucleotide primers from Biosan, Russia), 36 μl of buffer for reverse transcription, 40 units of revertase MoMLV (Vektor-Best, Novosibirsk, Russia), and 0.4 mM dNTP. The cDNA was synthesized at 37°C (1 h), 42°C (30 min), 50°C (10 min). The enzyme was inactivated by heating the mixture at 75°C for 5 min. Resultant cDNA (0.25–0.5 μl) was used for subsequent PCR.

Table 1. Primers used in the study

Gene	Nucleotide sequence of primers	T_{anneal}	T_{acq}
Ren	F: 5' – CCT GGG AGT CAA AGA GAA GA – 3' R: 5' – ACA GGT CAT CGT TCC TGA AG – 3'	64^{0}C	85^{0}C
Agt	F:_5'-CCT CGC TCT CTG GAC TTA TC-3' R:_5'-CAG ACA CTG AGG TGC TGT TG-3'	63^{0}C	87^{0}C
Ace	F: 5'- ATG GTA CAG AAG GGC TGG AA - 3' R: 5'- TTG TAG AAG TCC CAC GCA GA - 3'	62^{0}C	88^{0}C
Ace2	F: 5'- TGC CGA CCA AAG CAT TAA AG -3' R: 5'- TCT CTC ATG GCA TAG GCA AC -3'	63^{0}C	84^{0}C
Agtr1a	F: 5'- AAA TGA GCA CGC TTT CTT ACC G - 3' R: 5'- TGA GGC AGG GTG AAT GGT CC - 3'	63^{0}C	86^{0}C
Agtr2	F: 5'- ACA AAC CGG CAG ATA AGC AT - 3' R: 5'- GAG AGG AAG GGT TGC CAA AA -3'	63^{0}C	84^{0}C
PRR	F: 5'- ACT CTG TTC TCA ACT CGC TC -3' R: 5'- TCT TCT CCA TAA CGC TTC CC -3'	63^{0}C	84^{0}C
Rpl30	F: 5'- CAT CTT GGC GTC TGA TCT TG - 3' R: 5'- TCA GAG TCT GTT TGT ACC CC – 3'	62 – 64^{0}C*	84^{0}C

Note: T_{anneal} , annealing temperature; T_{acq} , temperature of fluorescence signal acquisition.
*–primer annealing for reference gene was performed at the same temperature as primer annealing for target gene.

Preparation of "Standard" cDNA

3 μl aliquots from each of the obtained cDNA samples from the same tissue were mixed together. The resulting "averaged" solution was used in PCR for plotting calibration curves.

Real-Time PCR

PCR (iQ5 amplifier, Bio-Rad Laboratories, USA) with SYBR Green I (Molecular Probes, USA) was used to determine the gene expression levels. The housekeeping gene *Rpl30* encoding ribosomal protein L30 was used as a reference gene.

The reaction mixture (20 μl) contained PCR buffer, 0.2 mM dNTPs, 1 unit of HotStart Taq polymerase (all reagents were from Vector-Best, Novosibirsk, Russia), SYBR Green I (1:20,000) (Molecular Probes, USA), 0.3 μM of each forward and reverse primer (nucleotide sequences of the primers used in this study are shown in Table 1; all primers were from Biosan, Novosibirsk, Russia). Real-time PCR was carried out under the following conditions: initial heating for 1 min at 95°C, then 35-40 cycles of 15 sec at 95°C, 20 sec at 65°C, 20 sec at 72°C, fluorescence signal acquisition for 10 sec at 83°C (for *Rpl30*), then fluorescence signal acquisition for target genes (table) for 10 s, followed by recording the melting curve from 65°C to 94°C. In each experiment, eight to ten cDNA samples with primers for a target gene (4 replicates per cDNA sample), the same samples with primers for the reference gene (4 replicates) and the standard cDNA (from 1:1 to 1:64 dilutions) with the same primers (2 replicates) were placed onto the same plate. For each cDNA sample, the PCR experiment was repeated at least twice. The relative amount of the tested cDNA was determined using calibration curves derived from the dilutions of the "standard" cDNA. This value for the target genes was further normalized against the qPCR level of the reference gene (*Rpl30*). This comparison allowed estimation of the differences in the expression levels of the studied genes in animals of different strains, or between rested rats and ones under stress.

Secretory Activity of Adrenal Cortex

The group of animals included 13 ISIAH males and 7 WAG males aged 5 – 6 months. Rats were anesthetized via intraperitoneal infusion of thiopental (50 mg/kg body weight). The vein of the left adrenal was ligated at the site of its confluence with the renal vein, a teflon catheter was then inserted into the adrenal vein. After closure of the operative wound, blood flowing from the adrenal vein was collected into heparinized tubes. Blood volume was 1.3 – 1.5 ml. After blood collection, the right adrenal was rejected for subsequent measurement of hormone concentration in gland tissue. Blood from the adrenal vein flowed freely into the tube, the sampling time was registered precisely, allowing to calculate blood flow volume through the adrenal. Plasma flow required for calculation of secretion of the adrenal hormones was calculated on the basis of venous hematocrit values. Concentration of cortico-steroid hormones in plasma and adrenal tissue was determined by using high pressure liquid chromatography (HPLC). Measurements were performed with an Agilent 1260 (USA) chromatograph equipped with a diode-matrix UV detector and a Zorbax Extend C18 column..

This technique allowed us to measure the concentration of aldosterone, corticosterone, 11-dehydrocorticosterone, and 11-deoxycorticosterone in blood flowing from the adrenal gland and in the adrenal tissue.

Response of Gluco- and Mineralocorticoid Hormones to Acute Emotional Stress

Rats of the second group (10 of each strain) were subjected to acute stress by placement into a large dessicator with cotton balls at the bottom wetted with ether. Seven min later, a blood sample was collected from the tail vein to measure corticosterone and aldosterone concentration.

Basal (control) concentration of corticosterone and aldosterone was measured in peripheral blood plasma from rats after their prompt decapitation. The peripheral plasma corticosterone concentration (PCC) and that of aldosterone (PAC) were determined with the immune-enzyme assay kits using an Aldosterone ELISA Kit (USA) and Corticosterone EIA Kit (USA).

Arterial Pressure Measurement

Arterial pressure was measured by the indirect tail-cuff method (BioPack, USA). Basal BP was measured under light ether anesthesia to eliminate the effect on the BP level of psychological stress produced by the measurement procedure in unanesthetized rats.

Immobilization Stress

Immobilization stress was provided by rat restriction in a narrow wire mesh cylinders, whose dimensions corresponded to rat body size. The tail was passed through an aperture in the back door. It was outside the cage so that stress-induced BP level could be measured. Rats were stress-exposed for 30 min.

Statistics

All statistical calculations were performed with software package Statistica v.5.5 (Statsoft, USA) using ANOVA/MANOVA for comparisons of group means and nonparametric methods such as Mann – Whitney U-test, Kruskal – Wallis ANOVA and median test. Differences were considered as statistically significant at $p < 0.05$. As a rule, parametric and nonparametric analysis gave consistent results. The few exceptional instances were considered as statistically insignificant. The data are presented as means and their standard errors ($M \pm S.E.M.$).

Correlation analysis was also used for treatment of data on gene expression in young 1.5 month old rats. Pearson's correlation coefficient was calculated. Because a group consisted of 6 individuals each, the nonparametric analog of this analysis, Spearman's range correlation coefficient, was applied as an additional control. The results were considered to be significant at $p < 0.05$. Results with significance of $p \leq 0.1$ according to both Pearson and Spearman were taken into consideration as suggestive.

Results and Discussion

Arterial Pressure

Basal BP in the ISIAH rats aged 1.5 months was moderately (not over 150 mm Hg), yet significantly increased compared with the WAG rats ($p < 0.005$) (Figure 1).

After emotional stress, caused by restriction, differences in BP increased in each strain both for the absolute value and increment under stress (Figure 1).

Notably, the increment of BP under stress correlated with the BP absolute value in rats of both strains ($p = 0.03$ for the WAG and $p = 0.04$ for ISIAH rats). However, the correlation between basal pressure and increment of BP under stress tended to be negative in the WAG rats only (Pearson's coefficient $R = -0.738$, $p = 0.094$). This meant that the greater was basal pressure, the weaker was its increase under stress. This relation was much less significant in the ISIAH rats.

In adult (7 months old) rats of both strains, the interstrain differences between basal and stress-induced BP became more prominent (Figure 2), although the increment of BP after stress, which occurred against the background of a rather high basal value in the ISIAH rats (around 180 mm Hg), did not differ by 7 months of age between the two strains ($p = 0.38$).

The positive correlation between the increment of BP and the absolute BP value under stress was retained by this age in ISIAH rats only ($R = 0.995$, $p = 0.011$).

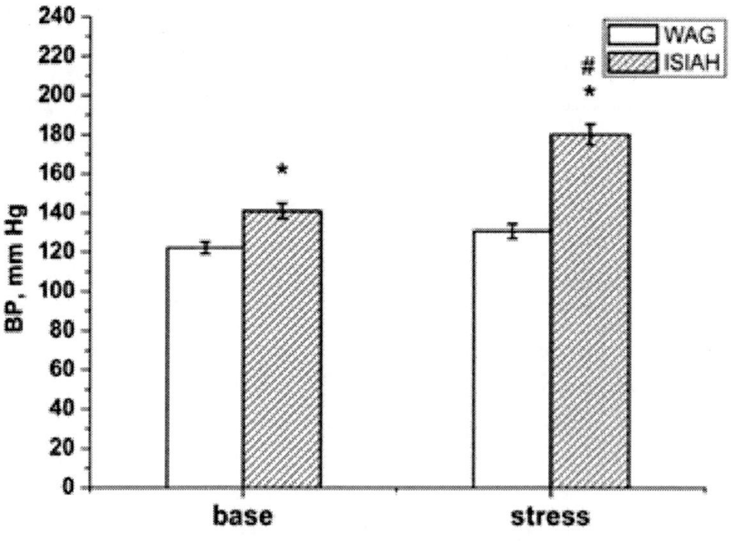

Figure 1. Arterial pressure, BP, in the young (1.5 months old) WAG and ISIAH rats in rest (basal level) and under emotional stress. Data are presented as $M \pm S.E.M.$ *, statistically significant inter-strain differences; #, statistically significant differences between the rats of the same strain in rest (control) and under stress.

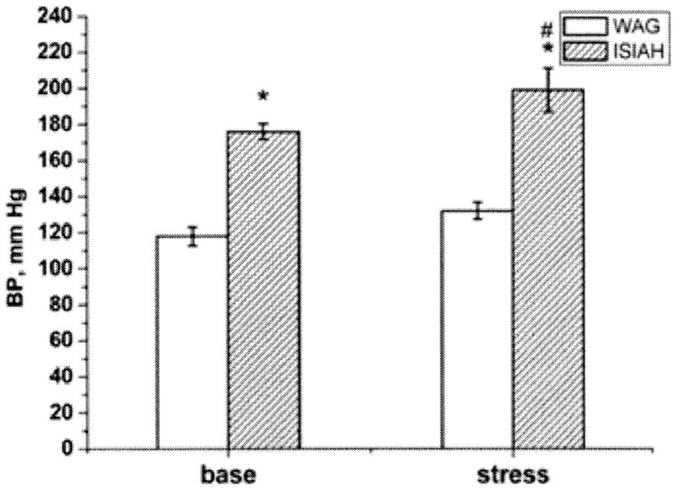

Figure 2. Arterial pressure, BP, in the adult (7 months old) WAG and ISIAH rats in rest and under emotional stress. Data are presented as $M \pm S.E.M.$ *, statistically significant inter-strain differences; #, statistically significant differences between the rats of the same strain in rest (control) and under stress.

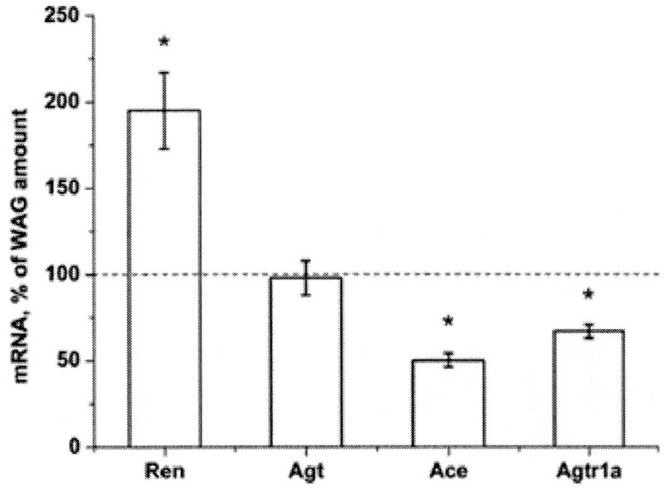

Figure 3. The RAS gene expression in the young ISIAH rat kidneys shown as percent of corresponding expression in control WAG rats. Data are presented as $M \pm S.E.M.$ *, statistically significant inter-strain differences, $p < 0.05$.

Kidneys

Study of the expression of the RAS genes involved in hypertension development in the kidneys of 1.5 month old ISIAH rats by semiquantitative Real-time PCR revealed that *Ace* mRNA level was decreased twofold and that of Ang II receptor 1A type (*Agtr1a*) by 33 % when compared with the normotensive WAG controls. The two strains did not differ by the expression of the *Agt* gene (Figure 3).

Table 2. Correlations between the levels of mRNA of RAS genes in the WAG rats

	1	2	3	4	5	6	7	8	9	10	11	12	13	14	15	16	17	18	19	20	21	22	23	24	25	26
1		--!	--!		+							++		+!					--					++		
2	--!		++			++!			-		-!			--!												
3	--!	++							-		-			--												
4								-				++!											+			
5	+						++!			++!		++	+				++				++!				--	-!
6		++!							--!		--!			--!												
7					++!											++	++!			++!	++!			+		
8				-					+													--!				
9		-	-			--!		+						++	-											
10					++!							+														--
11		-!	-			--!							++	+!								--	--!	+		
12	++			++!	++					+															--	-
13					+						++						++!							+		
14	+!	--!	--			--!			++		+!															
15									-							+!	+	+		++						
16							++								+!		++	+		++!	++			+		
17					++		++!						++!		+	++		++		++	+					
18															+	+	++			++!				++!		
19	--																									
20							++!								++	++!	++	++!			+					
21					++!		++!									++	+			+						
22								--!			--												++!		--!	
23				+							--!											++!			-	
24	++						+				+		+			+		++!								
25				--								++										--!	-			
26					-!					--		-														

Designations: 1 – *Ren*, 2 – *Agt*, 3 – *Ace*, 4 – *Agtr1a*, all – in the kidneys; 5 – *Ace*, 6 – *Ace2*, 7 – *Agtr1a*, all – in the myocardium; 8 – *Ren*, 9 – *Agt*, 10 – *Ace*, 11 – *Ace2*, 12 – *Agtr1a*, 13 – *Agtr2*, 14 – *PRR*, all – in the hypothalamus; 15 – *Ren*, 16 – *Agt*, 17 – *Ace*, 18 – *Ace2*, 19 – *Agtr1a*, 20 – *Agtr2*, 21 – *PRR*, all – in the medulla oblongata; 22 – *Agt*, 23 – *Agtr1a*, 24 – *Agtr2*, 25 – *Ace2*, all – in the adrenal glands; 26 – *Ace* in the lungs. " + " and " - ", Pearson's correlations with $0.05 \le p \le 0.1$, positive and negative, respectively; " ++ " and " - -", correlations with $p < 0.05$; " ! ", correlations detected according to both Pearson's and Spearman's analysis.

Table 3. Correlations between the levels of mRNA of RAS genes in the ISIAH rats

	1	2	3	4	5	6	7	8	9	10	11	12	13	14	15	16	17	18	19	20	21	22	23	24	25	26
1									++!	+	--!		++!			+		++		++		++!				++!
2								-																		
3						+																				
4					--!		--!			+					-	++	++!	+							-	
5				--!			+										--						++!		+	
6			+				++!														-!					
7				--!	+	++!				--!						--!					-					
8		-																			-					
9	++!										--							++				++				
10	+			+			--!						++		--	++!		+		+	+					-
11	--!								--				--!		+	-		--				-		-		--!
12																			--!			-			--!	
13	++!									++	--!				--!	+		++!								++!
14						+													+							
15				-						--	+		--!			--		--						-		
16	+			++			--!			++!	-		+		--		+	++						+		+
17				++!	--											+		+					-	++		
18	++			+					++	+			++!		--	++	+					++		++		+!
19												--!		+											+!	
20	++									+											+	+				++
21						-!	-	-		+										+						
22	++!								++		-	-					++			+						
23					++!												-									
24											-				-	+	++	++								
25				-	+							--!					-		+!							
26	++!									+	--!		++!			+		+!		++						

The genes and correlations are designated in the same way as in the Table 2.

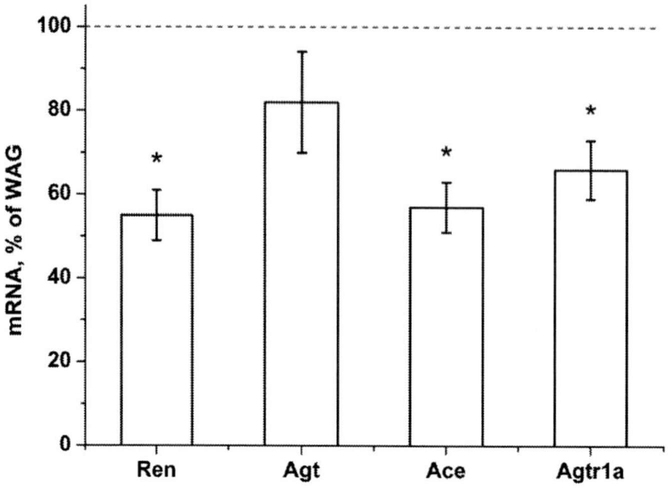

Figure 4. The RAS gene expression in the adult ISIAH rat kidneys shown as percent of corresponding expression in control WAG rats. Data are presented as $M \pm S.E.M.$

Concomitantly, there was an almost twofold rise in renin mRNA in the kidneys of young ISIAH rats relative to the normotensive WAG controls (Figure 4).

Search for correlations between the expression of the RAS genes in the kidneys of young rats revealed an essential difference between the compared strains. In the WAG rats (Table 2), there was a negative correlation between the levels of renin mRNA, on the one hand, and *Ace* and *Agt* mRNA, on the other hand (R = -0.883, p = 0.020 and R = -0.843, p = 0.035, respectively).

In contrast, no correlations were found between the expression of the RAS genes in the kidneys of the ISIAH rats (Table 3). The increase in *Ren* expression in the kidneys of the ISIAH rats at this age may be regulated independently of the other components of the renal RAS. This appears plausible because their expression is either reduced or of the same magnitude as in the controls.

It is of interest that *Ren* expression in the kidneys correlated with *Ace* mRNA level in the lung of the ISIAH rats only (R = 0.938, p = 0.006). The latter parameter reflected the *Ace* expression level in the circulation. The augmentation in Ang I content in the blood as a consequence of an almost twofold increase in expression (and secretion) of renal renin could possibly stimulate the increase in *Ace* expression in the vascular bed, although not to the extent detectable by our methods. In fact, we revealed no interstrain differences in *Ace* expression in the lungs of young rats.

As a result of search of the relation between the renal expression of the RAS genes and BP in young WAG rats, we disclosed a negative correlation between basal BP and the expression of the *Agt* gene (R = -0.9724, p = 0.001). Some increase in the level of intrarenal Agt, followed by that of Ang II, may be possibly mobilized the systemic BP to compensate the reduced renal blood flow and filtration rate. Furthermore, we found a negative correlation between the expression of the *Agtr1a* gene with both the absolute BP value under stress and its increment in the WAGs (R = -0.944, p = 0.005 and R = -0.8305, p = 0.041, respectively). To be precise, mRNA level was measured in resting rats and, for this reason, the correlation concerned rather the capacity to increase BP under stress. Appearing paradoxical at first sight, the negative correlation between the content of *Agtr1a* mRNA and capacity to increase BP under stress may be explained by the features of post-transcriptional regulation of these receptors. No such relations were found in the young ISIAH rats. However, they showed a positive correlation between basal *Ace* expression and the increment of BP under emotional stress ($R = 0.779$, $p = 0.068$; Spearman's coefficient $R_S = 0.886$, $p = 0.019$). In fact, the mean level of *Ace* expression in the ISIAH kidneys was decreased as a possible compensation already in young rats, whereas increased BP level was determined by other causes.

The expression levels of the RAS genes (*Ren, Ace*, *Agtr1a*) in the kidneys of the adult (4 months old) ISIAH rats in conditions of rest were significantly lower than in the WAG normotensives. The expression of the *Agt* was exceptional, like in young rats. The WAG and ISIAH rats did not differ by *Agt* expression (Figure 4).

Short-term (17 hrs) water deprivation did not alter mRNA content of the RAS components in the kidneys of both strains. We have demonstrated that such a water restriction raises the expression of the cyclooxigenase-2 (COX-2) gene (*Cox-2*) in the ISIAH kidneys, which affects the secretion level of renin. Under conditions of rest, *Cox-2* mRNA content in the ISIAH rats was decreased twofold compared with the WAG normotensives, however, under stressful water deprivation, *Cox-2* expression was significantly, by three times increased in the ISIAH rats and by 70 % only in the WAGs compared with the conventional conditions. As a result, *Cox-2* mRNA level in the ISIAH became close to the one in the WAG rats [42].

As it is known, 24 hr water deprivation increases the activity of renin in the ISIAH rats [43]. However, the COX-2 expression in renal tissue is activated when extracellular fluid volume is decreased and water-electrolyte balance is impaired [44]. COX-2-derived prostanoids play a role in the regulation of the renin secretion, not in its gene expression [45]. For this reason, it may be assumed that when water deprivation is relatively short-term, the increase in the activity of renin in plasma may be solely due to the COX-2 stimulated release from its stores in the juxtaglomerular cells.

The results provided evidence indicating that the activity of the RAS is attenuated in ISIAH rats. This should be considered in context of existing view-points on low-renin hypertension. In addition to a decrease in the activity of renin, the other specific features of low-renin hypertension include enhanced salt-sensitivity of BP, an increase in the extracellular fluid volume, also that of plasma, and sodium accumulation in the body. Furthermore, experimental data indicated that the low-renin salt-sensitive hypertension is associated with decreased level of NO synthesis and impaired endothelium-dependent vasodilatation [46, 47].The latter reinforced the idea that impairment in the vascular NO system is also involved in the development of the low-renin hypertension. A decrease in the kidney NO-synthase (NOS1) was observed earlier in the ISIAH rats [16].

Several models of the low-renin hypertension have been described. Exemplary are the Lyon genetically hypertensive rats (LH), whose levels of renin and prorenin both in plasma and kidneys are considerably lower than in the controls [48]. Dahl SS (DS) is another rat strain characterized by a low renin level. Not only the activity of plasma renin, but also the concentration of aldosterone in plasma is significantly lowered in DS rats fed a high-salt diet from the age of 7 weeks despite a corticosterone level not different from the control [49].

There is some inconsistency of the literary data, with most researchers referring SHRs to rats with the normal or low-renin form of hypertension [50]. However, at an early age of these rats a period when plasma renin activity is increased is distinguished [51]. A similar early surge of RAS activity was observed in the LH rats and in our experimental ISIAH rats. Thus, it is reasonable to expect that the increase in the functional activity of the renal renin system during early development may be a step required for the formation of the hypertensive state in at least certain rat strains; after the surge, BP may be maintained high even without enhanced renin production in the kidneys.

In the process of SHRs maturation and formation of the hypertensive status the renal renin activity reduces. This is observed at the levels of renin gene transcription, enzyme activity and BP measurement [50, 52]. During this period of BP surge a brief blockade of RAS in SHR pups induces a reduction in BP, which remains noticeable for some weeks after abolition of the blockade [53]. This state is characteristic also probably of the ISIAHs. In fact, blockade of the renin system during early development in the ISIAHs is followed by a delay in the formation of the hypertensive state and by a less pronounced increase in BP during aging [54, 55].

Earlier studies in the ISIAH rats showed that the activity of renin and aldosterone level in plasma did not exceed those in WAGs [16, 33]. Based on these data, we refer, with certitude, the ISIAH rats to models of the low-renin form of hypertension. The pattern of this form in the ISIAHs is classical as confirmed by the data on the small but significant increase in sodium concentration in plasma and much larger rise of the sodium concentration in connective tissue (a natural sodium store in the organism) in the ISIAH rats [56]. For a sodium store, such as connective tissue, this large difference between rat strains is obviously admissible, being much smaller for plasma, where ion concentration is under strict homeostatic control.

As it is known, the relation between the renal RAS and sodium level in the organism is reciprocal: the renin-aldosterone system is recruited to retain sodium, on the one hand; retention of sodium leads to inhibition of this system, on the other hand, and this was what we observed. Nevertheless, in this case sodium must be retained, but what is the mechanism? There are forms of arterial hypertension associated with sodium accumulation against the background of attenuated function of the renal RAS. A case in point is the syndrome of apparent mineralocorticoid excess [57]. In this syndrome, sodium retention is due to insufficiency of the enzyme converting corticosterone, which possesses mineralocorticoid activity, into dehydrocorticosterone with low affinity to mineralocorticoid receptors. In such a case, stimulation of the mineralocorticoid receptors occurs with corticosterone which concentration is two orders of magnitude higher than concentration of aldosterone, whose secretion may even diminish as a consequence of the renal RAS suppression. It was shown that WAGs and ISIAHs did not differ significantly by the corticosterone-dehydro-corticosterone ratio in blood flowing from the adrenal gland, also in the peripheral blood plasma and in adrenal tissue. This allowed us to exclude the assumption that enhanced mineralocorticoid effect may be resulted from corticosterone excess in the ISIAH rats [19]. Another explanation may be offered for enhanced sodium retention when the function of the renin system is suppressed: the retention may be explicable by change in the function of the transport ion channels, which are targets for aldosterone. This is characteristic of the Liddle's syndrome in which mutations in the genes encoding the synthesis of the epithelial sodium channel (ENaC) subunits were identified (4). Amstislavsky et al. [16] demonstrated increased renal expression of ENaC mRNA and also mRNA of other ion transport channels in the ISIAH rats. This specificity requires further study. It appears very likely that change in the function of the renal ion channels may underlie the formation of the low-renin arterial hypertension in the ISIAH rats.

Changes in the function of the arterial baroreflex are also may be involved in hypertension development. The baroreflex is responsible for control of the BP by maintaining it close to the set point. The baroreflex rapidly resets to higher pressure in response to its sustained increase [58]. The sensitivity of the arterial baroreflex is decreased in the SHR, LH and DS strains compared with the normotensives leading to a weaker baroreflex control over heart rate and activity of the sympathetic nervous system [59]. There are data indicating that the baroreceptor mechanism in the kidneys plays a dominant role in the regulation of renin production [60].

The frequent episodes of increase in BP in young ISIAH rats may be consequences of their sympathoadrenal system sensitivity to mild emotional stress and to the "stress of the life" [34]. These episodes can lead to resetting of the baroreflex, thereby affecting the activity level of the RAS.

Similarities and differences of ISIAHs with reference to the functioning of the sympathetic adrenomedullar and hypothalamic-pituitary adrenal systems of the widely used SHR hypertensives have been highlighted [34], as for the renin-angiotensin system, ISIAH have features common with SHR and other models of low-renin hypertension, also features making them different. This group of the hypertensive rat strains is assigned to the one distinguished by low renin activity in plasma and expression of the renin gene in the kidneys. In the SHR rats, the expression of the *Agt* gene in the kidneys is decreased [50]. In contrast, in the DS rats high-salt diet (the condition for the formation of the hypertensive status) causes a sharp increase in the content of intrarenal Agt [61], without altering concomitantly the expression of the AT1 receptor gene [62].

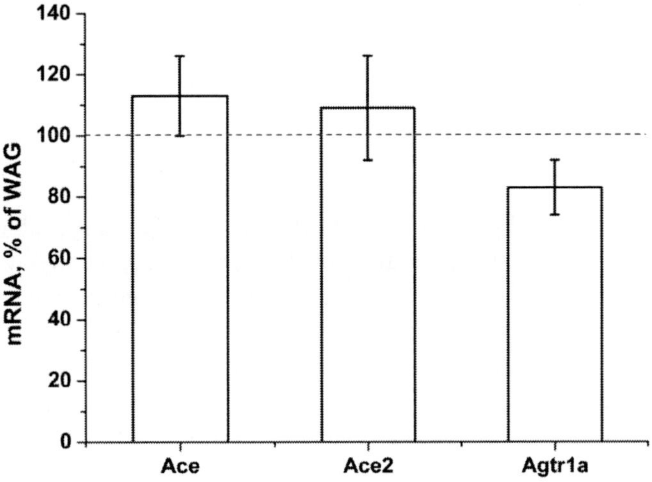

Figure 5. The myocardial RAS gene expression in the young ISIAH rats shown as percent of corresponding expression in control WAG rats. Data are presented as $M \pm S.E.M.$

Young, not adult SHRs showed increased expression of the AT1A receptors in the renal proximal tubule [63]. A decreased content of ACE in the kidneys compared with the controls was detected in the young SHR rats; this difference disappeared in adults [64]. As for the ISIAH rats we observed no significant differences in the expression of the *Agt* gene in the kidneys compared with normotensive controls, while the content of renal *Ace* mRNA and that of *Agtr1a* mRNA was reduced in both young and mature ISIAH rats.

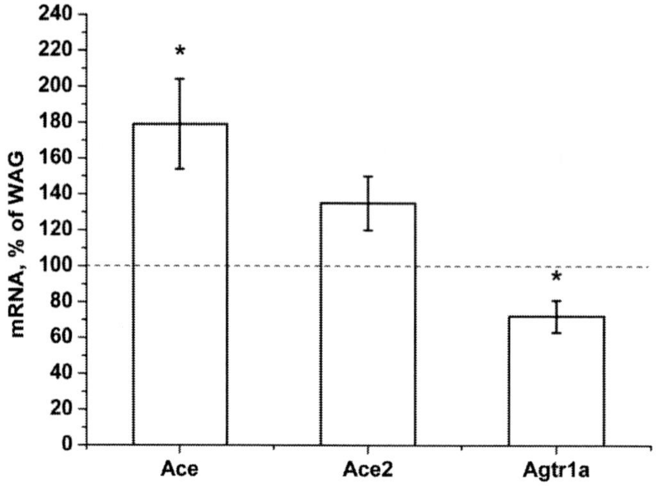

Figure 6. The myocardial RAS gene expression in the adult ISIAH rats shown as percent of corresponding expression in control WAG rats. Data are presented as $M \pm S.E.M.$ *, statistically significant inter-strain differences, $p < 0.05$.

Myocardium

The compared strains at the age of 1.5 months did not differ significantly by the expression of the analyzed RAS genes (*Ace*, *Ace2,* and *Agtr1a*) in the myocardium (Figure 7).

In the young WAG rats, the correlation between the *Ace* and *Agtr1a* mRNA levels in the myocardium was positive ($R = 0.896$, $p = 0.016$, $R_S = 0.8286$, $p = 0.042$); this correlation was lower in the ISIAH rats and did not reach significance ($R = 0.809$, $p = 0.051$, $R_S = 0.886$, $p = 0.019$) (Table 2).

We observed a positive correlation between the content of *Ace2* mRNA in the myocardium and that of *Agt* expression in the kidneys ($R = 0.852$, $p = 0.091$, $R_S = 0.943$, $p < 0.05$) and a less significant for renal *Ace* and (a negative) for *Ren* (Table 2). Furthermore, *Ace2* mRNA expression in the myocardium of the young WAGs correlated negatively with mRNA content of *Agt, Ace* and the *PRR* genes in the hypothalamus. In the young WAGs, the level of *Ace* mRNA in the myocardium was also positively correlated with *Ace* mRNA level in the hypothalamus also with PRR mRNA in the medulla oblongata; as for the content of *Agtr1a* mRNA in the myocardium, it was found to be positively correlated with the expression of the RAS genes (*PRR, Agtr2* and at a lower probability with *Ace*) in the medulla oblongata (Table 2). These correlations probably evidence that the expression of the *Ace* and the AT1A receptor genes in the myocardium is differently and independently regulated.

It should be also noted that the young ISIAH rats showed none of the above correlations (Table 3). In contrast to the WAG rats, the ISIAH hypertensives exhibited only a negative correlation between the levels of *Ace* and *Agtr1a* mRNA in the myocardium, on the one hand, and the *Agtr1a* mRNA level, on the other hand. The negative correlation between the level of *Agtr1a* mRNA in the myocardium and *Agt* mRNA in the medulla oblongata was significant according to Spearman's rank correlation ($p = 0.019$), whereas parametric analysis revealed a trend only ($p = 0.090$). As for the correlation of BP with the expression of the RAS genes in the myocardium, the WAG rats showed a negative correlation between basal BP and *Ace2* expression (R = -0.932, $p = 0.007$, $R_S = -0.986$, $p = 0.0003$). ACE2, an ACE homolog, cleaves Ang II to Ang (1–7) [65]. In contrast to ACE, ACE2 does not convert Ang I to Ang II. For this reason ACE2 may be effective as mediator for inhibition of Ang II formation through stimulation of alternative pathways for Ang I degradation.

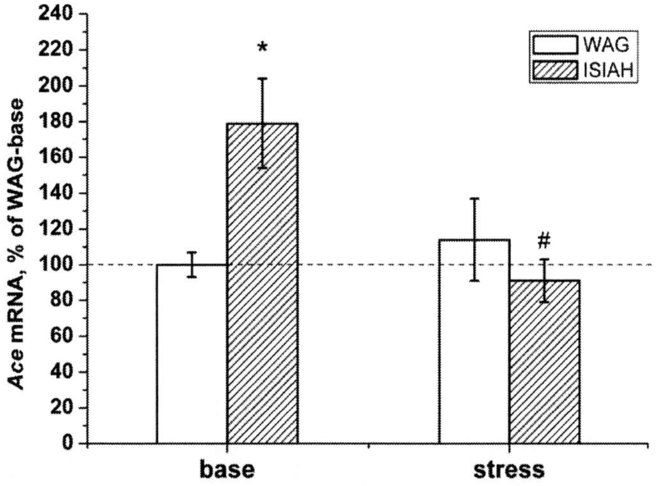

Figure 7. The relative myocardial content of *Ace* mRNA in the WAG and ISIAH rats at the age of 4 months in conditions of rest (base) and under water deprivation stress. The mRNA level in the WAG rats in rest is set at 100%. Data are presented as $M \pm S.E.M.$ *, the significant difference between the strains ($p < 0.05$); #, the significant difference between the control and experiment ($p < 0.05$).

The BP under stress correlated with the content of *Agtr1a* mRNA in the myocardium of the ISIAH rats. Moreover, the correlation between the increment of BP under stress and the *Ace2* expression was found to be positive in this strain (R = 0.857, $p = 0.029$, $R_S = 0.943$, $p = 0.005$). The absolute value of BP correlated with the expression of *Ace2* (R = 0.772, $p = 0.072$; $R_S = 0.880$, $p = 0.021$). This would seem to be at variance from the stated in the preceding paragraph. Nevertheless, ACE2 is capable not only metabolize Ang II to Ang (1 – 7), but also to cleave vasodilator bradykinin (BK) to inactive metabolite [des-Arg9]-BK [65]. However, the increase in *Ace2* expression in the ISIAH rats may be a compensation for smoothing the vasoconstrictive effect of factors, increasing their BP. The increase in the expression of Ang (1–7) in cardiac tissues and that of its producing enzyme ACE2 occurred at the same time. Low doses of Ang (1–7) improve cardiac output and counteract Ang II induced vasoconstriction; this indicated that Ang (1–7) may possibly have a protective role in reducing Ang II effects [66].

The expression level of the *Agtr1a* in the myocardium was reduced by 28% in 4 month-old ISIAH rats compared with the age-matched WAGs. *Ace* mRNA content in the myocardium of the ISIAH rats proved to be considerably increased, by 80 % (Figure 8).

The relation between cardiac hypertrophy and changes in expression of the members of the cardiac RAS has been noted in numerous reports. The *in vitro* and *in vivo* data confirmed that both local mechanical stimuli and increased salt loading are significant regulators of cardiac RAS activity. With reference to the heart of the dog with experimentally produced ventricular hypertrophy, Lee [67] by using PCR have demonstrated that this hypertrophy was associated with an elevation in *Ace* mRNA expression and a fall in the expression of the

Agtr1, while the expression level of the *Agt* and *Ren* genes remained unaltered. Thus, the ideas that the components of the cardiac RAS are regulated independently and differently and that opposite changes in their expression may manifest their various roles in the myocardial hypertrophy received support.

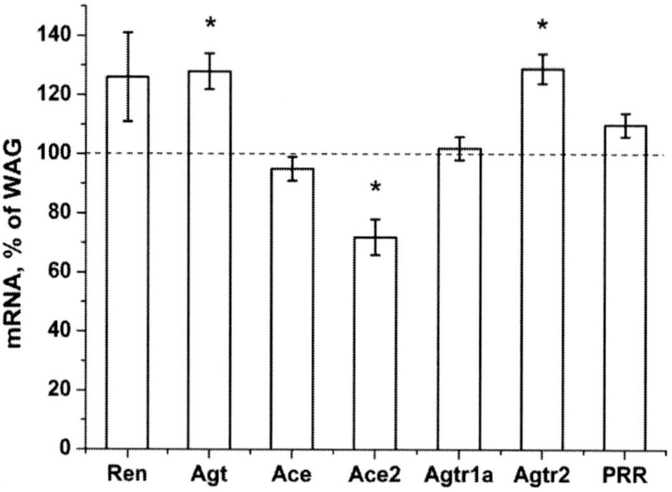

Figure 8. The RAS gene expression in the hypothalamus of the young ISIAH rats shown as percent of corresponding expression in control WAG rats. Data are presented as $M \pm S.E.M.$ *, statistically significant inter-strain differences, $p < 0.05$.

Both in the Wistar rats with hypertrophy of the left ventricle caused by aortic stenosis [68] and in humans [69] the ACE was related to formation of myocardial hypertrophy. In such a myocardium, conversion of Ang I to Ang II was increased and the content of *Ace* mRNA in the left ventricle was increased fourfold compared with the control [68].

Myocardial hypertrophy developed in the salt-sensitive Dahl (DS) rats on high-salt intake, which was, however, not proportional to the hypertension level. In such rats, the myocardial parameters (*Ace* gene expression and enzyme activity) increased compared with the DS rats on the control diet and Dahl R (salt-resistant strain) on either diet. Blockade of the sympathetic nerve activity prevented hypertension without affecting the expression and the activity of ACE and cardiac mass. High-salt intake did not increase cardiac Ang II in Dahl S, thereby suggesting that the increase in *Ace* mRNA and ACE activity may be pertinent to non-angiotensinergic mechanisms involved in cardiac hypertrophy. [70].

There are other lines of evidence indicating that high-salt diet increased not only *Ace* but also *Agtr1a* mRNA in the myocardium of DS rats on high-salt diet compared with the normotensive controls. In this model of the low-renin and low-aldosterone hypertension, glucocorticoid-mediated activation of the mineralocorticoid receptors may be contributors to the progression of cardiac hypertrophy and fibrosis, hypertrophy of coronary vascular walls, too [49].

Studies concerned with the cardiac RAS in the SHRs are numerous. Some data indicate that the mRNA content of the *Agt*, *Ace* and *Agtr1a* genes are increased in the SHR compared with the normotensive WKY controls; other studies have found no differences between the two strains (see [71] for reference). According to Naito et al. [71], these discrepancies arise from circadian fluctuations in the expression of the RAS genes. It is noteworthy that the diurnal variations in the cardiac RAS are characteristic of the SHR unlike WKY rats. Regulation of *Ace* and *Agtr1a* gene expression by Ang II at specific time points was observed also only in the SHR group [71].

Some researchers believe that hypertrophy of the cardiac muscle is caused by increased level of Ang II acting through the AT1A-dependent mechanism [72]. The *Agtr1a* gene promoter is active in the cardiac muscle, and the expression of this gene is induced by an increase in BP. It has been suggested that Ang II induces cardiac and vascular hypertrophy directly by activating the AT1 receptor and indirectly by stimulating the release of certain growth factors and cytokines [73]. There is substantial experimental evidence indicating that there is no direct correlation between cardiac hypertrophy and the AT1 receptors. Thus, the transgenic mRen-2 rats with enhanced renin expression were characterized by hypertension and cardiac hypertrophy. In this transgenic rats, the receptor AT1 was decreased in the aorta, atrials and ventricles by 40 – 50 % as compared with the Sprague-Dawley controls. This noticeably reduced the response of the heart and aortic wall to Ang II stimulation [74]. In contrast, in mice with the *Agtr1a* mutation showing sustained increased activation of the receptor, no marked myocardial hypertrophy was observed; moderate (by 20 mm Hg) and persistent elevation of BP, also enhanced BP response to Ang II were registered; other parameters (low renin and normal aldosterone production) were the same as in the low-renin hypertension [75].

In the AT1A receptor knockout mice, it has been shown that the hypertrophy in response to hemodynamic load can form independently of AT1 [76]. No changes were observed in the expression of the *Agtr1* gene in the altered human heart [77]. Finally, the renal AT1 receptor was shown to be the absolutely necessary condition for the development of the Ang II-dependent hypertension and cardiac hypertrophy. When these receptors are eliminated from the kidneys, the remaining extrarenal receptors do not suffice for causing hypertension and cardiac hypertrophy [78].

The truth lies midway. As shown by examination of the signaling pathways leading to the formation of cardiac hypertrophy, there exist both AT1-dependent and AT1-independent (via stimulation of the α1-adrenoreceptors or ET receptors for endothelin-1) pathways [79].

In contrast to the SHR and DS hypertensives, we observed a considerable increase in the expression of the *Ace* gene and a less conspicuous decrease in the *Agtr1a* gene in the adult ISIAHs. The young (1.5 months old) ISIAH rats did not differ in this regard from the normotensive controls, although evidence of myocardial hypertrophy was detected even at an earlier age [10].

True enough, the weaker correlation between mRNA levels of *Ace* and *Agtr1a* in the young ISIAH compared to WAGs may indicate that there existed differences in the expression of the local RAS genes already at this age; the RAS expression may be affected by the plasma level of Ang II, which may be increased in ISIAHs due to a high renal renin production at an early age. The expression level of *Agtr1a* in the kidneys of the young ISIAHs is probably reduced through a negative feedback mechanism presumably involving the renal baroreflex.

To accept the idea that the AT1A receptor in the myocardium of the young ISIAH rats is activated to some extent by plasma Ang II [73], namely a common effector (whose action is multidirectional in the different organs) made explicable the negative correlation between the expression of the cardiac RAS components and the renal *Agtr1a*. Morphological changes in the heart of the aging ISIAHs presumably arose regardless of the function of the local RAS in response to elevated BP, which already at four weeks of age significantly surpassed the control level. As for *Ace* expression in the heart, it markedly increased later to maintain probably the needed level of endogenous Ang II in conditions of decreased expression and activity of plasma renin. However, the lacking tendency to a negative correlation between *Ace* mRNA in the myocardium and in pulmonary tissue in the ISIAH rats (the latter corresponds to *Ace* expression in the circulation), the correlation observed for WAGs, may be indicative also of changes in the expression of cardiac *Ace* in the ISIAH rats.

Water deprivation for 17 hrs affected neither the expression level of the *Agtr1a* gene in the myocardium in both strains, nor the *Ace* expression in the control WAGs. However, elevated *Ace* mRNA level in the myocardium of ISIAHs decreased to the values measured in normotensives (Figure 9). The increase in the cardiac RAS is related to an increase in heart functional load and subsequent development of myocardial hypertrophy, while a decrease in ACE activity after water deprivation may be due to an opposite event, a decreased cardiac load due to reduced fluid (including plasma) volume and cardiac preload. Water deprivation of the same duration we used led to a 6 % reduction in the volume of circulating plasma [80].This was inevitably associated with a decrease in work required for the circulation of the reduced blood volume.

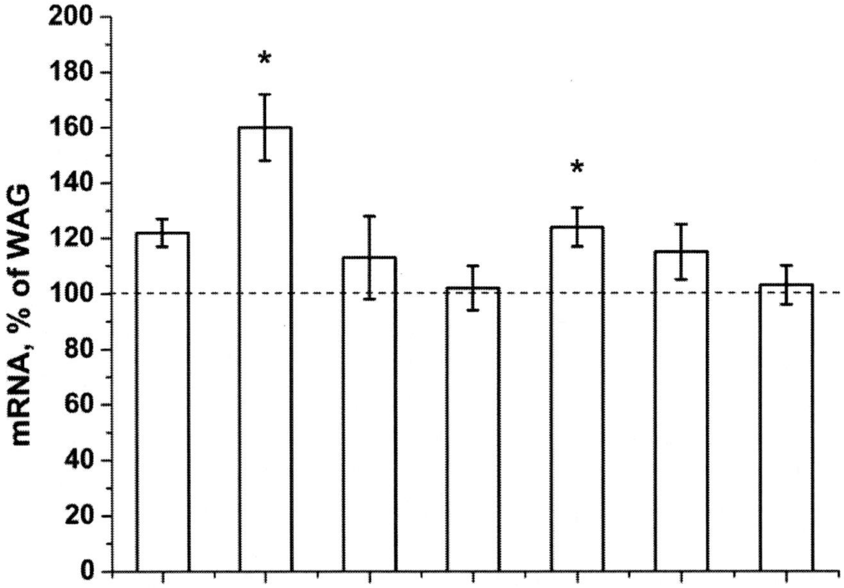

Figure 9. The RAS gene expression in the medulla oblongata of the young ISIAH rats shown as percent of corresponding expression in control WAG rats. Data are presented as *M* ± *S.E.M.* *, statistically significant inter-strain differences, $p < 0.05$.

To reiterate, in the kidneys of ISIAH rats subjected to the stress of water deprivation, the expression of the *Cox-2* gene, whose products stimulate renin secretion from the juxtaglomerular cells, was sharply augmented. It may be suggested that the increase in the activity of plasma renin, the key enzyme of the circulating RAS, detected under such dehydration [43] reduces the demand for increased activity of the cardiac RAS and, in this way, can also lead to the observed mitigation of *Ace* expression in the myocardium.

Brain Structures

The RAS gene expression in the brain was long and fruitfully studied in SHRs, rats with spontaneous hypertension. These animals are characterized by changes in RAS gene mRNA levels directly in the brain structures [81].The content and renewal of Ang II in the hypothalamus are elevated in SHR adults relative to the normotensive controls. SHR is characterized also by an increase in the number of binding sites for Ang II in some nuclei of the hypothalamus and medulla oblongata, also by a higher content of *Agtr1a* mRNA in the anterior hypothalamus). In addition, the concentration of the *Agtr1a* mRNA in the brainstem is higher in SHRs than in WKY rats [82]. *Agt* mRNA level started to raise from 4 weeks of age, particularly in the hypothalamus, this rise continued with aging of these hypertensives [83]. Renin-like activity in the anterior hypothalamus and some medulla oblongata nuclei during hypertension development was also higher in SHRs than in the WKY normotensive controls [84]. All this suggested that the brain RAS may participate actively in the mechanism increasing arterial pressure not only in SHR, but also in other hypertensive strains. However, no studies of the expression of the RAS genes in the brain structures of ISIAH rats have been reported so far.

A greater *Agt* mRNA content was detected both in the hypothalamus and medulla oblongata of the young ISIAH. Moreover, the mRNA level of the *Agtr1a* was found to be increased in the medulla oblongata and that of the *Agtr2* in the hypothalamus. The level of *Ace2* mRNA in the hypothalamus of ISIAHs proved to be lower by 30 % (Figures 8 and 9).

Based on our previous and current data, it was concluded that ISIAHs belong to the low-renin form of hypertension. However, although in the kidneys the expression of renin mRNA is increased in the young ISIAHs and, in contrast, significantly decreased in adult ISIAHs, in the brain structures it was at the level close to the one observed in the control WAGs. This is in agreement with other researchers who obtained data indicating that the activity of the brain RAS is regulated autonomously, independently of RAS regulation in the other organs [85]. The examined brain structures are isolated from the circulation by the blood brain barrier, which prevents plasma Ang II from acting on the receptors in the central nervous system. The local brain RAS can have an autonomous influence on BP regulation of thirst and salt and water consumption, influencing on the secretion of vasopressin and adrenal hormones and taking part in the central activation of the sympathetic nervous system [86]. The administration of pharmacological blockers of brain RAS can affect significantly BP level irrespectively of the activity of the peripheral RAS. Microinjections of captopril (an ACE inhibitor) into the brain ventricles of SHR and TGR mRen2 hypertensive rats led to a decrease in BP without affecting peripheral ACE activity. A similar injection of losartan, a blocker of the AT1A receptor, also led to a decrease in BP in the above hypertensive strain. In contrast, in normotensive rats these centrally administered drugs were not associated with changes in BP [87].

In the young ISIAHs, like in SHRs [83], the mRNA level of the Ang II precursor Agt was increased in both brain structures involved in BP regulation. Despite the absence of significant differences in *Ren* mRNA levels in these brain structures between WAGs and ISIAHs, it may be supposed that an increase in *Agt* expression is the first step to augmented Ang II content in the hypothalamus and medulla oblongata in the young ISIAHs.

Angiotensinogen Agt is the sole substrate for renin. It is synthesized not only in the liver, but also in some organs where local tissue RAS is present. Cleavage of Agt by renin is the first and rate-limiting step in the cascade of enzymatic events that make up the circulating renin-angiotensin system. Agt, whose concentration in plasma is 1000-fold that of renin [88], has been traditionally considered as a "reservoir" for renin action. However, according to the calculations of Corvol and Jeunemaitre [88], the plasma Agt concentration would have to be ten-fold greater for its hydrolysis to be a zero-order reaction; consequently, the large amount of Agt in the plasma probably does not provide an excess of substrate for renin. Hence, Agt, along with renin, can play a limiting role in RAS function. There was direct *in vivo* evidence from several independent sources [88].The same considerations are applicable to the local RAS where the rate of Ang I production may also be controlled by Agt concentration. Thus, a local increase in Agt concentration can lead to an increase in that of Ang II, even though renin content is constant in the examined region [89]. Ang II produced locally by tissue RAS may act as autocrine or paracrine regulator. These tissue systems may be regulated locally, independently of the circulating system. Thus, Agt synthesized by glial cells was shown to be secreted and then taken up by neurons, forming a paracrine renin-angiotensin system [90]. Agt synthesis was demonstrated also in astrocytes, the largest accumulations of Agt-containing astrocytes occurring in the nuclei of the hypothalamus, midbrain and brainstem. Moreover, the nuclei most actively participating in Agt synthesis (i.e. in the accumulation of its mRNA) proved to be the same as those also showing Ang II binding with high affinity [91]. It is of relevance that *Agt* mRNA is elevated not only in the liver, but also in the brain (not the kidney) tissues by glucocorticoids [91, 92]. Agt has been referred to "an acute-phase response protein", which means that its gene transcription is activated by cytokines, but in the presence of glucocorticoids only [91].

From the above body of evidence it may be inferred with respect to the young ISIAHs that the increase in Agt expression in the hypothalamus and medulla oblongata leads to Ang II augmentation in those brain structures that affect the activity of the sympathetic nervous system. An increase in Ang II production and enhanced AT1 activation reduce baroreflex sensitivity in the nucleus of solitary tract (NTS), as reported elsewhere [93, 94] and augment neuronal activity in the rostral ventrolateral medulla (RVLM) [95, 96], this may give rise to events presumably mediating neurogenic hypertension.

As it is known, the relation between Ang II and the sympathetic system is close [97]. Ang II exerts a strong effect on the central nervous system by regulating and modulating thirst, salt appetite, vasopressin release, and the sympathetic nerve activity. As a consequence, activation of the central RAS can contribute to hypertension pathogenesis. Ang II receptors have been identified in regions of the brainstem involved in the control of sympathetic activity. For example, Ang II binding was found in the NTS, also in the rostral and caudal regions of the VLM, and microinjections of Ang II into these brain regions enhanced sympathetic activity. These binding sites are the nuclei involved in the signal pathways of the arterial baroreflex.

It is believed that the multiplicity of the physiological effects of Ang II, including vasoconstriction and cellular growth, are mediated through the AT1 receptor. AT1A receptor is localized on the surface of the vascular smooth muscle cells, and its activation results in elevation in intracellular calcium, generation of reactive oxygen forms and cellular contraction [98].

The role of the Ang II type 2 (AT2) receptor remained unclear for a long time. It was assumed that it is in many aspects opposite to that of the AT1 receptor. The data obtained in mice deficient in the AT2 receptor gene, *Agtr2*, confirmed its involvement in sympathetic inhibition. While AT1 in the central nervous system is with confidence related to the processes of sympathetic excitation, the activation of AT2 is thought to produce an opposite effect on the sympathetic tone [99].

In recent years only it became clear that the AT2 receptors are expressed not only in the vascular wall, also in the thalamic regions, hypothalamus and specific brain stem nuclei [100]. AT2 stimulation is involved in axon regeneration, memory processes and behavior control. Stimulation of AT2 has a protective effect on ischemic damage of the brain, which is partly provided through modulation of the cerebral blood flow. There are data indicating that Ang II induces the differentiation of neurons and the growth of axons mediated through mitogen-activated protein kinase (MAPK) or nitric oxide via activation of the AT2 receptor, which in this way is included in brain development.

We showed that the expression of the *Agtr1a* is increased in the medulla oblongata of the young ISIAH rats. This can lead to sustained rise in the sympathetic tone and finally cause an increase in BP. As it is known, imbalance between the levels of the AT1A and AT2 receptors in the RVLM produce sympathetic excitation and hypertension in experimental animals [101]. As for the increase in the level of *Agtr2* mRNA in the hypothalamus of ISIAH, it looks to be compensatory. This appears plausible in view of the literary data indicating that the agonist of the AT2 receptor effectively attenuated norepinephrine excretion and BP in rats through signaling pathways of NO synthase in the paraventricular nucleus (PVN) of the hypothalamus [99]. Since AT2 increases the NO release and reduces potassium flow in neurons, its activation must suppress the sympathetic tone.

With respect to the decreased expression of ACE2 in the hypothalamus of the young ISIAHs, it must be remembered that the formation of its major product Ang (1 – 7), in particular, during long-term RAS activation, counterbalances or attenuates the vasoconstrictive and proliferative actions of Ang II [65, 102]. Ang (1 – 7) opposes mainly the action of Ang II, stimulating NO and the vasodilator prostaglandins [103]. There is evidence that Ang (1 – 7) can potentiate the effect of bradykinin (BK) on its receptor B2 by binding the active site (c-domain) of ACE [104, 105]. In addition to potentiation of BK, Ang (1 – 7) mediates NO release [106], vasodilatation, inhibition of cell growth in vessels and diminishment of Ang II induced vasoconstriction [24, 107]. ACE2 deficiency can, for this reason, produce an enhancement of Ang II action in this brain region. It is worthy to note that Ang II infusion decreases the expression of ACE2 in PVN [108]. Consequently, ACE2 deficiency may be due to Ang II excess in the tissue of the hypothalamus and, in turn, contribute to the formation of an increased content and greater influence of Ang II in the brain structures, also to activation of the sympathetic nervous system.

In WAGs, the expression of the *PRR* gene strongly correlated with basal BP, that of *Ace2* correlated weaker with it, *Agt* only tended to correlate (all the correlations were positive). A negative correlation was observed for the *Agtr1a* expression with the absolute value of BP under stress and with its increment. In ISIAHs, Pearson's correlation analysis revealed a positive correlation between the expression of the *PRR* and BP increment under stress, however, Spearman's analysis did not confirm this. The pattern was the same in the medulla oblongata of the ISIAHs (a weak correlation between *PRR* expression with the increment of BP according to Pearson, but not supported by nonparametric analysis). No correlation between BP and the expression of the RAS genes was detected in WAGs.

In 7 month-old WAG adults, the expression of the *PRR* gene in the hypothalamus correlated already with the increment of BP, the correlation being negative. Besides, the correlation tended to be positive ($p = 0.054$) between the expression of *Agtr2* and basal BP. In the ISIAH adults, the expression of *Ace2* and the increment of BP under stress correlated positively in the hypothalamus. There were no correlations with BP in the medulla oblongata of adults of both strains.

We searched for correlations between *Agtr2* mRNA in the brain structures of young rats: a negative correlation between mRNA levels of *Agtr2* and *Ace2* in the hypothalamus was found in ISIAHs (Table 3), also a tendency to a positive correlation between the expression of *Ace2* and *PRR* in the hypothalamus of WAGs (Table 2). A positive correlation linked the expression of the *Agtr1a* in the hypothalamus and of *Ren* in the kidneys of the young WAGs. This may be explained by the unidirectional action exerted by Ang II produced in this brain region. A strong negative correlation was observed in the WAG hypothalamus for genes such as *Agt, Ace2* and *PRR*, on the one hand, and *Ace2* in the myocardium, on the other hand. The *PRR* in the hypothalamus of the WAG rats in turn was positively correlated with the expression of *Ren* in the kidneys and negatively with renal level of *Agt* mRNA. In the WAG rats, virtually no correlations between the expression of the RAS genes in the hypothalamus and medulla oblongata were disclosed. The positive correlation between mRNA levels of *Agtr2* in the hypothalamus and *Ace* in the medulla oblongata was an exception. The negative correlation between *Ace2* in the hypothalamus and *Agtr1a* in the adrenals may be accounted for by the counteraction of the enzyme to Ang II formation in this brain structure, ultimately lowering the activation level of the RAS in the adrenals. Interestingly, a negative correlation was revealed also between the expression of *Ren* in the hypothalamus and *Agt* in the adrenals. A negative feedback mechanism cannot be excluded here. These correlations may be suppressed or masked in the ISIAH rats by other processes.

They showed quite a different pattern not revealed in the WAGs: a positive correlation between mRNA levels of the *Agt* and *Agtr2* in the hypothalamus, on the one hand, and *Ren* in the kidneys, on the other hand. An activation of the sympathetic nervous system by the elevated Ang II in the hypothalamus may possibly lead to an increase in renin expression in the kidneys. An increase in the expression of the *Agtr2* in the hypothalamus was stimulated also by an augmentation in Ang II. For this reason, hypothalamic *Agtr2* and *Ren* mRNA level in the kidneys were not linked by a cause-effect relation; this link reflected the consequence of same event, the high *Agt* expression in the hypothalamus. As for the correlation between the expression of *Ace2* in the hypothalamus and *Ren* in the kidneys, it proved to be negative. ACE2 activity opposes the increase in Ang II content and, in doing so, ANG II effects on the kidneys. It is of interest that in young ISIAHs similar correlations were detected for *Ace* expression in the lungs (reflecting, as already noted, *Ace* expression in the circulation): the correlation was positive for *Agtr2* and negative for *Ace2* in the hypothalamus. In addition, we observed a negative correlation between *Ace* expression in the hypothalamus and myocardium in the WAG rats. This correlation was not observed in the young ISIAHs, whose changes in cardiac *Ace* expression compelled by hypertensive remodeling of the myocardium became probably more consequential despite the fact that significant changes in this expression were as yet undetectable in the young ISIAHs. Concomitantly, a negative correlation between the expression of the *Agtr1a* in the myocardium and of *Ace* in the hypothalamus was found in the young ISIAHs only, although in terms of the group means no differences in the expression of these genes between the strains were found at the age of 1.5 months. As for links between the brain regions, only in the ISIAH rats the correlation was positive between mRNA levels of *Ace* in the hypothalamus and *Agt* in the medulla oblongata, it was negative between the expression of the *Agtr2* in the hypothalamus and *Ren* in the medulla oblongata, also between *Agtr1a* expression in these two brain regions. A positive correlation between *Agt* expression in the hypothalamus and adrenals was detected also in the ISIAH rats only.

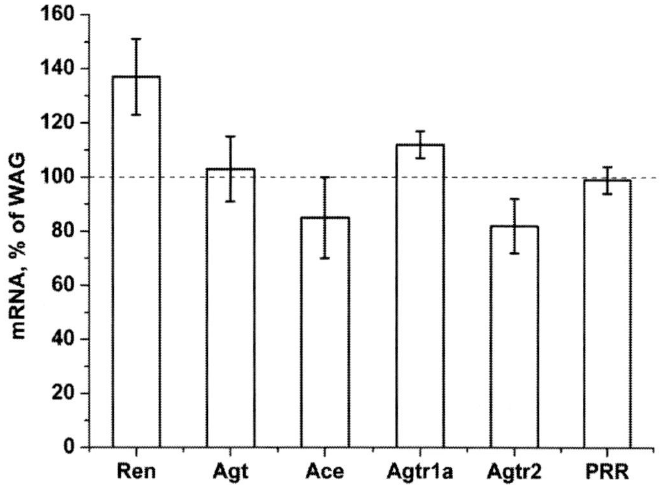

Figure 10. The RAS gene expression in the hypothalamus of the adult ISIAH rats shown as percent of corresponding expression in control WAG rats. Data are presented as $M \pm S.E.M.$

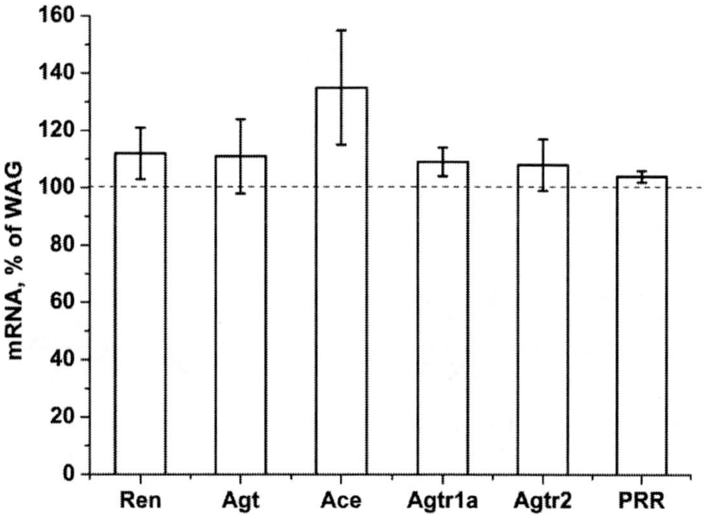

Figure 11. The RAS gene expression in the medulla oblongata of the adult ISIAH rats shown as percent of corresponding expression in control WAG rats. Data are presented as $M \pm S.E.M.$

A positive correlation between *Ren* and *Agt* expression in the medulla oblongata of the young WAGs was quite expected. The positive correlation between the expression of *Agt* and *Agtr2* also met expectation, because the latter is modulated by its ligand, Ang II. The correlation between mRNA levels of *Agtr2* and *Ace2*, also *Ace* and *PRR* in this brain region was positive. Not one of these correlations was revealed in the medulla oblongata of the ISIAH rats.

With regard to the expression of the RAS genes in the other regions and organs, no correlations were found between these genes in the medulla oblongata and in the kidneys or adrenals of the WAGs (Table 2). The *Agtr1a* gene showed positive correlations at the same time with three genes, *Ace*, *Agtr2*, and *PRR,* in the medulla oblongata. The same correlation was demonstrated for *PRR* in the MO with *Ace* in the myocardium. In contrast to the WAGs, the ISIAHs exhibited positive correlations between the RAS genes in the medulla oblongata and genes in the adrenals: for *Ace2* with *Agtr2* and a weaker for *Agtr1a* with *Ace2* (Table 3). *Ace2* in the medulla oblongata of the ISIAHs was positively correlated with *Agtr1a* in the kidneys, while *Agt* was negatively correlated with *Agtr1a* in the myocardium. The correlations between the expression of the RAS genes in the medulla oblongata and hypothalamus were considered above.

Judging by the data on the mRNA expression in the brain structures, differences between ISIAH hypertensives and control normotensives were found for 1.5 month-old animals only. In resting adults, there were no differences in the expression of the genes under study (Figures 10 and 11).

The *Ace2* gene was exceptional in that its expression was increased in the hypothalamus (Figure 12) and decreased in the medulla oblongata (Figure 13) in the ISIAH rats.

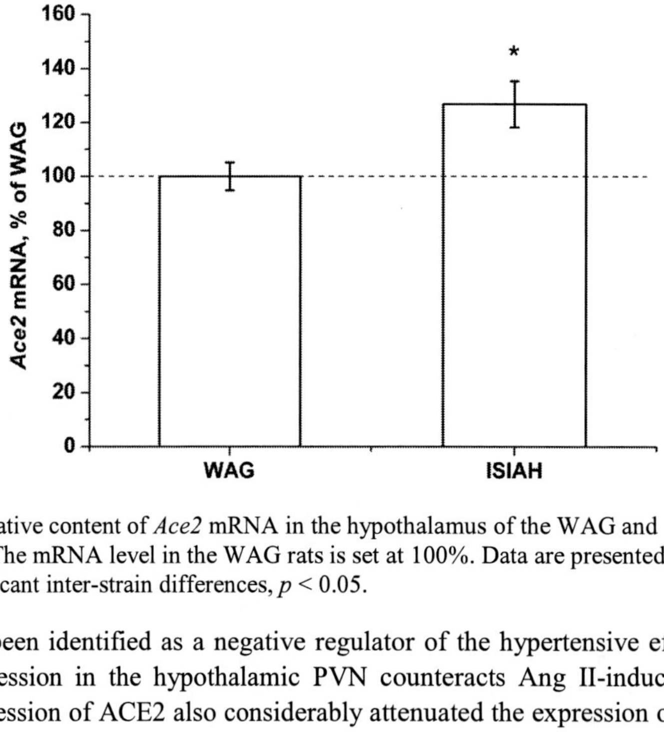

Figure 12. The relative content of *Ace2* mRNA in the hypothalamus of the WAG and ISIAH rats at the age of 7 months. The mRNA level in the WAG rats is set at 100%. Data are presented as $M \pm S.E.M.$ *, statistically significant inter-strain differences, $p < 0.05$.

ACE2 has been identified as a negative regulator of the hypertensive effects of Ang II. ACE2 overexpression in the hypothalamic PVN counteracts Ang II-induced hypertension [108]. Overexpression of ACE2 also considerably attenuated the expression of AT1 and ACE and enhanced that of AT2 and Mas [the receptor for Ang (1 – 7)] in the PVN. In addition to this, overexpression of ACE2 in the PVN attenuated the Ang II-induced increase in the expression of proinflammatory cytokines: the tumor necrosis factor-α (TNF-α), interleukin (IL)-1β, and IL-6 in the PVN. Attenuation of proinflammatory cytokines in the PVN, in combination with shift of RAS to the antihypertensive axis [ACE2/Ang (1 – 7)/Mas] may be responsible for the protective effect of the higher expression of ACE2 in the PVN to the Ang II-induced hypertensive response [108].

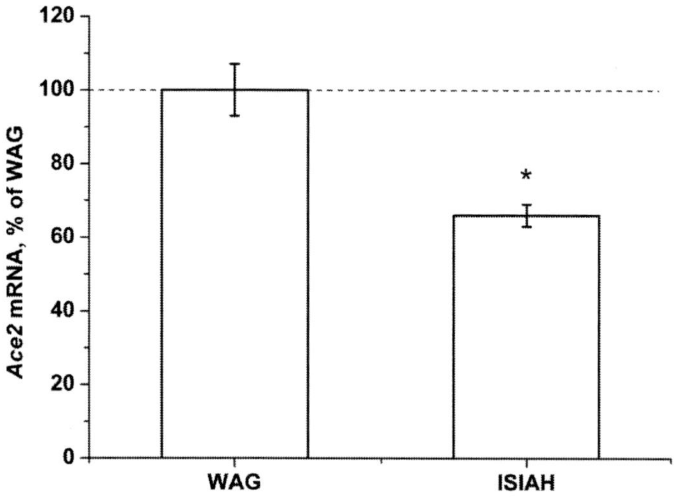

Figure 13. The relative content of *Ace2* mRNA in the medulla oblongata of the WAG and ISIAH rats at the age of 7 months. The mRNA level in the WAG rats is set at 100%. Data are presented as *M* ± *S.E.M.* *, statistically significant inter-strain differences, $p < 0.05$.

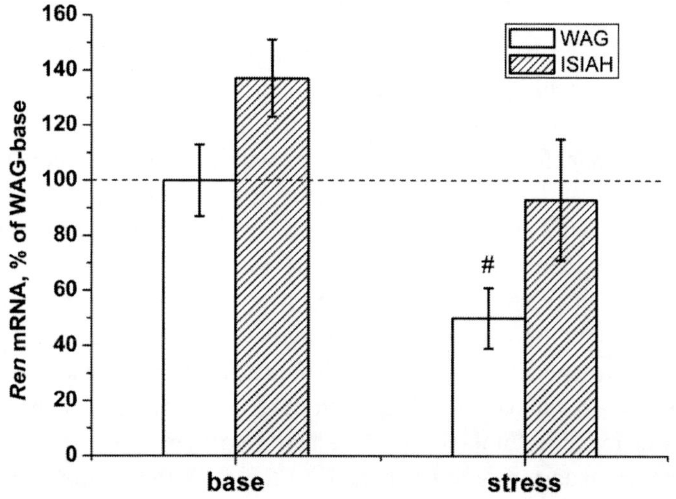

Figure 14. The relative content of *Ren* mRNA in the hypothalamus of the WAG and ISIAH rats at the age of 4 months in conditions of rest (base) and under water deprivation stress. The mRNA level in the WAG rats in rest is set at 100%. Data are presented as *M* ± *S.E.M.* #, the significant difference between the control and experiment ($p < 0.05$).

However, the expression of *Ace2* gene was decreased in the medulla oblongata in the adult, not the young ISIAHs. This expression level possibly lowered in response to normalization of Agt content in this brain region.

A stress of a brief 17 hr water deprivation produced virtually no changes in the expression of the RAS genes (*Ren* and *Ace*) in the ISIAHs as oppose to the WAG normotensives (Figures 14 and 15). A decrease in the level of *Ren* mRNA in the hypothalamus was observed in the mildly stressed WAGs.

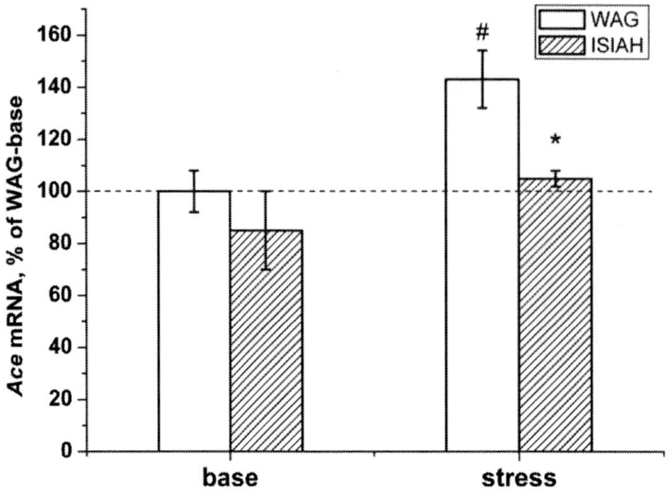

Figure 15. The relative content of *Ace* mRNA in the hypothalamus of the WAG and ISIAH rats at the age of 4 months in conditions of rest (base) and under water deprivation stress. The mRNA level in the WAG rats in rest is set at 100%. Data are presented as $M \pm S.E.M.$ *, statistically significant inter-strain differences; #, the significant difference between the control and experiment ($p < 0.05$).

The decrease was probably indirectly related to the increased renin activity in the circulation (the impermeability of the blood-brain barrier for renin was evidence against a direct relation). The decrease in the expression of renin in the ISIAHs did not reach significance. One reason for that were the large within group individual differences. *Agt* mRNA level remained almost unaltered in each rat strain during these experiments. This allowed us to suggest that Ang I content in this brain region also did not change significantly. True, we observed an increase in *Ace* mRNA in the hypothalamus of the water-deprived WAGs. However, the increase may be attributed to the non-angiotensinergic mechanisms of the ACE actions. In conditions of decreased volume of circulating fluids, i.e., hypotensive, the ACE ability to proteolysis of vasodilators (bradykinin) may come to the foreground. In the ISIAH rats, BP remained increased through other systems and mechanisms, and transcription of *Ace* remained at the level of the control group.

From the literary data it is known that SHR, the most thoroughly studied hypertensive strain, retain, when adults, a high level of *Agt* and *Agtr1a* mRNA in the brain structures. The SHR adults may differ even more in this respect than young SHRs from the control strain. There is an important difference to be remembered here. An elevated expression of the *Agtr1a* is characteristic of many tissues in SHR rats (the myocardium, in particular), an ubiquitous elevation, whereas *Agtr1a* expression level was decreased in the myocardium and kidneys of the ISIAH adults. Based on the obtained results, there appears to be age-dependent differences in the time course of changes in the RAS gene expression between the SHRs and ISIAHs. A lowering of RAS activity with age occurred not only in the kidneys, also in brain structures such as the hypothalamus and medulla oblongata despite the formation of the hypertensive status. The differences in the expression of the *Agt* and *Agtr1a* between SHR and ISIAH adults demonstrated that the roles of the control systems of BP may change in the ISIAHs and that different systems can maintain the hypertensive status in the mature SHRs and ISIAHs (an enhancement of the mineralocorticoid function, or water and sodium retention may be causative). In the ISIAH adults, an increase in the activity of the sympathetic adrenal and adrenocortical hormonal systems is accredited a central role, being directly in charge of also enhanced stress reactivity [34]. We believe that an initial mechanism in the formation of a hormonal background in ISIAH adults may be an increase in the activity level of the RAS genes in the brain structures at an early age.

Adrenal Glands

In the adrenal glands of young 1.5 months old rats the levels of *Agt* and *Ace2* mRNA, those of *Agtr1a* and *Agtr2* were revealed to be high enough to be detectable by semiquantative PCR. We found no differences in the expression of the *Agt, Ace2,* and *Agtr1a* genes between the ISIAH and WAG rats. The level of *Agtr2* mRNA was decreased by 37 % in the ISIAH rats (Figure 16). Correlations were not found between BP and gene expression in the adrenals of resting and stressed young and adult rats of each strain.

Spearman's rank correlation analysis revealed a positive correlation between the levels of *Agt* and *Agtr1a* mRNA (R_S = 0.8857, p = 0.019) in young WAGs (although Pearson's coefficient was R = 0.7923, p =0.060, i.e., it did not reach significance). This may indicate that angiotensin peptides perform autocrine or paracrine functions in the adrenal glands (Table 2). However, this correlation was not observed for the ISIAH rats.

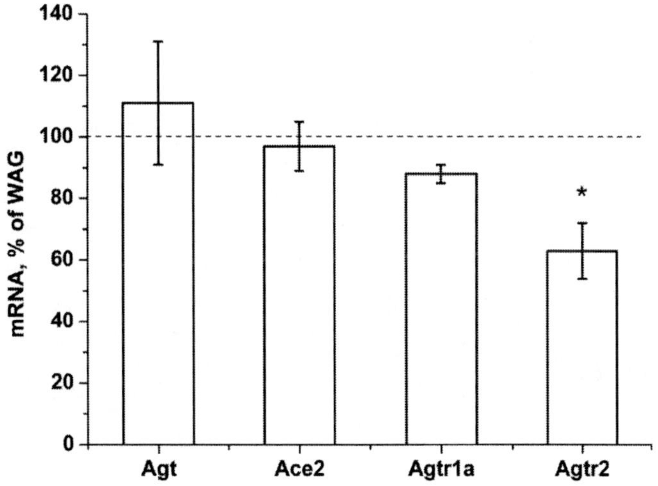

Figure 16. The adrenal RAS gene expression in the young ISIAH rats shown as percent of corresponding expression in control WAG rats. Data are presented as $M \pm S.E.M.$ *, statistically significant inter-strain differences, $p < 0.05$.

The situation was the similar in the WAG rats with a negative correlation between gene expression of the *Ace2* and *Agt* in the adrenals: it was significant according to Spearman only (R_S = -0.829, p = 0.042); however, Pearson's analysis disclosed a tendency only without significance (R = -0.735, p = 0.096). The correlation pattern was also similar for *Agtr1a* in the adrenals and *Ace2* in the hypothalamus. The ISIAH rats showed a similar correlation between the expression of the *Ace2* in the adrenals, on the one hand, and *Agtr1a* in the hypothalamus and medulla oblongata, on the other hand (Table 3). The correlations between the expression of the adrenal genes and those of the other organs were discrepant in the WAG and ISIAH rats. Thus, for the adrenals of the WAGs, a single significant correlation (negative) was demonstrated, between expression of the *Agt* in the adrenals and *Ren* in the hypothalamus. Not one of the above correlations was detected in the ISIAHs, not even trends. The content of *Agt* mRNA in the adrenals of the young ISIAHs correlated with the one in the hypothalamus and the content of *Ren* mRNA in the kidneys. The expression level of the *Agtr1a* in the adrenals showed a positive correlation with the level of *Ace* mRNA in the myocardium. Taken together, these observations evidenced that substantial regulatory changes in the expression of the analyzed genes took place in the hypertensive animals.

An imbalance of the Ang II receptors was observed in the adrenal glands of the young ISIAHs, like in the brain structures: a decreased *Agtr2* expression with a virtually unaltered of *Agtr1a*. From the literary data it is known that to "knockdown" the AT2 receptor by injection of a retroviral vector containing full-length AT2 antisense cDNA into normotensive rats sufficed for resistant effect of the enhanced systolic BP and pressor responses to Ang II [109]. The expression of *Agtr2* can be supressed by glucocorticoids [110]. There are data indicating that the density of the AT2 receptors in the adrenals was decreased when the concentration of aldosterone was increased [111]. It is relevant, that enhancement of the glucocorticoid function of the adrenal cortex and a tendency to higher aldosterone secretion were observed in 5 month-old ISIAH rats (19). They might have been the causes of the observed reduction in the expression of the *Agtr2*. However, there is as yet no information about increased secretion of corticosterone or aldosterone in the ISIAHs at an age earlier than 5 months. Understanding of the role of the AT2 receptor is far from complete. This is mainly because dealing with the "active" receptors which positively evoke actions [112]. Analysis becomes "a matter of love and hate" for the inhibitory or modulatory receptors, such as AT2 appears to be in most cases. Modulation is a pivotal property of the fine tuning of a wide spectrum of effects extending, in the case of AT2, from natriuresis, body temperature regulation, BP, reproduction, embryonic development, cell differentiation, recovery of damaged tissues, to programmed cell death [112]. To clarify the role of the AT2 receptor in the progression of the hypertension in ISIAH, analysis of its expression must be confined not only to the brain and adrenals, it must be extended to the kidneys and heart. The pattern changed somewhat during maturation so that the strains did not differ by the age of 4 months in conditions of rest in anyone of the adrenal RAS genes (Figure 17).

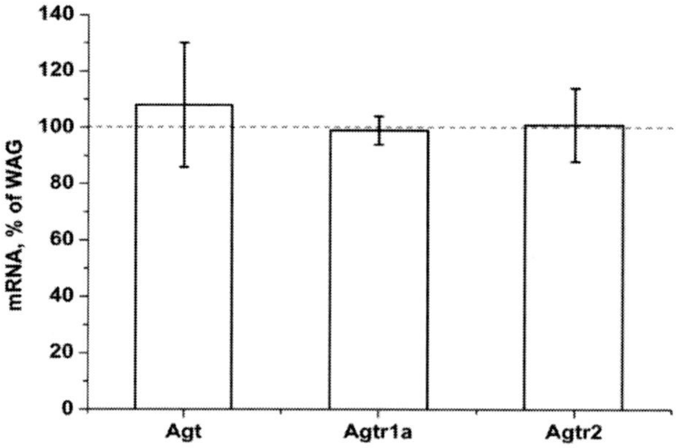

Figure 17. The adrenal RAS gene expression in the adult ISIAH rats shown as percent of corresponding expression in control WAG rats. Data are presented as $M \pm S.E.M.$

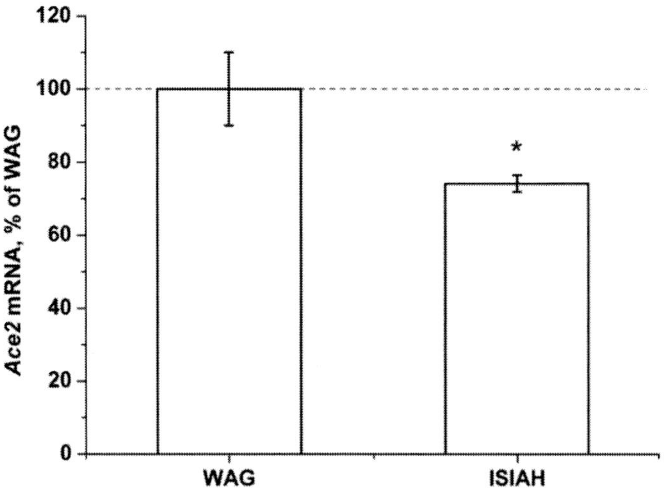

Figure 18. The relative content of *Ace2* mRNA in the adrenals of the WAG and ISIAH rats at the age of 7 months. The mRNA level in the WAG rats is set at 100%. Data are presented as $M \pm S.E.M.$ *, statistically significant inter-strain differences, $p < 0.05$.

We succeeded in detecting a significant decrease in the content of *Ace2* mRNA only by the age of 7 months in the ISIAH rats (Figure 18).

However, dehydration stress caused an increase in the content of *Agtr1a* mRNA in the adrenals of adult WAG controls, whereas it remained unaltered in the ISIAH rats (Figure 19). Water deprivation stress was concomitantly without effect on the mRNA level of the other adrenal RAS genes. It may be supposed that the increase in the *Agtr1a* expression is directed at augmenting aldosterone secretion in the WAG rats. This mechanism proved to be suppressed in the ISIAH rats.

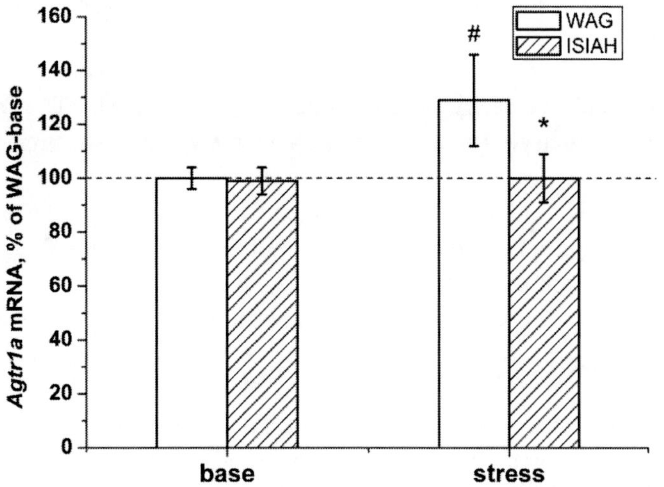

Figure 19. The relative content of *Agtr1a* mRNA in the adrenals of the WAG and ISIAH rats at the age of 4 months in conditions of rest and under water deprivation stress. The mRNA level in the WAG rats in rest is set at 100%. Data are presented as $M \pm S.E.M.$ *, the significant difference between the strains ($p < 0.05$); #, the significant difference between the control and experiment ($p < 0.05$).

Table 4. The mass of adrenal glands, the content of hormones in the adrenal tissue (ng) and their secretion level (ng/min), measured in anesthetized WAG and ISIAH rats [*M* ± *S.E.M. (n)*]

Index	WAG rats	ISIAH rats	The significance of interline differences
Right adrenal gland mass	20.4 ± 0.7 (16)	24.4 ± 1.3 (15)	$p < 0.05$
The content of corticosteroid hormones in the adrenal tissue, ng			
Aldosterone	11.8 ± 2.0 (14)	18.3 ± 2.7 (15)	NS (not significant)
11-dehydrocorticosterone	27.3 ± 2.5 (14)	30.7 ± 4.8 (15)	NS
Corticosterone	690 ± 56 (14)	755 ± 41 (15)	NS
11-deoxycorticosterone	175 ± 12 (14)	201 ± 11 (15)	NS
Secretion of corticosteroids by the adrenal cortex, ng/min			
Aldosterone	2.1 ± 0.4 (7)	2.3 ± 0.2 (13)	NS
11-dehydrocorticosterone	14.4 ± 3.1 (7)	29.1 ± 5.4 (13)	$p < 0.05$
Corticosterone	519 ± 61 (7)	769 ± 83 (13)	$p < 0.05$
11-deoxycorticosterone	45.6 ± 6 (7)	87 ± 12 (13)	$p < 0.01$

In the course of studies of the secretory activity of the adrenal cortex we noted that adrenal mass in significantly greater in the ISIAH rats than in WAG normotensives (Table 4). Thus, it may be believed that selection for enhanced response of BP to stress is associated with a general increase in the functional activity of the adrenals.

This is supported by estimates of secretory activity of the adrenal cortex measured in rats under surgical anesthesia during cannula insertion into the suprarenal vein (Table 4). A considerable and significant enhancement of the secretion of corticosterone, 11-dehydroxycorticosterone, and 11-deoxycorticosterone were observed. The secretion of the corticosterone and 11-deoxycorticosterone was increased by two times in the ISIAHs compared to WAGs.

The secretion levels of aldosterone in the compared strains were the same, however. As for the content of hormones in adrenal tissues, the estimates for all the four we analyzed were higher in the ISIAH than WAG rats, the difference, however, did not reach significance. This observation is obviously explained by the fact that the hormones synthesized in the adrenal cortex virtually are not stored there, being secreted into the circulation as they are synthesized.

Survey of the hormonal response of the ISIAHs and WAGs to 7 min stress disclosed a characteristic pattern (Figures 20 and 21). The basal control values of the concentrations of both corticosterone and aldosterone were almost the same in peripheral blood plasma. Stress produced an increase in the concentrations of both hormones in each strain. This was in agreement with the previous data (34). The response had certain noteworthy features. Firstly, the increment of the concentration of corticosterone in plasma was significantly greater in the ISIAHs than WAG rats; secondly, in the WAG normotensives the elevation in the major mineralocorticoid aldosterone in response to acute stress, which was mainly emotional, was expressed poorer than corticosterone response, whereas the stress response of aldosterone in the ISIAH hypertensives was quite substantial, significantly surpassing the observed for WAGs.

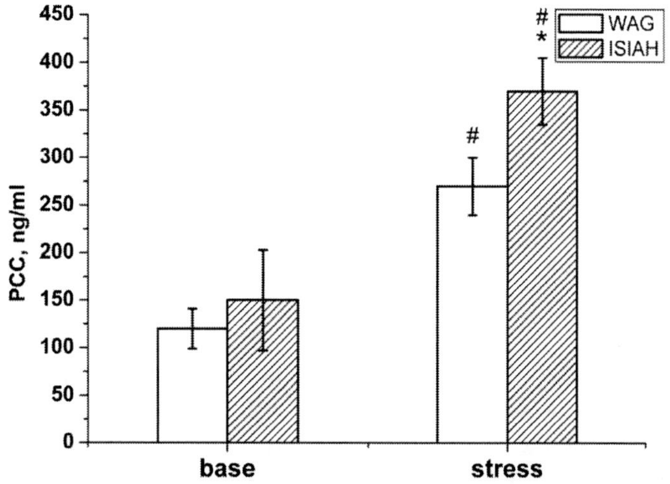

Figure 20. Plasma corticosterone concentration in the adult (5 – 6 months old) WAG and ISIAH rats in rest (basal level) and under acute stress. Data are presented as *M* ± *S.E.M.* *, statistically significant inter-strain differences; #, statistically significant differences between the rats of the same strain in rest (control) and under stress.

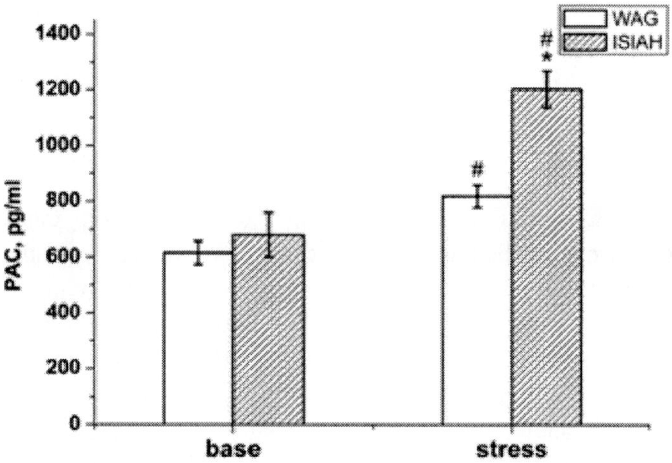

Figure 21. Plasma aldosterone concentration in the adult (5 – 6 months old) WAG and ISIAH rats in rest and under acute stress. Data are presented as *M* ± *S.E.M.* *, statistically significant inter-strain differences; #, statistically significant differences between the rats of the same strain in rest (control) and under stress.

The enhancement of the mineralocorticoid response to stress in the hypertensives may evidence in favor of the idea that aldosterone possibly plays a very important role in the pathogenesis of stress-dependent arterial hypertension. Enhancement of the mineralocorticoid function in the ISIAH rats may also be supported by increased secretion of 11-

deoxycorticosterone, which we detected. As indicated above, there is increasing evidence in the literature confirming the significance of increased aldosterone level in the pathogenesis of EH. As for our experiments, the rather impressive response to stress of the ISIAH rats highlighted the significance of this pathogenetic mechanism in the development of the stress-dependent form of the hypertensive disease.

Our current results agree with those obtained in humans. An increase in the hormonal, including the mineralocorticoid response to psychological stress has been reported for patients with hypertension, also in normotensives whose parents were affected with the hypertensive disease [113]. Tomaschitz et al. [29] have established that, even in the absence of classical evidence of aldosteronism, an increase in aldosterone inadequate to other parameters of RAS activity is involved in the pathogenesis of primary hypertension. An increase in the concentration of aldosterone that does not exceed the upper limit of the norm, along with that in the aldosterone-renin ratio, was implied here. In this current study, we showed that the expression of the renin gene in renal tissue of ISIAH rats is reduced in adulthood (Figure 4).

In our view, this shift of the balance between the levels of renin and aldosterone in favor of the latter may be evidence of the significant role of the ACTH in the stimulation of aldosterone secretion in the stress-dependent hypertension. The conclusion is obvious: analysis of a variety of corticosteroid hormones in the ISIAH rats with the stress-sensitive hypertension corroborated the idea that an increase in the mineralocorticoid function of the adrenal cortex contributes greatly to this form of hypertension. A similar mechanism of the formation of the hypertensive status may be possibly operative in humans with an enhanced response to stressful stimuli.

Conclusion

"Happy is he who knows the causes of things..." (Virgil)

Not all the correlations, similarities-differences emerging from this current study are readily explicable. Some may be introduced by chance. Whatever the random factors were, it is undeniable that the transcription of the RAS genes is significantly modified in the ISIAH rats. The conclusion is drawn primarily from the almost complete absence of correlations between gene expression of an organ (as observed for the kidneys and adrenals of ISIAHs), also from changes in the correspondence between the expression of a gene in one organ and an entire gene group in another organ (between *PRR* in the hypothalamus and a number of genes in the kidneys of WAGs or between *Agtr1a* in the kidneys and a number of genes in the medulla oblongata of ISIAHs). At the same time, interrelations with gene expression are more clear-cut at the body level in the young ISIAH rats: the elevated *Agt* mRNA in the hypothalamus providing evidence of increased Ang II content correlated with higher level of renin mRNA in the kidneys of young animals from where it enters the circulation, also the relation between the expression of renin in the kidneys and ACE in the circulation, as evidenced by the positive correlation between *Ren* mRNA in the kidneys and *Ace* mRNA in the lungs of the ISIAH rats.

To summarize, the development of the stress-sensitive arterial hypertension is associated with changes in the activity of the renin-angiotensin-aldosterone system. The rearrangements in the functioning of the RAS pass through at least two steps during the progression of the pathogenesis of stress-sensitive hypertension. At the first step, during the establishment of the hypertensive status, the activation of the initial limb of the RAS is related to the conversion of Agt in the brain (namely, in the hypothalamus and medulla oblongata) and kidneys. This is possibly due to the increased reactivity of the sympathoadrenal system in the ISIAH rats. Subsequently, as hypertension reaches a high level and stabilizes, the functional tension of the renin mechanism reduces. The hypertensive status at the second step of pathology is stable and corresponds to the low-renin hypertension but with enhanced in relation to the low renin level aldosterone. Aldosterone level in resting conditions in the ISIAH rats does not differ from the control, but under emotionsl stress it raises to levels much exceeding the control. An enhanced plasma aldosterone response to ACTH also was revealed in the ISIAH rats. The reactivity of the sympathoadrenal system concomitantly remains elevated. The model we generated, the ISIAH rats, support the following: first, stress and increased stress-reactivity can initiate the formation of stable arterial hypertension; second, the subsequent development of the pathogenesis of the stable arterial hypertension proceeds with the involvement of the RAS. The enhanced response of the aldosterone system to emotional stress may also be of great importance.

Acknowledgments

This work was supported by a research grant from RFBR (№08-04-00533) and the Ministry of Education and Science of the Russian Federation (State contracts № 02.740.11.0705 and 3N-319-09).

References

[1] Chobanian AV, Bakris GL, Black HR, Cushman WC, Green LA, Izzo JL, Jr et al Seventh report of the Joint National Committee on Prevention, Detection, Evaluation, and Treatment of High Blood Pressure: Complete report. *Hypertension.* 2003;42:1206–52.

[2] National Center for Health Statistics. *Health, United States, 2011: With special feature on socioeconomic status and health.* Hyattsville, MD; 2012.

[3] World Health Organization (WHO). *Global atlas on cardiovascular disease prevention and control* [online]. 2012 [cited 2012 Oct 02] Available from: http://www.who.int/cardiovascular_diseases/en/.

[4] Rosskopf D, Schürks M, Rimmbach C, Schäfers R. Genetics of arterial hypertension and hypotension. *Naunyn Schmiedebergs Arch. Pharmacol.* 2007;374:429–69.

[5] Longini IM, Higgins MW, Hinton PC, Moll PC, Keller JB. Environmental and genetic sources of familial aggregation of blood pressure in Tecumseh, Michigan. *Am. J. Epidemiol.* 1984;120:131–44.

[6] Garcia EA, Newhouse S, Caulfield MJ, Munroe PB. Genes and hypertension. *Curr. Pharm. Des*. 2003;9:1679–89.

[7] Rassler B. The renin-angiotensin system in the development of salt-sensitive hypertension in animal models and humans. *Pharmaceuticals*. 2010; 3:940-60.

[8] Gross DR. Iatrogenic, congenic, and transgenic models of hypertension. In: *Animal models in cardiovascular research*. Springer; 2009. p. 259-305.

[9] Bader M. Rat models of cardiovascular diseases. *Methods Mol. Biol*. 2010; 597: 403-14.

[10] Markel AL, Maslova LN, Shishkina GT, Bulygina VV, Machanova NA, Jacobson GS. Developmental influences on blood pressure regulation in ISIAH rats. In: McCarty R, Blizard DA, Chevalier RL, editors. *Development of the hypertensive phenotype: basic and clinical studies: Handbook of hypertension*, 19. Amsterdam: Elsevier Science Publishers BV, 1999. p. 493-526.

[11] Markel AL. Development of a new strain of rats with inherited stress-induced arterial hypertension. In: Sassard J, editor. *Genetic hypertension*, 218. Colloque INSERM. London: John Libbey Eurotext Ltd; 1992. p. 405–407.

[12] Markel AL, Dymshits GM, Shmerling MD, Jacobson GS. Genes, stress and hypertension. *Biulleten Sibirskogo otdeleniia Rossiĭskoĭ akademii meditsinskikh nauk (Bulletin SO RAMN)* 2002;104(2):35-40.

[13] Markel AL, Kalashnikova EV, Goryakin SV, Sakharov DG, Moreva TA, Dymshits GM et al. Functional activity of the sympathoadrenal system in hypertensive NISAG rats. *Bull .Exp. Biol. Med*. 2006; 141(3):275-277.

[14] Buzueva II, Shmerling MD, Filiushina EE, Markel AL, Iakobson GS. Structural features of the rat adrenal cortex with inherited stress-induced arterial hypertension in the early period of postnatal ontogenesis. *Morfologiia*. 1998(2):84-8.

[15] Buzueva II, Shmerling MD, Filiushina EE, Markel AL, Iakobson GS. Structural characteristics of the adrenal cortex from rats with inherited stress-induced hereditary arterial hypertension in the late postnatal ontogenesis. *Morfologiia*. 2000(6):61-5.

[16] Amstislavsky S, Welker P, Fruhauf JH, Maslova L, Ivanova L, Jensen B et al. Renal and endocrine changes in rats with inherited stress-induced arterial hypertension (ISIAH). *Histochem. Cell Biol*. 2005;8:1-9.

[17] Buzueva II. Effect of enalapril injected in the early period of postnatal ontogeny on structure of adrenal glands in mature hypertensive NISAG rats. *Bull. Expl. Biol. Med*. 2006;141(2):175-7.

[18] Buzueva II, Filiushina EE, Shmerling MD, Kudryashova DR, Markel AL, Jacobson GS. The delayed effect of losartan and terazosin injections in prepubertate period of ontogenesis on the structure of the glomerular zone of adrenal cortex in the ISIAH rats. *Biulleten Sibirskogo otdeleniia Rossiĭskoĭ akademii meditsinskikh nauk (Bulletin SO RAMN)* 2007;125(3):98-102.

[19] Antonov EV, Moreva TA, Cherkasova OP, Gilinsky MA, Markel AL, Jacobson GS. Investigation of the adrenal cortex secretory activity in the ISIAH hypertensive strain of rats. *Biulleten Sibirskogo otdeleniia Rossiĭskoĭ akademii meditsinskikh nauk (Bulletin SO RAMN)* 2010;30(4): 68-75.

[20] Khvorostova YuV, Filipenko ML, Dymshits GM, Markel AL. Expression of the proopiomelanocortin gene in the pituitaries of rats of the hypertensive strain NISAG. *Russ. J. Genet*. 2001;37(5):523-7.

[21] Khvorostova YuV, Kalashnikova EV, Cherkasova OP, Fedoseeva LA, Redina OE, Dymshits GM et al. Glucocorticoid receptor gene expression in ISIAH hypertensive rat strain. *Ross. Fiziol. Zh. Im. I. M. Sechenova*. 2003; 89(12):1523-8.
[22] Khvorostova YuV, Goryakin SV, Petrova GV, Filipenko ML, Shikhevich SG, Redina OE et al. Function of hypothalamic-pituitary-adrenocortical system in ISIAH hypertensive rat strain. *Ross. Fiziol. Zh. Im. I. M. Sechenova.* 2002;88(11):1423-32.
[23] Haulica I, Bild W, Serban DN. Angiotensin peptides and their pleiotropic actions. *J. Renin. Angiotensin. Aldosterone Syst.* 2005;6:121–31.
[24] Carey RM, Siragy HM. Newly recognized components of the renin-angiotensin system: potential roles in cardiovascular and renal regulation. *Endocr. Rev.* 2003; 24: 261–71.
[25] Donoghue M, Hsieh F, Baronas E, Godbout K, Gosselin M, Stagliano N et al. A novel angiotensin-converting enzyme related carboxypeptidase (ACE 2) converts angiotensin I to angiotensin (1–9). *Circ. Res.* 2000; 87:1–9.
[26] Tipnis SR, Hooper NM, Hyde R, Karran E, Christie G, Turner AJ. A human homolog of angiotensin-converting enzyme: cloning and functional expression as a captopril-insensitive carboxypeptidase. *J. Biol. Chem.* 2000;275:33238–43.
[27] Santos RA, Simoes e Silva AC, Maric C, Silva DM, Machado RP, de Buhr I et al. Angiotensin-(1-7) is an endogenous ligand for the G protein-coupled receptor Mas. *Proc. Natl. Acad. Sci. USA*. 2003; 100(14): 8258-63.
[28] Moeller I, Chai SY, Smith I, Lew R, Mendelsohn FA. Haemorphin peptides may be endogenous ligands for brain angiotensin AT4 receptors. *Clin. Exp. Pharmacol. Physiol. Suppl.* 1998;25:S68–71.
[29] Tomaschitz A, Pilz S, Ritz E, Obermayer-Pietsch B, Pieber TR. Aldosterone and arterial hypertension. *Nat. Rev. Endocrinol.* 2010;6(2): 83-93.
[30] Freel EM, Connell JMC. Mechanisms of hypertension: the expanding role of aldosterone. *J. Am. Soc. Nephrol.* 2004;15(8):1993–2001.
[31] Kubzansky LD, Adler GK. Aldosterone: A forgotten mediator of the relationship between psychological stress and heart disease . *Neurosci. Biobehav. Rev.* 2010;34(1):80-6.
[32] Antonov AR, Khidirova LD, Markel AL, Letyagina VV, Jacobson GS. Changes in the gluco- and mineralocorticoid adrenal function in experimental myocardial infarction of rats. *Advances in current natural sciences.* 2009(9):190.
[33] Cherkasova OP, Fedorov VI, Markel AL. Activity of angiotensin-converting enzyme in hereditary stress-induced arterial hypertension. *Bull. Exp. Biol. Med.* 2005; 140(10): 381-3.
[34] Markel AL, Redina OE, Gilinsky MA, Dymshits GM, Kalashnikova EV, Khvorostova YuV et al. Neuroendocrine profiling in inherited stress-induced arterial hypertension rat strain with stress-sensitive arterial hypertension. *J. Endocrinol.* 2007; 195: 439–50.
[35] Cuadra AE, Shan Z, Sumners C, Raizada MK. A current view of brain renin-angiotensin system: Is the (pro)renin receptor the missing link? *Pharmacol. Ther.* 2010; 125(1): 27-38.
[36] Yim HE, Yoo KH. Renin-angiotensin system - considerations for hypertension and kidney. *Electrolyte Blood Press.* 2008;6:42-50.
[37] Rosivall L. Intrarenal renin–angiotensin system. *Mol. Cell Endocrinol.* 2009; 302(2): 185-92.

[38] Paul M, Mehr AP, Kreutz R. Physiology of local renin-angiotensin systems. *Physiol. Rev*. 2006;86:747–803.

[39] Bader M, Ganten D. Update on tissue renin–angiotensin systems. *J. Mol. Med*. 2008; 86: 615–21.

[40] Johnson RJ, Rodriguez-Iturbe B, Kang D-H, Feig DI, Herrera-Acosta J. A unifying pathway for essential hypertension. *Am. J. Hypertens*. 2005; 18:431–440.

[41] Chattopadhyay N, Kher R, Godbole M. Inexpensive SDS/phenol method for RNA extraction from tissues. *Biotechniques*. 1993;15(1):24-6.

[42] Fedoseeva LA, Dymshits GM, Markel AL, Jakobson GS. Renin system of the kidney in ISIAH rats with inherited stress-induced arterial hypertension. *Bull. Exp. Biol. Med*. 2009; 147(2):177-80.

[43] Cherkasova OP, Fedorov VI. Renin activity in kidney and plasma at hereditary stress-induced arterial hypertension. *Vestn. Tomsk. Gos. Univ*. 2006(21):167-8.

[44] Yang T, Singh I, Pham H, Sun D, Smart A, Schnermann JB et al. Regulation of cyclooxygenase expression in the kidney by dietary salt intake. *Am. J. Physiol*. 1998; 274: F481–9.

[45] Kammerl MC, Nüsing RM, Seyberth HW, Riegger GAJ, Kurtz A, Krämer BK. Inhibition of cyclooxygenase-2 attenuates urinary prostanoid excretion without affecting renal renin expression. *Pflügers Arch*. 2001;442: 842–7.

[46] Duffy SJ, Biegelsen ES, Eberhardt RT, Kahn DF, Kingwell BA, Vita JA. Low-renin hypertension with relative aldosterone excess is associated with impaired NO-mediated vasodilation. *Hypertension*. 2005; 46:707-13.

[47] Yugar-Toledo JC, Tacito LHB, Ferreira-Melo SE, Sousa W, Consolin-Colombo F, Irigoyen MC et al. Low-renin (volume dependent) mild-hypertensive patients have impaired flow-mediated and glyceryl-trinitrate stimulated vascular reactivity. *Circ. J*. 2005; 69:1380–5.

[48] Sassard J, Lo M, Liu K-L. Lyon genetically hypertensive rats: an animal model of "low renin hypertension". *Acta Pharmacol. Sin*. 2003;24 (1):1-6.

[49] Nagata K, Obata K, Xu J, Ichihara S, Noda A, Kimata H et al. Mineralocorticoid receptor antagonism attenuates cardiac hypertrophy and failure in low-aldosterone hypertensive rats. *Hypertension*. 2006; 47:656-64.

[50] Nakamura A, Johns EJ. Renal nerves, renin, and angiotensinogen gene expression in spontaneously hypertensive rats. *Hypertension*. 1995; 25:581-6.

[51] Gomez RA, Lynch KR, Chevalier RL, Wilfong N, Everett A, Carey RM et al. Renin and angiotensinogen gene expression in maturing rat kidney. *Am. J. Physiol. Renal. Physiol*. 1988;254: F582-87.

[52] Samani NJ, Swales JD, Brammar WJ. A widespread abnormality of renin gene expression in the spontaneously hypertensive rat: modulation in some tissues with the development of hypertension. *Clin. Sci. (Lond*). 1989; 77:629–36.

[53] Harrap SB, Van der Merwe WM, Griffin SA, Macpherson F, Lever AF. Brief angiotensin converting enzyme inhibitor treatment in young spontaneously hypertensive rats reduces blood pressure long-term. *Hypertension*. 1990;16(6):603-14.

[54] Filiushina EE, Shmerling MD, Lazarev VA, Buzuyeva II, Markel AL, Yakobson GS. Delayed effects of hypotensive drugs on structural characteristics of the renal glomerular system in hypertensive NISAG rats. *Bull. Exp. Biol. Med*. 2007; 143(6): 749-52.

[55] Korostyshevskaya LM, Maximov VF, Markel AL, Shmerling MD, Buzueva II, Filushina EE et al. Cardiovascular peculiarities in hypertensive rats (ISIAH strain) after antihypertensive drug intervention duting juvenile period of life. *Ross. Fiziol. Zh. Im. I. M. Sechenova*. 2007; 93(2):169-79.

[56] Fedoseeva LA, Ryazanova MA, Antonov EV, Dymshits GM, Markel AL. Expression of the renin angiotensin system genes in the kidney and heart of ISIAH hypertensive rats. *Biochemistry (Moscow) Suppl. Series B, Biomedical chemistry*. 2011; 5(1):37–43.

[57] Wilson RC, Dave-Sharma S, Wei J-Q, Obeyesekere VR, Li K, Ferrari P et al. A genetic defect resulting in mild low-renin hypertension. *Proc. Natl. Acad. Sci. USA*. 1998;95:10200–5.

[58] Andresen MC, Yang M. Arterial baroreceptor resetting: contributions of chronic and acute processes. *Clin. Exp. Pharmacol. Physiol*. 1989; 15(Suppl): 19–30.

[59] Veerasingham SJ, Raizada MK. Brain renin–angiotensin system dysfunction in hypertension: recent advances and perspectives. *Brit. J. Pharmacol*. 2003; 139: 191–202.

[60] Crowley SD, Gurley SB, Oliverio MI, Pazmino AK, Griffiths R, Flannery PJ et al. Distinct roles for the kidney and systemic tissues in blood pressure regulation by the renin-angiotensin system. *J. Clin. Invest*. 2005; 115:1092–9.

[61] Kobori H, Nishiyama A, Abe Y, Navar LG. Enhancement of intrarenal angiotensinogen in Dahl salt-sensitive rats on high salt diet. *Hypertension*. 2003;41(3):592–7.

[62] Nishiyama A, Yoshizumi M, Rahman M, Tamaki T, Kobori H, Abe Y. Effects of AT1 receptor blockade on MAPK activities and renal injury in Dahl salt-sensitive rats. *FASEB J*. 2002;16:A418–9.

[63] Cheng H-F, Wang J-L, Vinson G P, Harris RC. Young SHR express increased type 1 angiotensin II receptors in renal proximal tubule. *Am. J. Physiol*. 1998;274 (Renal Physiol. 43): F10–7.

[64] Correa FM, Viswanathan M, Ciuffo GM, Tsutsumi K, Saavedra JM. Kidney angiotensin II receptors and converting enzyme in neonatal and adult Wistar-Kyoto and spontaneously hypertensive rats. *Peptides*. 1995; 16(1):19-24.

[65] Chappell MC. Role of ACE, ACE2 and neprilysin in the kidney. In: Po Sing Leung, editor. *Frontiers in research of the renin-angiotensin system on human disease: Proteases in biology and disease*, Vol. 7. Springer; 2008. p. 1–20.

[66] Keidar S, Kaplan M, Gamliel-Lazarovich A. ACE2 of the heart: from angiotensin I to angiotensin (1–7). *Cardiovasc. Res*. 2007;73:463–9.

[67] Lee Y-A, Liang C-S, Lee M-A, Lindpainter K. Local stress, not systemic factors, regulate gene expression of the cardiac renin-angiotensin system *in vivo*: a comprehensive study of all its components in the dog. *Proc. Natl. Acad. Sci. USA*. 1996;93(20):11035-40.

[68] Schunkert H, Dzau VJ, Tang SS, Hirsch AT, Apstein CS, Lorell BH. Increased rat cardiac angiotensin converting enzyme activity and mRNA expression in pressure overload left ventricular hypertrophy effects on coronary resistance, contractility, and relaxation. *J. Clin. Invest*. 1990; 86:1913-20.

[69] Schunkert H, Hense HW, Muscholl M, Luchner A, Kurzinger S, Jan Danser AH et al. Associations between circulating components of the renin-angiotensin-aldosterone system and left ventricular mass. *Heart*. 1997;77:24-31.

[70] Zhao X, White R, Van Huysse J, Leenen F. Cardiac hypertrophy and cardiac renin-angiotensin system in Dahl rats on high salt intake. *J. Hypertens.* 2000;18(9):1319-26.

[71] Naito Y, Tsujino T, Fujioka Y, Ohyanagi M, Iwasaki T. Augmented diurnal variations of the cardiac renin-angiotensin system in hypertensive rats. *Hypertension.* 2002; 40: 827-33.

[72] Herzig TC, Jobe SM, Aoki H, Molkentin JD, Cowley AW, Izumo S et al. Angiotensin II type1a receptor gene expression in the heart: AP-1 and GATA-4 participate in the response to pressure overload (hypertrophy DNA injection). *Proc. Natl. Acad. Sci. USA.* 1997;94:7543–8.

[73] Oparil S, Zaman MA, Calhoun DA. Pathogenesis of hypertension. *Ann. Intern. Med.* 2003; 139:761-76.

[74] Nickenig G, Laufs U, Schnabel P, Knorr A, Paul M, Boehm M. Down-regulation of aortic and cardiac AT1 receptor gene expression in transgenic (mRen-2) 27 rats . *Br. J. Pharmacol.* 1997;121:134-40.

[75] Billet S, Bardin S, Verp S, Baudrie V, Michaud A, Conchon S et al. Gain-of-function mutant of angiotensin II receptor, type 1A, causes hypertension and cardiovascular fibrosis in mice. *J. Clin. Invest.* 2007; 117(7):1914–25.

[76] Harada K, Komuro I, Shiojima I, Hayashi D, Kudoh S, Mizuno T et al. Pressure overload induces cardiac hypertrophy in angiotensin II type 1A receptor knockout mice. *Circulation.* 1998;97(19):1952–1959.

[77] Urata H, Healy B, Stewart RW, Bumpus FM, Husain A. Angiotensin II receptors in normal and failing human hearts. *J. Clin. Endocrinol. Metab.* 1989;69:54-66.

[78] Crowley SD, Gurley SB, Herrera MJ, Ruiz P, Griffiths R, Kumar AP et al. Angiotensin II causes hypertension and cardiac hypertrophy through its receptors in the kidney. *Proc. Natl. Acad. Sci. USA.* 2006; 103(47): 17985–90.

[79] Dorn II GW, Force T. Protein kinase cascades in the regulation of cardiac hypertrophy. *J. Clin. Invest.* 2005;115:527–37.

[80] De Luca LA, Xu Z, Schoorlemmer GHM, Thunhorst RL, Beltz TG, Menani JV et al. Water deprivation-induced sodium appetite: humoral and cardiovascular mediators and immediate early genes. *Am. J. Physiol. Regul. Integr. Comp. Physiol.* 2002; 282: R552–9.

[81] Tamura K, Umemura S, Nyui N, Yamakawa T, Yamaguchi S, Ishigami T et al. Tissue specific regulation of angiotensinogen gene expression in spontaneously hypertensive rats. *Hypertension.* 1996;27:1216 –23.

[82] Komatsu C, Shibata K, Fururkawa T. The developmental increase of the AT1A, but not the AT1B, receptor mRNA level at the preoptic area in spontaneously hypertensive rats. *Life Sci.* 1996;58: 1109–21.

[83] Shibata K, Komatsu C, Misumi Y, Furukawa T. Developmental differences of angiotensinogen mRNA in the preoptic area between spontaneously hypertensive and age-matched Wistar-Kyoto rats. *Mol. Brain Res.* 1993;19:115–20.

[84] Phillips MI, Mohuczy-Dominiak D, Coffey M, Galli SM, Kimura B, Wu P et al. Prolonged reduction of high blood pressure with an in vivo, nonpathogenic, adeno-associated viral vector delivery of AT_1-R mRNA antisense. *Hypertension.* 1997; 29: 374 – 80.

[85] Ruiz P, Basso N, Cannata MA, Tauquini AC. The rennin-angiotensin system in different stages of spontaneous hypertension in the rat (SHR). *Clin. Exp. Hypertens.* 1990; 12:63–81.
[86] Schinke M, Baltatu O, Bohm M, Peters J, Rasher W, Bricca G et al. Blood pressure reduction and diabetes insipidus in transgenic rats deficient in brain angiotensinogen. *Proc. Natl. Acad. Sci. USA*. 1999; 96:3975 – 80.
[87] Park CG, Leenen FH. Effects of centrally administered losartan on deoxycorticosterone-salt hypertension rats. *J. Korean Med. Sci.* 2001; 16(5):553–7.
[88] Corvol P, Jeunemaitre X. Molecular genetics of human hypertension: role of angiotensinogen. *Endocr. Rev*. 1997;18(5): 662–77.
[89] Campbell DJ. Circulating and tissue angiotensin systems. *J. Clin. Invest*. 1987; 79:1–6.
[90] Deschepper CF, Bouhnik J, Ganong WF. Colocalization of angiotensinogen and glial fibrillary acidic protein in astrocytes in rat brain. *Brain Res*. 1986; 374: 195–8.
[91] Lynch KR, Peach MJ. Molecular biology of angiotensinogen. *Hypertension*. 1991;17:263-9.
[92] Kalinyak JE, Perlman AJ. Tissue-specific regulation of angiotensinogen mRNA accumulation by dexamethasone. *Biol. Chem*. 1987;262:460-4.
[93] Averill DB, Diz DI. Angiotensin peptides and baroreflex control of sympathetic outflow: pathways and mechanisms of the medulla oblongata. *Brain Res. Bull.* 2000;51:119−28.
[94] Boscan P, Allen AM, Paton JF. Baroreflex inhibition of cardiac sympathetic outflow is attenuated by angiotensin II in the nucleus of the solitary tract. *Neuroscience*. 2001;103(1):153−60.
[95] Li YW, Guyenet PG. Angiotensin II decreases a resting K+ conductance in rat bulbospinal neurons of the C1 area. *Circ. Res*. 1996;78:274−282.
[96] Tagawa T, Fontes MA, Potts PD, Allen AM, Dampney RA. The physiological role of AT1 receptors in the ventrolateral medulla. *Braz. J. Med. Biol. Res*. 2000;33:643−52.
[97] Malpas SC. Sympathetic nervous system overactivity and its role in the development of cardiovascular disease. *Physiol. Rev*. 2010;90:513–57.
[98] Mattson MP, Maudsley S. Live longer sans the AT1A receptor. *Cell Metab*. 2009; 9(5):403–5.
[99] Gao L, Zucker IH. AT2 receptor signaling and sympathetic regulation. *Curr. Opin. Pharmacol*. 2011;11:124–30.
[100] Horiuchi M, Mogi M, Iwai M. The angiotensin II type 2 receptor in the brain. *J. Renin. Angiotensin. Aldosterone Syst*. 2010;11:1-6.
[101] Gao L, Wang W-Z, Wang W, Zucker IH. Imbalance of AT1R and AT2R in the RVLM: potential mechanism for sympathetic overactivity in heart failure. *Hypertension*. 2008; 52(4):708–14.
[102] Chappell MC, Ferrario CM. Angiotensin-(1-7) in hypertension. *Curr. Opin. Nephrol. Hypertens*. 1999;88:231–5.
[103] Sampaio WO, Santos RA, Faria-Silva R, Mata Machado LT, Schiffrin EL, Touyz RM. Angiotensin-(1-7) through receptor mas mediates endothelial nitric oxide synthase activation via Akt-dependent pathways. *Hypertension*. 2007;49:185–92.
[104] Paula RD, Lima CV, Khosla MC. Angiotensin (1–7) potentiates hypotensive effect of bradykinin in conscious rats. *Hypertension*. 1995; 26:1154–1159.

[105] Broshinan KB, Li P, Ferrario CM. Angiotensin (1–7) dilates canine coronary arteries through kinins and nitric oxide. *Hypertension*. 1996; 27:523–8.

[106] Li P, Chappell MC, Ferrario CM, Broshinan KB. Angiotensin (1–7) augments bradykinin-induced vasodilation by competing with ACE and releasing nitric oxide. *Hypertension*. 1997;29:394–400.

[107] Ueda S, Masumori-Maemoto S, Ashino K, Nagahara T, Gotoh E, Umemura S et al. Angiotensin (1–7) attenuates vasoconstriction evoked by angiotensin II but not by noradrenaline in man. *Hypertension*. 2000; 35:998–1001.

[108] Sriramula S, Cardinale JP, Lazartigues E, Francis J. ACE2 overexpression in the paraventricular nucleus attenuates angiotensin II-induced hypertension. *Cardiovasc. Res*. 2011;92 (3):401-408.

[109] Wang HW, Gallinat S, Li H, Sumners C, Raizada MK, Katovich MJ. Elevated blood pressure in normotensive rats produced by 'knockdown' of the angiotensin type2 receptor. *Exp. Physiol*. 2004;89(3):313–22.

[110] Matsubara H. Pathophysiological role of angiotensin II type 2 receptor in cardiovascular and renal diseases. *Circ. Res*. 1998;83:1182-91.

[111] Wang DH, Qiu J, Hu Z. Differential regulation of angiotensin II receptor subtypes in the adrenal gland. Role of aldosterone. *Hypertension*. 1998; 32:65-70.

[112] Steckelings UM, Kaschina E, Unger T. The AT2 receptor – a matter of love and hate. *Peptides*. 2005;26:1401–9.

[113] Hollenberg NK, Williams GH, Adams DF. Essential hypertension: abnormal renal vascular and endocrine responses to a mild psychological stimulus. *Hypertension*. 1981;3(1):11-7.

In: Renin-Angiotensin System
Editors: Ayako Himura and Takeshi Sato
ISBN: 978-1-62417-788-0

Chapter II

Renin-Angiotensin System Activation: Implications for Eye Diseases

Maria E. Marin-Castaño*
Department of Ophthalmology, Bascom Palmer Eye Institute,
University of Miami, Miami, Florida, US

1. Abstract

The goal of this chapter is to review the most relevant scientific evidence supporting the role of the renin-angiotensin system (RAS) activation, in the pathogenesis of age-related macular degeneration (AMD) and diabetic retinopathy (DR), two leading causes of blindness in elderly and people of working age respectively, and highlight the importance of Angiotensin II (Ang II), prorenin, and prorenin receptor in the etiology of these diseases. Early AMD, include the presence of waste material in the form of focal deposits named drusen below the retinal pigment epithelium (RPE) and within Bruch's membrane, a stratified extracellular matrix situated between the choriocapillaris and RPE. Late (wet) AMD is characterized by inflammation and the growth of leaky new abnormal blood vessels under the RPE from the subjacent choroid known as choroidal neovascularization. The early stage of DR, non-proliferative diabetic retinopathy is identified by deposits forming in the retina. Proliferative diabetic retinopathy is characterized by neovascularization on or adjacent to the optic nerve and vitreous, pre-retinal hemorrhage, which occurs in the vitreous humor or front of the retina and ischemia. Extracellular matrix turnover (ECM), inflammation, and neovascularization are key cellular processes that play a central role in the pathogenesis of these deaseases. The scientific evidence to support the proposed role of Ang II, prorenin, and prorenin receptor-mediated cellular effects on subretinal deposits formation, inflammation and neovascularization is reviewed in depth.

* Reprint requests: Maria E. Marin-Castaño, M.D., PhD, William L. McKnight Vision Research Center, 1638 N.W. 10th Avenue, Miami, FL 33136, Tel.: (305) 482-5142, E-mail: mcastano@med.miami.edu.

Keywords: System renin-angiotensin, Age-related Macular Degeneration, diabetic retinopathy, Angiotensin II, Angiotensin II receptors, prorenin, prorenin receptor, sub-RPE deposits, extracellular matrix turnover, inflammation, neovascularization

2. The System Renin Angiotensin

Knowledge of the renin–angiotensin system (RAS) has advanced remarkably over recent years from that of a classical endocrine system that explained homeostasis for maintenance of circulating intravascular volume and thereby restoration of arterial pressure to a newer concept including a number of local RASs that operate independently within several organs. Classically, the systemic RAS basically depends upon its rate-limiting enzyme renin which is produced in the juxtaglomerular apparatus of the kidney. Thus, with the release of renin from the juxtaglomerular apparatus, it gains access to the circulation where it acts on its protein substrate angiotensinogen (an alpha-2 globulin synthesized by the liver) to generate the decapeptide angiotensin I. In turn, angiotensin I is converted by the angiotensin converting enzyme 1 (ACE1), which is predominantly expressed in high concentrations on the surface of endothelial cells in the pulmonary circulation [1], into the octapeptide angiotensin II (Ang II) by cleavage of the terminal dipeptide from the parent decapeptide. The result is freely circulating Ang II, the most important hormone associated with hypertension (Figure 1). Ang II effects are mediated by the type 1 (AT1) a type 2 (AT2) Ang II cell surface receptors which belong to a group of seven-transmembrane domain G-protein coupled receptors and have a 30% sequence similarity and different functional properties and signal transduction mechanisms [2, 3]. In rodents, AT1 receptors can be subdivided into AT1a and AT1b subtypes [4, 5], which share 95% sequence homology and exhibit similar ligand binding affinities and signal-transduction properties, but differ in their tissue expression.

RAS acts as a feedback system, in which Ang II is traditionally considered the main regulatory peptide and ACE1, the main regulatory enzyme and AT1 receptor, the main regulatory receptor. In view of controlling blood pressure, the most important actions of Ang II are vasoconstriction, sympathetic nervous stimulation, increased aldosterone biosynthesis and renal actions [6]. These Ang II effects elicit tissue responses mainly via AT1 receptors. In fact, according to recent evidence, the circulating RAS is not thought to be directly responsible for the rise in blood pressure especially in essential hypertension in elderly people, but there are more important non-circulating "local" renin-angiotensin autocrine or paracrine systems, which have important roles in adjusting blood pressure and regional blood flow [7].

As mentioned above, in addition to the circulatory RAS, there is a tissue-localized system which has been known for some time and which is known to regulate long-term changes in a variety of organs like kidneys, adrenals, brain, reproductive organs and vasculature [8-10]. In tissues, Ang II is derived either from the circulation or from local production. Local Ang II formation can also be catalyzed by enzymes other than the classical ACE. These actions are called renin-independent or ACE-independent pathways for Ang II production e.g. via chymase or cathepsin G, but they may have a minor role and evidence-based studies are warranted [10]. By blocking the activity of these enzymes, Ang II production can be reduced. In addition to these ACE-independent enzymes, there is an important, recently found RAS component: angiotensin-converting enzyme 2 (ACE2). ACE2 can degrade Ang I to Ang [2-10] and Ang II to form the biologically active Ang [1-7], which in turn and in many respects acts oppositely to Ang II [11]. Ang [1-7] mainly acts via a novel angiotensin receptor type, Mas receptor. Mas receptor is a G-protein-coupled receptor encoded by the Mas protooncogene found first in the mouse kidney [12]. The activation of Mas receptor causes effects opposite to the AT1 receptor activation, such as vasodilatation, antiproliferation, antifibrosis and it plays a role in fluid volume homeostasis [13]. All of these alternative pathways for Ang II production and for degradation are important both physiologically and pathophysiologically. In addition to these above-mentioned alternative pathways of local RAS activatory and inhibitory components, there is an interesting receptor type, a tissue (pro)renin receptor (PRR) which seems to act in the kidney, the heart and in the retina [14, 15]. PRR-bound renin and prorenin display increased enzymatic activity, and binding activates intracellular signalling, up-regulating the expression of profibrotic proteins. According to experimental studies, it is involved (independently of renin) in adult and embryonic stem cell biology, embryonic development and diseases including diabetic retinopathy [14, 15].

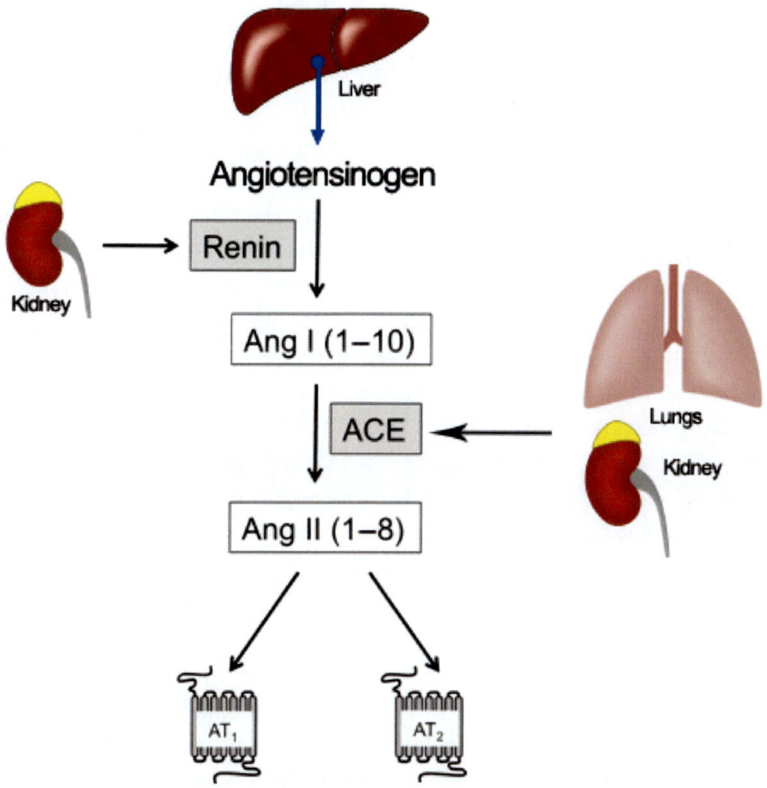

Figure 1. The renin–angiotensin system (RAS). The juxtaglomerular apparatus of the kidney produces renin. Renin cleaves its protein substrate angiotensinon, which is synthesized by the liver, generating the decapeptide Ang I. In turn, Ang I is converted by the ACE in the pulmonary circulation and renal endothelium into the octapeptide Ang II by cleavage of the terminal dipeptide from the parent decapeptide. ACE, angiotensin-converting enzyme; Ang, angiotensin; AT1, angiotensin receptor type 1; AT2, angiotensin receptor type 2.

3. Prorenin Receptor and Prorenin Binding

In recent years, evidence has revealed that prorenin, a RAS precursor molecule, may participate in pathological events at tissue level after binding to the so-called (pro)renin receptor (PRR) [16-20]. Prorenin has long been considered as having no biological activity in the classical RAS. Prorenin only recognized function has been as a precursor of the hormone renin which is generated after cleavage of the pro-segment, a process known as proteolytic activation of prorenin. However, the observation that normal physiological plasma levels of prorenin are approximately 10-fold higher than renin [21] has long intrigued researchers, who have been looking for a role to be played by prorenin other than being a mere inactive precursor. The riddle seems to have finally been unraveled by Nguyen et al [22] who first identified and cloned the PRR from cultured human mesangial cells. PRR is able to bind and activate both renin and prorenin [22, 23]. However, a detailed kinetic study showed evidence that prorenin appears to be the only relevant PRR ligand under physiological conditions [24]. After binding to PRR, prorenin undergoes a conformational change that renders this protein fully active, aside of triggering an intracellular signaling response [23].

Expression and function of PRR has not been well determined in tissues other than kidney or heart, where this receptor has been proposed to intervene in certain pathological events [16-20]. Although prorenin synthesis has been confirmed in the eye, little is known about the expression of PRR and prorenin action(s) in this organ. Pioneering studies in the eye have revealed PRR expression in the retinal microvascular endothelium and have focused on pathological neovascularization in animal models of ischemic retinopathy and endotoxin-induced uveitis [25, 26]. Evidence by these studies suggests that nonproteolytic activation of prorenin may play a role in pathological neovascularization.

Receptor-associated prorenin system (RAPS) refers to the pathogenic mechanisms whereby prorenin binding to (pro)renin receptor (PRR) dually activates tissue renin RAS and RAS independent intracellular signaling through the receptor.

PRR, also called ATP6AP2, was identified as a single transmembrane protein consisting of 350 amino acids. The fragment PRR has been shown to be associated with vacuolar-type H+-ATPase (V-ATPase) and required for Wnt/ß-catenin signaling pathway [27]. In addition to its role for vesicular acidification, PRR interacts with its ligand prorenin to exert renin activity through the conformational change of the prorenin molecule instead of the conventional proteolysis of the prorenin prosegment basically achieved by processing enzymes (Figure 2A). Since the membranebound PRR is reported to exist in the major organs but not in the circulation [28], the nonproteolytic activation of prorenin is hypothesized to play a critical role in the activation of tissue, but not circulatory, RAS. In addition, prorenin binding to its receptor is shown to cause RAS-independent signal transduction via phosphorylation of ERK (extracellular signal-regulated kinase) 1/2 in cells bearing PRR [28-31]. Thus, the nomenclature "receptor-associated prorenin system (RAPS)" for the dual activation of tissue RAS and RAS independent signaling pathway was proposed [32]. In streptozotocin (STZ)-induced diabetes, blockade of prorenin binding to its receptor led to complete suppression of proteinuria, glomerulosclerosis and renal production of angiotensin I and II without affecting circulatory RAS, indicating acritical contribution of RAPS to the pathogenesis of diabetic nephropathy (DR) [30, 33-35].

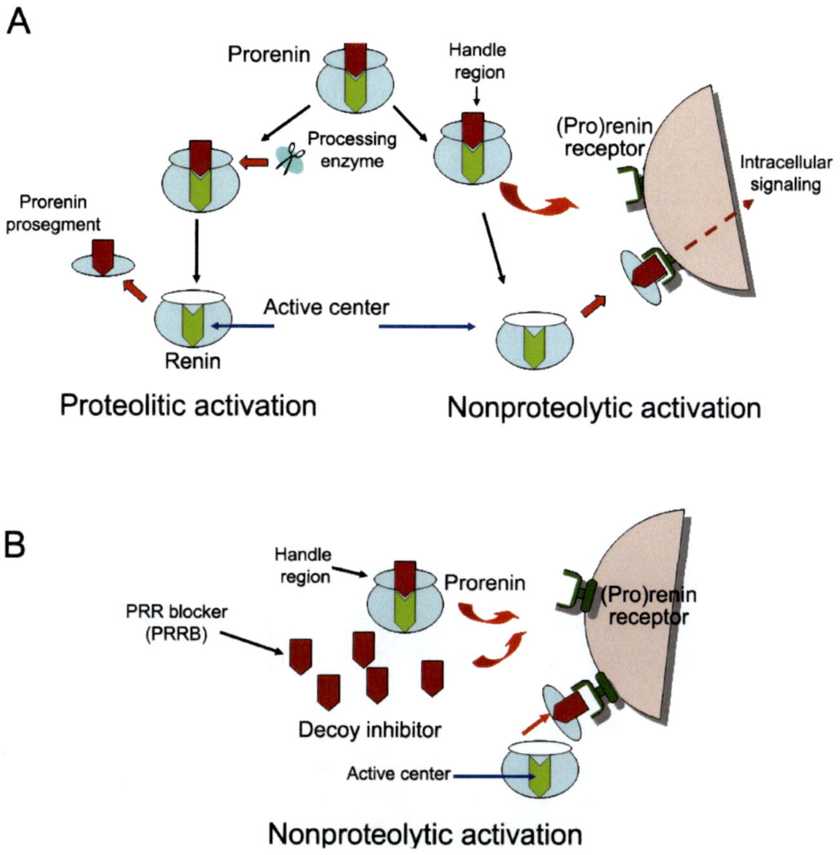

Figure 2. Major pathways of prorenin activation and PRRB as a decoy for prorenin. (A) Proteolytic activation of prorenin by processing enzymes versus nonproteolytic activation by (pro)renin receptor binding to the handle region of the prorenin prosegment. (B) Nonproteolytic activation of prorenin is blocked by a decoy peptide, PRRB, which competitively binds to (pro)renin receptor.

To cover the handle region (positions 11-15) of the prorenin molecule, which is the binding site of PRR [36], PRR blockers (PRRBs) were designed respectively by Satofuka et al [32] (Figure 2B). The specific inhibitory action of PRRB against prorenin binding with PRR and subsequent ERK activation as well as the specific inhibitory action of PRRB against tissue RAS or RAPS *in vivo* were confirmed in recent studies [27, 30-32, 34-39].

4. Local Ocular Renin Angiotensin System

The classical view of the RAS as a systemic regulator of blood pressure has been extended, and a substantial number of studies have highlighted the importance of local RAS in a variety of extra-renal tissues, including adrenal glands [40], thymus [41] and recently in the eye [42, 43]. Ophthalmic literature concerning the RAS started in 1977 with a study by Igic and coworkers [44] on the detection of ACE activity in homogenates of the retina. Since then, expression and localization of all components of the RAS have been well determined in adult eye tissues (Figure 3) including the retinal pigment epithelium (RPE), Müller cells, amacrine cells, and photoreceptors (Table I), where the mediators of the RAS are locally released, conferring the molecular basis for a biological function of these mediators in the eye [45-48]. However, whether intraocular mediators such as Ang II and renin are originated from local production or from the blood compartment has been debated. Studies in rat retinal tissues suggested local synthesis of both renin and ACE [49]. Along this line, Milenkovic et al. (2010) demonstrated that the RPE expresses renin and secretes it towards the retinal side. It has been also shown that neither Ang I, Ang II nor angiotensinogen are able to pass the blood-brain barrier and the barriers between eye and circulating blood are comparable to this [50, 51]. On the other hand, Ang II levels in the eye are higher than in plasma, indicating that there is a local production of Ang II in the eye [51, 52]. Therefore, increased local or tissue Ang II formation in the retina in the absence of elevated circulating Ang II may indeed be deleterious.

The RPE plays an important role in maintaining retinal function by transporting nutrients, isomerizing alltrans to 11-cis retinal, and phagocytosing shed photoreceptor outer segments [53]. By its anatomical location, the RPE forms the interface between the retina and the blood supply from the choroid and represents a part of the blood-retinal barrier. This makes the RPE suitable to serve as a mediator for transfer of molecules and signals between the blood and the outer retina. The fact that AT1R is localized at the basolateral membrane [54], which faces the blood side of the epithelium, suggests that the activity of the systemic RAS is a part of that signaling. Interestingly, it has been shown that modulation of the systemic RAS (e.g. by systemic application of ACE inhibitors) changes neuronal activity within the retina, mainly of bipolar cells and amacrine cells as monitored by electroretinography [55-57]. Moreover, modulators of the systemic RAS alter renin expression in the RPE [54] and plasma AngII can not cross the intraocular space [43]. These findings suggest that the systemic RAS most likely influences the intraocular RAS through the RPE.

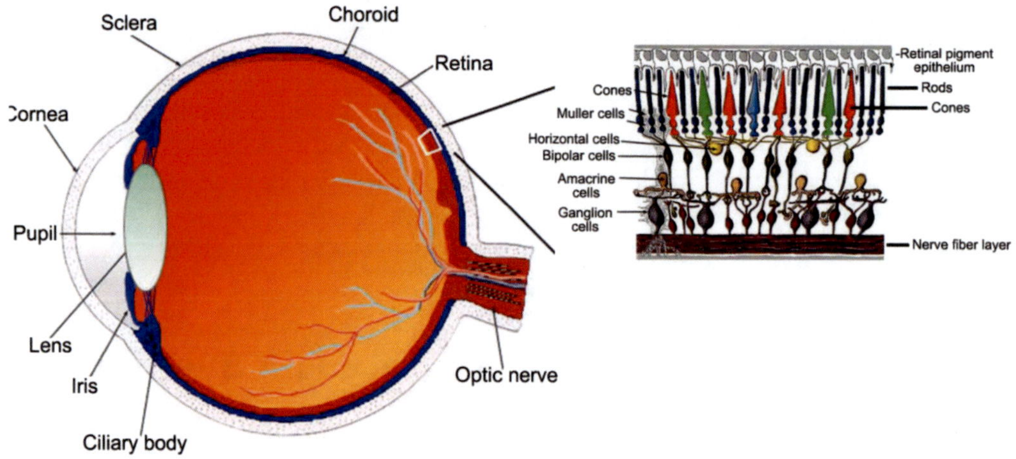

Figure 3. A drawing of a section through the human eye with a schematic enlargement of the retina.

The presence of the most important RAS components in the retina implies a physiological function of RAS within the eye. However, despite the considerable evidence for local RAS in the retina, its exact role and its possible relationship with the systemic RAS remain poorly understood.

Table 1. Localization of RAS components in ocular tissues in different species

RAS molecule	***Eye part***	***Species***	***References***
Prorenin	Retina	Human	Sramek et al., 1988
	Ciliary body	Human	Danser et al., 1989
	Vitreous body	Human	
Renin	Retina	Human, rabbit	Danser et al., 1989
	Ciliary body	Rabbit	Wagner et al., 1996
	Choroid	Human, rabbit	Ramirez et al., 1996
	Iris	Rabbit	
	Vitreous body	Human, rabbit	
	Aqueous humor	Rabbit	
Angiotensinogen	Retina	Human, rabbit	Sramek et al., 1992
	Ciliary body	Human, rabbit	Ramirez et al., 1996
	Choroid	Human, rabbit	Wagner et al., 1996
	Iris	Human, rabbit	
	Vitreous body	Human, rabbi	
	Aqueous humor	Rabbit	
	Retina	Dog, monkey, human	Vita et al., 1981
ACE1		Rabbit, porcine	Weinreb et al., 1985
	Ciliary body	Human, rabbit, porcine	Immonen et al.1987
	Choroid	Dog, monkey, human	Ramirez et al., 1996
		Rabbit, porcine	Wagner et al., 1996
	Sclera	Dog, monkey	Shiota et al., 1997
	Iris	Rabbit, porcine	Geng et al., 2003
	Cornea	Human	Savaskan et al., 2004
	Vitreous body	Dog, monkey, rabbit	
	Aqueous humor	Human, dog, monkey, rabbit	
	Tear fluid	Human, rabbit	
ACE2	Retina	Rodent	Tikellis et al., 2004
		Human	Senanayake et al., 2007
Chymase	Choroid	Dog	Shiota et al., 1997
	Sclera	Dog	Maruichi et al., 2004
	Vitreous body	Human	
AT1 receptor	Retina	Human	Savaskan et al., 2004
	Cornea	Human	Senanayake et al., 2007
	RPE	Human	Striker et al., 2008
	RPE	Rodent	Praddaude et al., 2009
AT2 receptor	Retina	Human	Senanayake et al., 2007
	RPE	Human	Striker et al., 2008
	RPE	Rodent	Praddaude et al., 2009
Ang I	Retina	Porcine	Danser et al., 1994
	Choroid	Porcine	
	Vitreous body	Porcine, human	
	Aqueous humor	Human	
Ang II	Retina	Human, porcine, rabbit	Danser et al., 1994
	Ciliary body	Human, rabbit	Ramirez et al., 1996
	Choroid	Porcine, human, rabbit	Savaskan et al., 2004
	Iris	Rabbit	Senanayake et al., 2007
	Cornea	Human	
	Vitreous body	Porcine, human, rabbit	
	Aqueous humor	Human, rabbit	
Ang 1-7	RPE	Rodent	Praddaude et al., 2009
	Retina	Human	Senanayake et al., 2007

5. Pathologic Role of Local Renin-Angiotensin System in the Eye

5.1. Age-Related Macular Degeneration

Age-related macular degeneration (AMD) is a pathological condition of the retina where vision becomes impaired to the extent of ultimately causing blindness. AMD is considered a public health problem, affecting nearly 10 million people in the US alone (Research to Prevent Blindness, NISE, NSF).

Histopathological signs of dry AMD, the early stage of the disease, include the presence of waste material in the form of focal deposits named drusen and other lipid rich extracellular deposits below the RPE and within Bruch's membrane (BrM) (Figure 4B), a stratified extracellular matrix situated between the choriocapillaris and RPE [58, 59]. During aging, deposits initially accumulate between the RPE and its basement membrane (called basal laminar deposit or BLD), but progression into AMD requires additional deposit formation within BrM, (called basal linear deposit (BLiD) and "nodular" drusen). Drusen increase in size and number as the disease progresses. Geographic atrophy represents the advanced stage of dry AMD and is characterized by progressive destruction of RPE cells and photoreceptors. Only a fraction of patients with drusen will develop wet AMD, the most rapidly progressing form which accounts for 80 to 90% of cases of severe vision loss related to the disease. The presence, size and area covered by drusen confer a significant *risk* for the development and progression to wet AMD [60-62]. Wet AMD is characterized by the growth of leaky new abnormal blood vessels under the RPE from the subjacent choroid (Figure 4C) known as choroidal neovascularization (CNV). Wet AMD is always preceded by early disease. Death or dysfunction of retinal photoreceptors is the ultimate cause of vision loss. However, the initial pathogenic target of AMD is the RPE, its ECM (called BrM), and the subjacent vascular bed (called choriocapillaris), the blood supply for the outer retina.

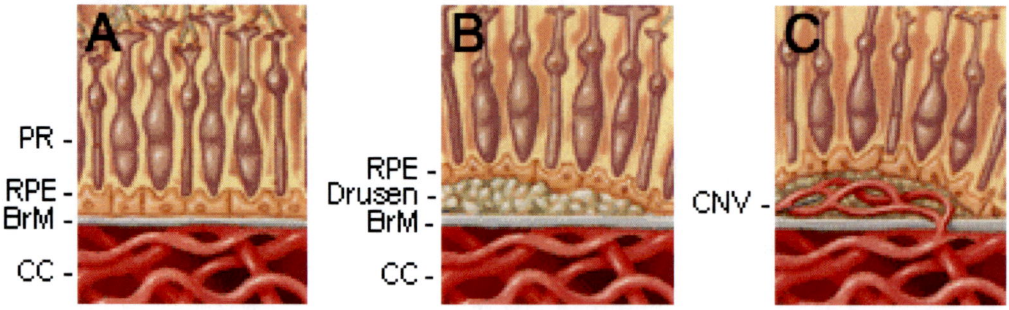

Figure 4. The pathologic changes to the retina and choroidal blood vessels typical of dry AMD (B) and early wet AMD (C) respectively. PR, *photoreceptors*; *RPE*, retinal pigment epithelium; BrM, Brusch's membrane; CC, choriocapillaries; CNV, choroidal neovascularization.

The formation of drusen is an active process with distinct biological pathways. However, lack of scientific consensus exists regarding the origin of drusen. Research from different groups has been based on the conceptually innovative RPE injury hypothesis which proposes that deposit formation and accumulation is secondary to chronic, repetitive but nonlethal RPE injury. Irrespective of the injury, this model proposes that all stimuli result in a final common pathway of cellular responses that cause the actual deposits. Repetitive injury ultimately can kill RPE leading to late dry AMD. *Our understanding of the two forms of AMD has increased substantially, yet there is still much debate as to why and how the disease progresses and what sequence of cellular events lead to the progression of dry to wet AMD. Overall,* the mechanism by which drusen might elicit CNV remains undefined.

Even though age is the major determinant for developing AMD, clinical studies have revealed a number of systemic and environmental risk factors [63-67]. Among them, activation of the RAS shows special relevance due to the increasing incidence of hypertension in Western societies. The discovery of a local RAS in the retina has opened new ways of understanding patho-physiological processes leading to extracellular (ECM) turnover disregulation, inflammation or neovascularisation. However, the mechanism(s) by which RAS activation may affect AMD remains unclear. In recent years, evidence has revealed that Ang II, AT1R signaling, and prorenin, may play a significant role in the mentioned pathologic processes [16-20, 68]. Moreover, recent observations point also to the participation of AT2R and AngI reaction products such as Ang1-7 [55].Thus the exploration of the local RAS of the retina will open new ways in the development of therapies.

5.1.1. Dysregulation of Extracellular Matrix Turnover, Inflammation, CNV and Tissue RAS

5.1.1. A. Dysregulation of Extracellular Matrix Turnover

An injury response relevant to early AMD is imbalance in ECM turnover. The normal anatomy and physiology of ECM in most tissues requires continuous turnover of matrix components by a tightly regulated balance in the production of matrix molecules like collagen, laminin, MMPs, and TIMPs [69, 70]. It has been shown that relatively small dysregulation in the relative production of MMPs, TIMPs, and collagen types I and IV [69, 70] may lead to net changes in the ECM, including thickening and deposit formation [70, 71]. Accordingly, dysregulated turnover of ECM is a major mechanism of disease pathogenesis in many tissue sites, including renal disease, atherosclerosis, lung disease, and others [70-73]. Unfortunately, minimal information is available concerning normal turnover in healthy BrM or imbalanced turnover in AMD.

Numerous biochemical and anatomical changes occur in BrM as part of aging retina in the absence of apparent disease, including collagenous thickening, calcification and lipid infiltration [74]. However, the accumulation of specific deposits composed by RPE-derived blebs from the basolateral RPE surface and other debris between the RPE basement membrane and BrM is a very prominent histopathologic feature of eyes with AMD [74-77]. In addition, recent studies performed on AMD patient eyes examined by electron microscopy have reported that RPE-derived debris from the basolateral RPE surface traversed the RPE basement membrane and deposited in the inner and outer collagenous layers of BrM [78]. However, the mechanism(s) by which these sub-RPE deposits accumulate and traverse the RPE basement membrane remains unexplored. In this regard, ample evidence supports the idea that MMPs and their TIMPs play an important role in AMD.

The RPE actively contributes to sustain a normal ECM turnover by two different mechanisms: synthesis of matrix metalloproteinase (MMP) enzymes and structural proteins (e.g. collagens and laminin). MMP-2 is the most abundant and significant MMP enzyme synthesized by the RPE, and there is evidence that this protein plays a crucial role in the ECM remodeling of the retina. The RPE is capable of producing many ECM components such as MMP-2, MMP-14, Basigin, also known as EMMPRIN (extracellular matrix metalloproteinase inducer) or CD147, collagen types I and IV, and TIMP-2 [79-82]. MMP-14 and basigin proteins are of special relevance to the AMD pathology as they promote MMP-2 activation. MMP-2 and MMP-14 are the major RPE enzymes synthesized for the degradation of matrix type IV and I collagens, laminin, and fibronectin, which are components found in BrM [81, 83]. MMP-2 is the key enzyme for ECM turnover in BrM and is synthesized as an inactive zymogen pro form (pro-MMP-2) [84]. The transmembrane metalloproteinase MMP-14 is well known to activate MMP-2 in a specific manner [83]. On the other hand, TIMP-2 may inhibit the cleavage of pro-MMP-2 into MMP-2 [70]. Based on these data our research focuses on MMP-2, MMP-14, and basigin, and propose that dysregulation of MMP-2 is the primary cause for the accumulation of sub-RPE deposits that become basal laminar deposits (BLD) and drusen. Thus, we propose that the progression of the sub-RPE deposits into BrM requires degradation of ECM proteins such as type IV and I collagens and laminin, which are critical components of RPE basement membrane and adjacent BrM [84, 85], and that ECM turnover upregulation via MMP-2 activation and MMP-14 is necessary for the breakdown of these physical barriers.

As mentioned previously, hypertension is of special interest as a potential link between cardiovascular pathologies and AMD [86-89] and Ang II is the most important hormone associated to hypertension which plays a pivotal role in pathological complications [90, 91]. Expression of Ang II, as well as other components of the RAS, has been demonstrated in the RPE and other eye tissues [45, 92-94]. Aside from the evidence supporting the existence of a local RAS in the adult eye, the expression of Ang II receptor types AT1 and AT2 has been demonstrated in the retina and the RPE [45-48] which provides the molecular basis for a biological function of Ang II in the eye.

Ang II-mediated regulation of genes, which are expressed in RPE and are important for the ECM turnover, might contribute to subRPE deposit formation and provide a pathogenic mechanism to explain the link between hypertension and AMD. Among its many actions, Ang II promotes interstitial ECM turnover by regulation of the ECM proteins [95-102]. For example, Ang II has been shown to stimulate synthesis of fibronectin, collagen, TIMP-2, and MMP-2 in mesangial and proximal tubule cells through activation of transforming growth factor-ß secretion (TGF-beta) [103, 104]. Ang II also activates TGF-beta-mediated MMP-2 release in endothelial cells [105]. In addition, Ang II increases collagen type I and III production via NADPH oxidase complex in cardiac fibroblasts [106], MMP-14, MMP-2 and MMP-9 expression and activity in MKN-28 cells, arteries, and aorta [99, 100, 107], as well as TIMP-1 expression and concentration in smooth muscle cells and coronary endothelial cells [79, 108]. The RPE actively contributes to maintain a normal turnover of ECM components. However, until now, the regulatory effects of Ang II on ECM proteins expression in the RPE were unknown. Therefore, our work aimed at characterizing the expression and function of Ang II receptors in the RPE and at investigating Ang II contribution to the development of early AMD. Our study confirmed that both Ang II receptor subtypes were expressed and upregulated by Ang II in human RPE and showed that stimulation of the AT1 receptor by Ang II is transduced into an intracellular signal, in particular an increase in the levels of intracellular calcium [48, 68]. This result constitutes clear evidence that the AT1 receptor expressed in human RPE is functionally active and might be efficiently coupled to the PLC-transduction pathway. Compared to these results, stimulation of the AT2 receptor by Ang II was not accompanied by mobilization of intracellular calcium. These data suggest differences in AT2 receptor coupling in human RPE cells. AT2 receptor could be specifically coupled to the cytosolic phospholipase A2 (cPLA2) as it has been shown recently in renal mesangial and proximal tubular epithelium cells and not to the PLC pathway [109]. Therefore, selective up or down-regulation of only AT2 receptor transduction pathway remains a possibility to be investigated.

Ang II also increased MMP-2 activity MMP-14, and basigin as well as type IV collagen degradation [48, 110]. These Ang II effects were abolished in the presence of the AT1 receptor antagonist candesartan. In contrast, Ang II decreased type IV collagen via both AT1 and AT2 receptors, suggesting a synergistic effect of the two receptor subtypes. Therefore, Ang II through MMP-2, MMP-14, and basigin regulation could stimulate RPE basement membrane breakdown allowing the migration of BLD and buildup of basal linear deposits or drusen.

The majority of intracellular actions of Ang II in most tissues are mediated by the activation of MAPKs, which are a group of serine/threonine kinases [111-113] which can be divided into three major groups: ERK, p38, and Jun N-terminus kinase (JNK) and participate in a wide array of cellular responses including proliferation, differentiation, migration, and stress responses among others [114-116]. We explored the involvement of MAPK signaling pathways as a potential key intracellular modulator of Ang II-induced increase in MMP-2 activity, MMP-14 and basigin protein expression in the RPE. We found that Ang II stimulates phosphorylation of ERK and p38 MAPK in RPE cells [110]. These effects were mediated by AT1 receptors. Blockade of ERK or p38 MAPK abrogated the increase in MMP-2 activity and MMP-14 and basigin proteins in RPE cells. Given that MMP-14 and basigin are major inducers of MMP-2, our results lead us to speculate that MMP-14 and basigin might regulate Ang II-induced MMP-2 activity through MAPKS- and AT1 receptor-dependent signaling pathways in the RPE. These original observations highlight the potential importance of this signaling pathway as a potential mediator of RPE response to Ang II-induced ECM dysregulation and breakdown of the RPE basement membrane believed to be involved in sub-RPE deposits progression in the pathogenesis of AMD. Based on our observations, MAPKs inhibitors and AT1 receptor blockers may prevent these ECM changes essential in early AMD development and provide a potential future clinical tool for the prevention of this disease that causes a great deal of discomfort and disability.

In order to elucidate potential pathogenic mechanism(s) linking the RAS and early (dry) AMD, we also evaluated the action of prorenin-activated PRR on relevant molecules for ECM turnover, such as MMP-2, type I and IV collagens and laminin, in the RPE, which is a cell type of pivotal importance in AMD. Therefore, we investigated and characterized the expression and function of PRR in human RPE cells. Our study demonstrated for the first time that human RPE expresses the PRR, and provides evidence that activation of this receptor elicits an intracellular response in RPE cells [117].

Isolated RPE cells from donor human eyes as well as freshly isolated human retinas demonstrated expression of PRR at mRNA and protein levels (Figure 5A). Moreover, we demonstrated that PRR expressed in the RPE cells is functional, as shown by prorenin-induced increases in Erk1/2 phosphorylation (Figure 5B). PRR expressionwas also shown to be regulated by its main physiological agonist prorenin (Figure 6).We found evidence that the PRR may be involved in ECM-remodeling processes through a prorenin-induced upregulation of type I collagen. Immunostaining analysis of human retinas revealed higher PRR and type I collagen expression in the RPE of eye donors with dry AMD and hypertension (Figure 7), supporting the in vitro findings using human-isolated RPE cells. Taken together, the present study demonstrated for the first time that the PRR is expressed in human RPE and suggests a molecular mechanism by which the RAS may exacerbate the pathology of dry AMD.

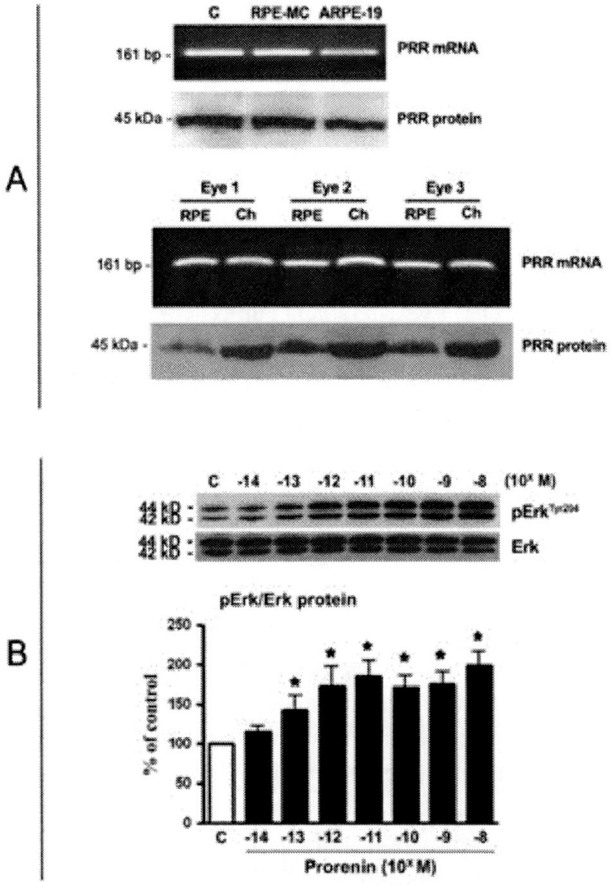

Figure 5. PRR expression in retina-isolated RPE and cell lines (A). (*Top*) PRR mRNA evaluated by RT-PCR and protein analyzed in total cell lysates by Western blot from human RPE-MC and ARPE-19 cells. Cultured mesangial cell samples were used as control (C). (*Bottom*) PRR mRNA and protein expression in RPE and choroids (Ch) from freshly isolated retina of three human eye pair donors. Total RNA was isolated and used as template for a PCR using primers specific for human PRR. Total protein was extracted from cell lysates and 40 μg loaded. Thenumber on the left represents either the molecular size in base pairs (bp) or the molecular weight of the protein in kilo Daltons (kDa). (B): Phosphorylation of the mitogen-activated protein kinase ErK1/2 in response to prorenin in RPE-MC cells. Cellswere pre-treated with 10^{-5} M AT1-receptor blocker (candesartan) and AT2-receptor blocker (PD123319) for 1 h, and then treated with increasing concentrations of prorenin (10^{-14}–10^{-8} M) for 10 min. *Top:* A representative Western blot for evaluation of phosphorylated Erk1/2 protein in cell lysates. Numbers on the left represent the molecular mass of the marker. Total Erk1/2 protein is shown as the loading control. *Bottom:* Bar graph showing the average results of three independent experiments normalized to the loading control. Results are expressed as means±SEM. *$p<0.05$ compared to untreated control cells.

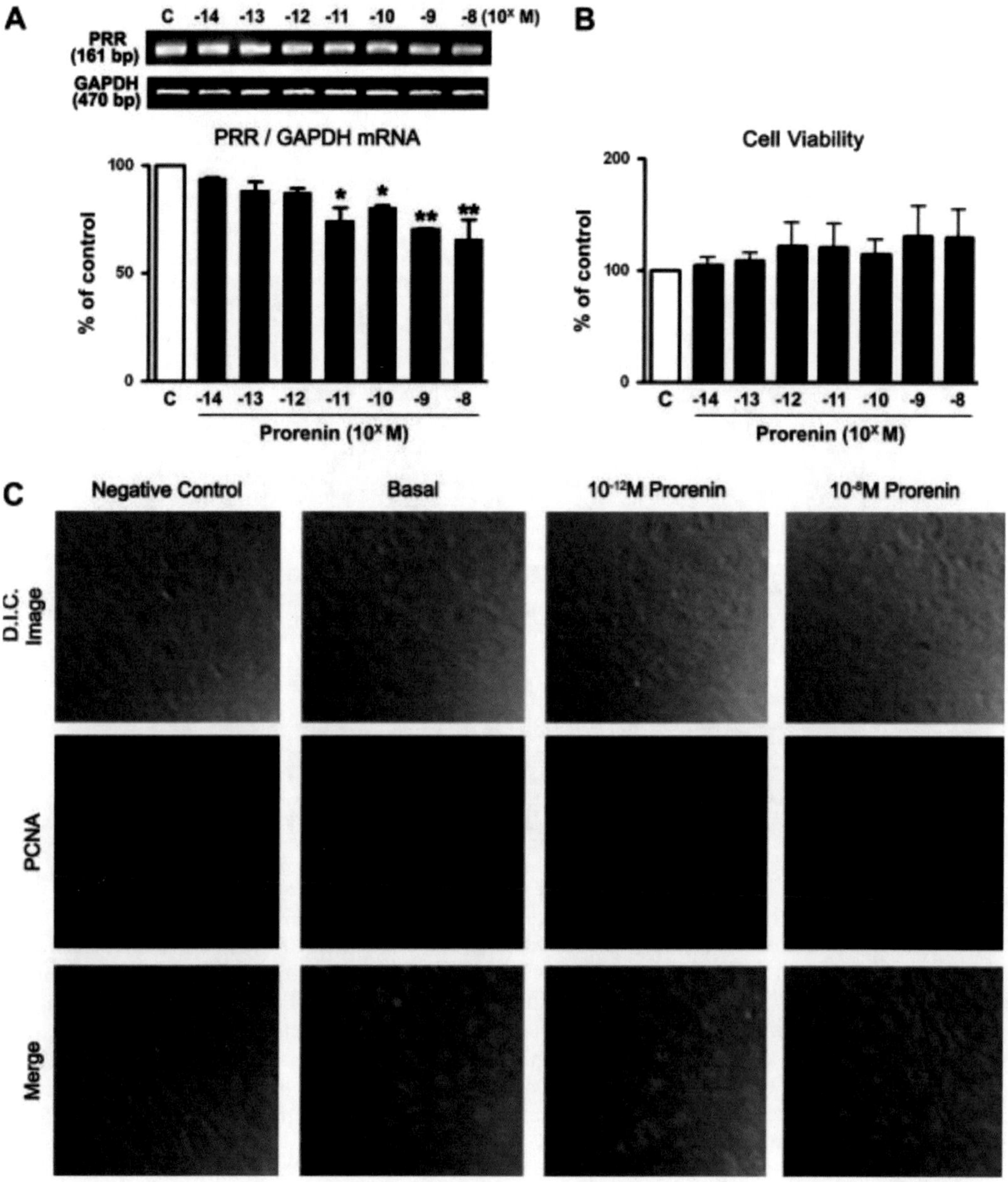

Figure 6. PRR mRNA and cell viability and proliferation in RPE-MC incubated with prorenin. RPE-MC cells were stimulated with different prorenin concentrations (10^{-14}–10^{-8} M) for 24 h. (A) Total RNA was isolated and PRR transcript levels evaluated by RT-PCR. *Top:* 2% agarose gel from a representative experiment showing amplicons for PRR (161 bp) and the house-keeping gene product GAPDH (470 bp). *Bottom:* Bar graph showing averages of PRR values normalized to GAPDH in three independent experiments. (B) Cell viability evaluated by count of cells in five independent experiments. (C) Immunocytochemical analysis of PCNA in cells incubated in the absence or presence (10^{-12} or 10^{-8} M) of prorenin. Composite image of cells stained with with mouse anti-PCNA analyzed under confocal microscope using magnification ×40. Secondary antibody was conjugated to Alexa-488 and the negative control was generated in the absence of primary antibody. Results are expressed as means ± SEM.*$p < 0.05$, **$p < 0.01$ compared to untreated control cells.

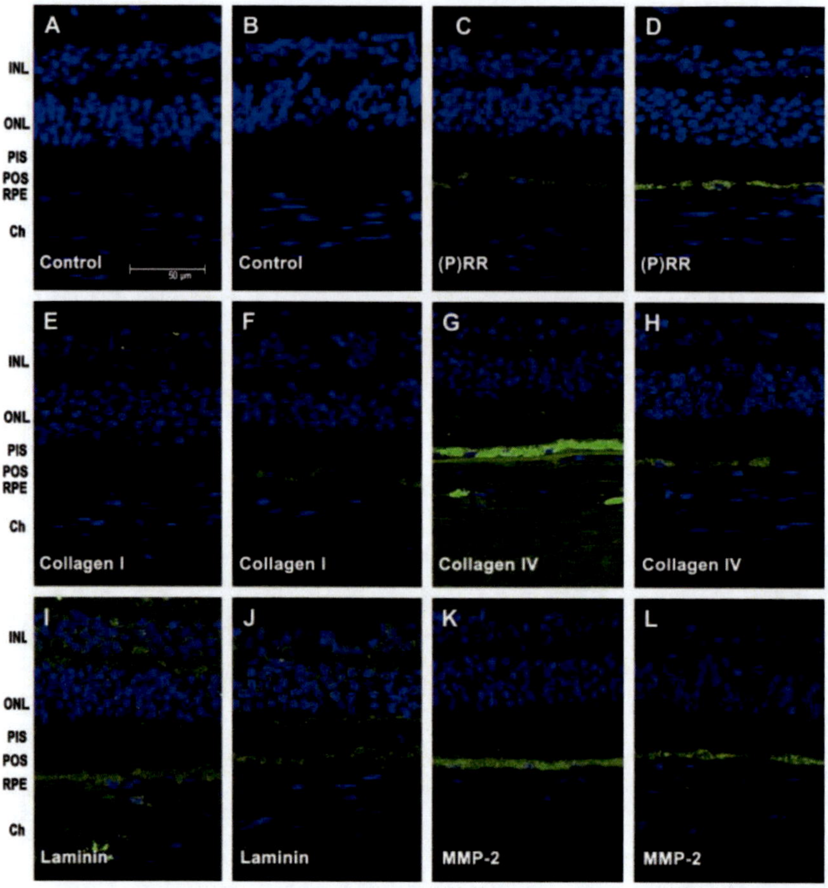

Figure 7. Immunohistochemical analysis of PRR and various ECM molecules in human retina. Composite image of retina sections from a human donor eyes with no known eye disease (A, C, E, G, I, and K), and from a human donor eyes with dry AMD and hypertension (B, D, F, H, J, and L). Sections were stained with rabbit polyclonal anti-PRR (C, D), goat polyclonal anti-type I collagen (E, F), mouse monoclonal anti-type IV collagen (G, H), rabbit polyclonal anti-laminin (I, J), or mouse monoclonal anti-MMP-2 (K, L), as indicated. Negative controls were generated by omission of the primary antibody (A, B). Secondary antibodies were coupled to Alexa-488. Nuclei were stained with DAPI. Sections were analyzed under confocal microscope using magnification x40 INL, inner nuclear layer; ONL, outer nuclear layer; PIS, photoreceptor inner segments; POS, photoreceptor outer segments; RPE, retinal pigment epithelium; Ch, choroid.

5.1.1. B. Inflammation

The formations of drusen as well as the mechanism(s) of how drusen might elicit CNV remain undefined. Recently, inflammatory-derived injury stimuli have been implicated, including oxidants, complement, immune complexes and factors produced by macrophages [80, 118, 119]. Inflammatory cells might be responsible for drusen progression into CNV by secretion of growth factors and cytokines that will damage the choriocapillaris and stimulate the invasion of neovessels into the subretinal space [120-122]. The mechanism of how drusen might elicit CNV remains undefined. However, a growing collection of evidence suggests that inflammation is an important component in the pathogenesis of both dry and wet AMD [123-127].

While it is largely recognized that macrophages accumulate in AMD lesion [128-134], there is ambiguity surrounding their role in the disease process with conflicting evidence regarding whether they might be helpful by scavenging accumulated debris and therefore protecting against CNV or harmful by stimulating CNV [135]. This might be due to the largely observational nature of human samples but also probably reflects different functions macrophages serve during distinct phases of the disease.

Inflammation is a complex process that involves local secretion of pro-inflammatory cytokines (leukocyte adhesion molecules, ICAM-1 and VCAM-1) [136, 137], MCP-1 [138-142] NFκB [143-145], and growth factors (tumour necrosis factor, TNF-α, TGF-β). The key inflammatory molecule in initiating inflammatory responses may be MCP-1 [138-144] a powerful chemokine, expressed at sites of injury. Indeed, the importance of MCP-1 in inflammatory diseases is highlighted by a careful MEDLINE search for MCP-1, which readily returns more than 3000 citations following its characterization in the late 1980s.

NFκB appears to control expression of MCP-1 [143-145]. After release, it activates the CCR2 chemotactic receptor to induce chemotactic responses that mediate monocyte and macrophage migration into sites of active inflammation in various diseases [146, 147]. MCP-1 is postulated to be responsible for the recruitment of macrophages early in repair processes. The RPE plays a pivotal role in the maintenance of the outer retina by secreting several cytokines including MCP-1 [148, 149], which has been suggested to be implicated in the pathogenesis of AMD [150, 151]. RPE cells can secrete MCP-1 in the direction of choroidal blood vessels during inflammatory responses therefore suggesting that RPE cells might promote macrophage recruitment to the choroid from circulating monocytes [152]. Thus, we have speculated that MCP-1 produced by the RPE is a relevant molecule in dry AMD and its progression.

Previous observations made using mouse animal models suggest that MCP-1 and chemokine receptor–2 might be involved in the etiology of AMD and that macrophage dysfunction may have a central role in the early stage of AMD development [150, 151]. Indeed, it has been proposed that the spontaneous disappearance of drusen in patients with AMD may be explained by phagocytosis of debris thereby indicating a beneficial role of macrophages [152]. However, on the other hand, macrophages recruited into the choriocapillaris, which upon scavenging debris and blebs, could release additional cytokines and mediators to amplify matrix turnover and deposit formation, induce RPE cytotoxicity or damage the choriocapillaris promoting complications, especially CNV formation.

Ang II, is known as a vasoconstrictor, however, several studies have shown its role as a potent mediator in the activation of inflammatory mechanisms involved in age-related diseases [153, 154]. Ang II plays a critical role in the pathogenesis of a wide spectrum of diseases [136, 137, 144, 155-159]. At physiological levels (fentomoles), Ang II is an important physiological regulator of blood pressure, cardiac function and body salt and fluid homeostasis [155]. However, increased local or tissue Ang II formation in target organs may indeed be very deleterious [136, 155-158]. Ang II is not only a potent vasoconstrictor which elevates arterial blood pressure, but also a powerful pro-inflammatory cytokine, chemokine and growth factor [136, 143-145, 160], which mediates the activation of inflammatory mechanisms involved in age-related diseases [153,154]. There is accumulating evidence that Ang II can cause target organ damage by facilitating inflammatory and growth responses through activation of NFκB [136, 143-145], the key nuclear transcription factor in inflammatory and fibrotic diseases. Activation of NFκB by Ang II may stimulate transcription of numerous inflammatory genes, including MCP-1, RANTES (Regulated on Active Normal T cell Expressed and Secreted) and interleukin (IL)-6, TNF-α and TGF-β [136, 143-145]. The view that MCP-1 is one of the most important chemokines in Ang II-induced inflammatory responses is supported by numerous studies, although the mechanisms by which Ang II increases MCP-1 expression and production are still not well understood [136, 143-145]. In a rabbit model of atherosclerosis, ACE1 inhibitor quinapril inhibited NFκB activity, expression and production of MCP-1 and neointimal macrophage infiltration at the injured sites [143]. In Ang II-induced hypertensive rats, vascular MCP-1 mRNA expression increased almost four-fold, which was significantly reduced by normalization of hypertension by the non-specific vasodilator hydralazine, but the effects of AT1 receptor blockade were not studied [140]. However, in a different study, Ang II enhanced expression of MCP-1 mRNA and protein production in rat vascular smooth muscle cells in a dose- and time-dependent fashion, and these effects were mediated by AT1 receptors involving the Rho-kinase pathway [161]. In mice, Wu *et al.* [162] showed that the AT1 receptor antagonist valsartan, at a dose that did not influence systolic blood pressure, significantly reduced the expression of MCP-1 along with other inflammatory genes such as TNF-α, IL-6, IL-1β and monocyte/macrophage infiltration in injured vessels. Interestingly, the effects of valsartan on MCP-1 expression were attenuated in AT2 receptor-deficient mice, suggesting that both AT1 and AT2 receptors are involved. The advantage of using a lower dose of AT1 receptor blockers is that the treatment does not reduce systolic blood pressure to the normotensive level, but retains clinical efficacy in inhibiting MCP-1 expression and improving cardiac function and mortality. Accordingly, the beneficial effects of the AT1 receptor blockers may be explained by a mechanism other than high blood pressure. A direct effect of Ang II on MCP-1 expression and production may be implicated [160].

Finally, the signalling mechanisms by which Ang II increases MCP-1 expression and production and induces end-organ damage remain to be elucidated. As mentioned previously, there is mounting evidence that NFκB may be one of the most important nuclear transcription factors that mediates Ang II-stimulated MCP-1 expression and production [136, 143-145]. However, the signalling pathways by which Ang II directly or indirectly activates NFκB, which is then translocated into the nucleus to mediate MCP-1 transcription and synthesis, remain largely unknown. A local RAS may be activated in most, if not all, diseases with consequently increased tissue or intracellular Ang II. Binding of extracellular Ang II to cell surface AT1 receptors may stimulate MCP-1 mRNA expression through activation of different intracellular signalling cascades, likely involving protein kinase C-activated intracellular calcium mobilization [163], tyrosine kinase and mitogen-activated protein kinase [164], phospholipase A_2 [165] and redox-sensitive NADH/NAD(P)H oxidase [164]. Future studies further addressing these important issues could improve our understanding of the potential role of pro-inflammatory cytokines and chemokines in mediating Ang II-induced target organ damage and assist in further development of novel drugs to prevent and treat these diseases.

Even if it has been suggested that increased MCP-1 expression may be a key mediator between Ang II and retinal damage in hypertensive patients, MCP-1 expression has not been investigated in RPE from hypertensive patients with AMD nor has been the regulation of RPE-derived MCP-1 expression following Ang II-mediated injury.

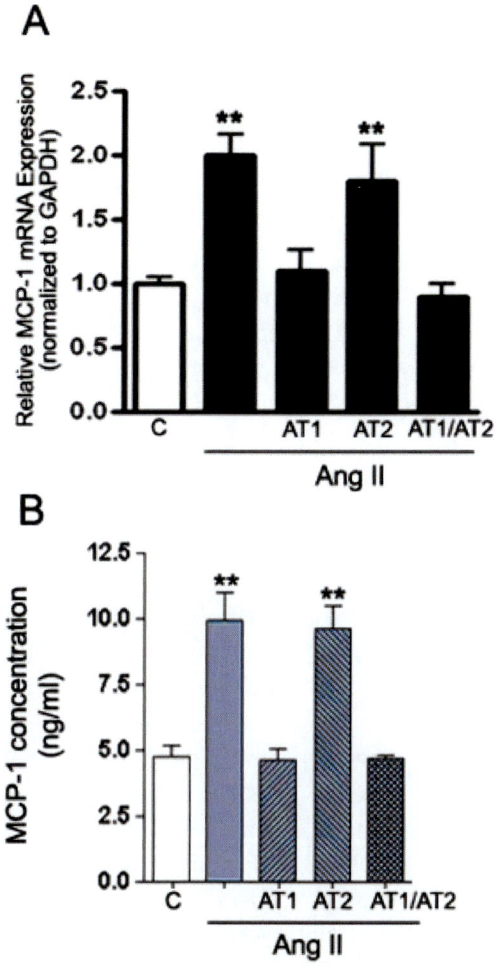

Figure 8. Ang II upregulated MCP-1 protein expression (A) and secretion (B) through Ang II receptor 1 (AT1) activation in RPE cells. Human ARPE-19 cells were incubated with Ang II alone (100 nM) for 24 hours or in combination with candesartan (CD, 100 nM), an AT1 receptor antagonist, or PD123319 (PD, 100 nM) an Ang II type 2 receptor antagonist for 30 min before Ang II stimulation, then washed with PBS and incubated in assay medium (0.1% FBS) for 24 hours. Supernatants and cell homogenates were collected to assess MCP-1 mRNA expression by real-time PCR and protein secretion by ELISA. Results are expressed as mean±SEM. **P<0.01, statistically significant difference compared with the control.

On the basis of our preliminary data and those of others, we have proposed a molecular inflammatory hypothesis for AMD that describes a central role for the redox-sensitive NF-κB in modulating the gene expression of MCP-1. Many studies have provided experimental evidence indicating that NF-κB can be activated by oxidative stress [166-169] and that the anti-oxidant may have beneficial effects on vascular inflammation that occurs in other age-related diseases [170, 171]. Thus, we proposed that Ang II will active RPE MCP-1 production leading to recruitment of macrophages to sub-RPE deposit areas, where they will scavenge, release more cytokines and mediators, and amplify the process promoting complications, especially CNV formation. Our preliminary data indicate that expression of MCP-1, key mediators pertinent to inflammation is markedly increased *in cultured human RPE cells in response to Ang II (Figure 8).* Moreover, our data indicate that the increase in MCP-1 mRNA and protein secretion by RPE was through AT1 receptors activation (Figure 8), highlighting such pro-inflammatory role of Ang II and their mechanism. These observations may have strong implications for the drusen progression to CNV in hypertensive patients with dry AMD. Future studies addressing whether or not Ang II directly or indirectly activates NFκB and the signalling pathways could improve our understanding of the potential role of Ang II in the progression of dry AMD to CNV.

Because hypertension has been unequivocally linked to the pathogenesis of AMD, it can be speculated that increase in RPE-derived MCP-1 production resulting from exposure to Ang II may be an important factor that could accelerate and promote the progression of early AMD to CNV. This theory is put forth bearing in mind the complexity of underlying cellular and *molecular mechanisms involved* in the inflammatory response.

5.1.1. C. Choroidal Neovascularization

As mentioned previously, AMD, is complicated by CNV leading to severe vision loss due to hemorrhage and exudation from the immature new vessels [172, 173]. Therefore, the discovery of a local RAS in the retina has opened new ways of understanding patho-physiological processes leading to neovascularisation. CNV proved to be an inflammatory disorder depending on intercellular adhesion molecule (ICAM)-1, MCP-1 and vascular endothelial growth factor (VEGF) [174]. It was showed that AT1R mediated upregulation of these inflammatory and angiogenic molecules is required for the development of CNV [175]. Moreover, several important findings concerning the role of PRR in CNV generation were revealed [38]. First, CNV development was associated with upregulation of prorenin mRNA expression, but not PRR, in the retinal RPE-choroid complex and PRRB treatment showed a significant decrease in the CNV volume, indicating that prorenin binding with its receptor contributes to CNV. Second, the cellular and molecular mechanisms in the PRRB-induced suppression of CNV included the inhibitory effects on macrophage infiltration into CNV, Ang II generation and the upregulated expression of inflammatory and angiogenic molecules such as ICAM-1, MCP-1, VEGF, VEGF receptor (VEGFR)-1 and VEGFR-2, all of which were downstream molecules of Ang II [175]. Although the detailed molecular and cellular mechanisms underlying CNV are not fully clarified, ICAM-1 expression [176, 177] and macrophage infiltration [174, 175] were observed in CNV tissues from human eyes with AMD and the laserinduced murine model, suggesting the close association of inflammation with the progression of CNV. Pharmacologic depletion of macrophages [122, 178] or genetic ablation of CCR2 [179], was shown to result in the reduction of CNV, suggesting that macrophages, recruited by MCP-1 released from RPE or vascular endothelial cells, facilitate the development of CNV by producing VEGF. PRRB-induced suppression of CNV indicates that tissue RAS is activated during CNV by (P)RR-mediated nonproteolytic activation of prorenin, leading to AT1-R signaling-mediated upregulation of CNV-related inflammatory molecules [175].

In order to elucidate the involvement of RAPS comprising both PRR-mediated signal transduction and tissue RAS activation, the role of RAS independent PRR signaling in CNV generation was recently studied by Satofuka et al [31]. The significant role of intracellular signaling via PRR in the development of CNV was confirmed when PRRB was administered to CNV mice which were treated with the AT1R blocker losartan or genetically deficient in AT1R or angiotensinogen (AGT). These data showed that macrophage infiltration into CNV was suppressed by PRRB in AGT-deficient mice [31]. Moreover, PRRB application to AT1-R-deficient mice with CNV led to significant suppression of ERK activation. Out of the CNV-related molecules, the expression of which was inhibited by PRRB, MCP-1 and VEGF , but not ICAM- 1, VEGFR-1 or VEGFR-2, were also regulated by PRR signaling per se [31]. These results revealed that molecular and cellular mechanisms mediated by RASindependent intracellular signaling via PRR is involved in CNV generation. Moreover, it was reported that nonproteolytic activation of prorenin selectively accelerates pathologic, but not physiologic, retinal neovascularization via the inflammatory processes in ischemia-induced retinal neovascularization [26]. Recently, PRRB was also shown to exert anti-angiogenic and anti-inflammatory effects in ischemia-induced retinal neovascularization [15], however, PRRB-induced injury to retinal neurons was simultaneously observed in contrast with its protective effect on the retinal vasculature.

5.2. Diabetic Retinopathy

The incidence of diabetic retinopathy is frightening with a recent study highlighting that the worldwide health burden includes 93 million people having diabetic retinopathy, and 17 million the proliferative and blinding form of the disease [180]. Almost all individuals with type I diabetes will develop retinopathy over a 15–20 year period, and approximately 20–30% will advance to the blinding form of diabetic retinopathy [181]. Greater than 60% of individuals with type 2 diabetes will have retinopathy. The main treatment for diabetic retinopathy is laser photocoagulation, which is directed to late stages of the disease process in order to reduce retinal neovascularization and vascular leakage. Although laser photogagulation is beneficial, it does not prevent the progression of vascular pathology, and visual outcome can still remain poor.

Diabetic retinopathy is classified according to the severity of vascular lesions, and is generally categorized into non-proliferative diabetic retinopathy, which comprises the early stages of the disease, and proliferative diabetic retinopathy, which is the most serious and vision-threatening stage [182]. Non proliferative diabetic retinopathy features thickening of capillary basement membranes, apoptosis of pericytes, microaneurysms, intraretinal hemorrhages and cotton-wool spots. The gradual closure of retinal vessels results in localized areas of tissue ischemia giving rise to venous beading and intraretinal microvascular abnormalities, increasing retinal hemorrhage and exudation. Tissue ischemia may also be worsened by endothelial cell apoptosis resulting in acellular capillaries (devoid of both pericytes and endothelial cells). Adherent leukocytes can also contribute to vessel closure. The advancement to proliferative diabetic retinopathy is viewed to be a consequence of tissue ischemia and the subsequent up-regulation of angiogenic growth factors such as VEGF, which stimulate new blood vessel growth over the optic disc or elsewhere in the retina. These new vessels can advance into the vitreous cavity leading to hemorrhage and tractional retinal detachments due to the contraction of associated fibrous tissue. Neovascularization and fibrosis can develop in the iris, leading to rubeosis iridis, which affects the outflow of aqueous humor resulting in neovascular glaucoma and an elevation in intraocular pressure which compromises vision. Diabetic macula edema occurs when fluid and hard exudates accumulate in the central area of the retina resulting in compromised clear central vision.

5.2.1. The RAS and Diabetic Retinopathy

Observations that components of the RAS's pathway were elevated in situations of retinal pathology led to study the role of the RAS in the retina. For instance, prorenin, renin, ACE and Ang II are increased in the plasma and eyes of individuals with diabetic retinopathy [47, 183, 184]. To date, most studies evaluating a causal role for the RAS in retinopathy have focused on the microvasculature, given that retinal vascular pathology is a major contributor to vision loss. There is evidence that Ang II influences both endothelial cells and pericytes in the retinal microvasculature. In cultured retinal endothelial cells, Ang II modulates both survival and proliferation. For instance, Ang II induced retinal endothelial cell apoptosis [185] and reduced the expression of pigment epithelium derived growth factor (PEDF) mRNA, an anti-angiogenic factor in the retina [186]. Ang II has mitogenic effect on retinal endothelial cells [185-187], and Ang II has been reported to enhance VEGF-stimulated endothelial cell proliferation, which involves angiopoeitin2, Tie2 and protein kinase C [187, 188].

The direct effects of Ang II on the retinal microvasculature have perhaps best been studied in retinal pericytes. Pericytes are considered to be the vascular smooth muscle cell counterpart for microvessels, and thereby are implicated in the regulation of capillary tone [189]. Pericytes may have additional functions including the maintenance of microvascular homeostasis [188]. For example, in diabetes their demise is considered to be an early sign of diabetic retinopathy. There is convincing evidence that Ang II directly influences retinal pericytes, by uncoupling them from the microvasculature, via the activation on non-specific cation and calcium-activated chloride channels [190, 191]. Tissue culture studies have revealed that via the AT1R, Ang II can stimulate pericyte migration which involves both transforming growth factor-β and platelet derived growth factor (PDGF) [192, 193]. Additionally, Ang II can also influence pericyte survival, by augmenting pericyte apoptosis, which may involve the advanced glycation end-product pathway [185, 194]. Overall, it is clear that Ang II influences the retinal microvasculature.

The report that prorenin is elevated in the plasma and vitreous of patients with diabetic retinopathy, lead to the suggestion that the RAS may play a causal role on the development of diabetic retinopathy [195]. Studies in experimental animals indicate that prorenin and other RAS components (e.g. angiotensinogen, ACE, ACE2, AT1R) are increased in the retina with diabetes [36, 196, 197]. Furthermore, Ang II may directly influence glucose uptake into retinal microvascular cells and retinal tissue [198, 199]. Studies in diabetic rodents have indicated that ACE inhibitors and AT1R blockers reduced retinal microvascular damage with reductions in vascular leakage, decreased the formation of acellular capillaries and decreased the expression of angiogenic factors such as VEGF [185, 201-204]. Retinal leukostasis and the upregulation of adhesion molecules are also reduced with ACE inhibition and AT1R blockade [185, 204-207]. Similar benefits on the retinal microvasculature and inflammation are observed in diabetic transgenic Ren-2 rats treated with the renin inhibitor, aliskiren [208], diabetic Long-Evans rats treated with a putative PRR inhibitor [36], and diabetic Sprague Dawley rats following the intraocular gene delivery of ACE2 [197]. The study of the proliferative form of diabetic retinopathy is not possible in rodents due to their failure to develop retinal neovascularization even after 1–2 years of diabetes. Even the overexpression of prorenin and renin in the transgenic Ren-2 rat with streptozotocin diabetes does not promote retinal neovascularization; however new blood vessel growth in the iris (rubeosis iridis) does develop and can be reduced with ACE inhibition with a concomitant reduction in VEGF expression [201].

Diabetes may also induce neuronal and glial deficits in diabetic retinopathy. The resident immune cells of the retina, microglia, may contribute to the inflammatory status of the retina in diabetes [209], by releasing proinflammatory factors. It has been suggested that in this situation, activated microglia contribute to the death of retinal neurons [210]. In terms of RAS blockade, AT1R inhibition has been reported to attenuate nuclear factor-κβ and microglia accumulation in animals with both diabetes and hypertension [206]. The diabetic retina may also exhibit a loss of dopaminergic and cholinergic amacrine cells [211], apoptosis of ganglion cells [212], glial dysfunction [213] and decreased number and length of photoreceptors [214]. This neuroglial pathology translates to electrophysiological deficits, which measured with the electroretinogram gives a global indication of retinal function [215, 216]. Diabetes induces a decrease in the b-wave amplitude, oscillatory potentials and a delay in oscillatory potential latency [215-217]. Diabetes also compromises color vision, contrast sensitivity and dark adaption rates [218, 219]. These functional deficits may occur before the observable presence of any vascular pathology [219]. In diabetic animals, ACE inhibition and AT1R blockade has been reported to attenuate these deficits in retinal function [220-224], indicating that the benefits of RAS blockade extend to non-vascular cells. Of interest is a study showing that AT1R blockade reduced diabetes-related changes in the electroretinogram with a concomitant reduction in the synaptic vesicle protein, synaptophysin, indicating a direct effect of the AT1R on retinal neuronal cells in diabetes [221].

Hypertension is a risk factor for the development of diabetic retinopathy. Some experimental studies of diabetes have attempted to determine whether hypertension per se contributes to diabetic retinopathy, or whether Ang II simulates retinal pathology via blood pressure-independent effects. This is a difficult pursuit, given that ACE inhibition, renin inhibition and AT1R blockade reduce both blood pressure and the cellular effects of Ang II. Studies in the hypertensive Ren-2 rat have indicated that both AT1R blockade (valsartan) and β-adrenergic blockade (atenolol) normalize blood pressure in this model [202, 223]. However, only valsartan improved retinal vascular pathology and deficits in the electroretinogram. Certainly, further evaluation of the blood pressure-independent effects of the RAS blockade in diabetic retinopathy are warranted given the possible application of these agents to patients who are both diabetic and normotensive.

5.2.2. Cellular Mechanisms Involved in the Effects of the Retinal RAS

The cellular mechanisms by which the RAS exerts its effects in the retina are still under investigation. It is likely that reactive oxygen species (ROS) are important given Ang II's ability to increase ROS production [224, 225], and the contribution of ROS to cellular damage in both ROP and diabetic retinopathy [226, 227]. A major source of ROS is nicotinamide adenine dinucleotide phosphate (NADPH, NOX). Six homologs of the cytochrome subunit of the phagocyte NOX (NOX2/gp91phox) are known and include, NOX1, NOX3, NOX4, NOX5, DUOX1, and DUOX2, which together comprise the NOX family [228]. ROS derived from NOX are implicated in the development of both ROP and diabetic retinopathy. For example, in experimental ROP, global inhibition of NOX reduced retinal neovascularization and VEGF expression, and the area of avascular retina [229, 230]. In experimental diabetes, NOX inhibition and a deficiency of NOX2 reduced retinal inflammation, ICAM-1 expression and vascular leakage [231]. Other NOX isoforms may also participate in diabetic retinopathy, with inhibition of NOX4 reported to reduce retinal vascular leakage, ROS generation and VEGF expression in db/db mice [232]. It is well known that Ang II and aldosterone influence NOX to generate ROS [224, 235]. Although the relationship between the RAS and NOX in retinopathy is not fully elucidated, there is evidence that the administration of Ang II to diabetic animals induced retinal leukostasis and superoxide formation which was inhibited by apocynin, a global NOX inhibitor [233]. Furthermore, candesartan reduced the expression of the p22phox subunit of NOX in diabetic retina, and Ang II infusion increased retinal VEGF and p22phox levels [234]. Clearly, the relationship between the RAS and NOX in ROP and diabetic retinopathy warrants further study.

5.2.3. The RAS and Clinical Diabetic Retinopathy

There is clear evidence from clinical trials such as the Diabetes Control and Complications Trial (DCCT) [235] and the United Kingdom Prospective Diabetes Study (UKPDS) trial [236] that controlling both blood glucose and blood pressure reduces the risk of severe diabetic retinopathy. The contribution of Ang II to diabetic retinopathy was evaluated in the EURODIAB Controlled trial of Lisinopril in Insulin-dependent Diabetes (EUCLID) trial. After 2 years, lisinopril reduced the progression of diabetic retinopathy by 50% and progression to proliferative diabetic retinopathy by 80% [237]. The study's limits include a short follow-up period of 2 years and differences in baseline glycaemic levels between groups. The largest study to date to evaluate the effects of RAS blockade with retinopathy as the primary endpoint is the DIabetic REtinopathy Candesartan Trial (DIRECT). This study involved over 5000 patients recruited from 309 centers worldwide, and involved a follow-up of individuals for five years [238, 239]. DIRECT reported that the AT1R blocker candesartan elicited a modest prevention of the onset of retinopathy in normotensive people with type 1 diabetes of 18%, which on post hoc analysis was 35%. In type 1 diabetic individuals there was no effect of candesartan on progression. On the other hand, in people with type 2 diabetes, candesartan treatment resulted in a 34% regression of retinopathy. Further findings from DIRECT indicated that the presence of microaneurysms predicted the increased risk of retinopathy progression in type 1 and type 2 diabetes, and candesartan reduced the risk of microaneurysm progression [240]. A greater benefit for RAS blockade has been reported in the Renin–angiotensin System Study (RASS) of 258 normotensive and normoalbuminuric individuals with type 1 diabetes, which after a 5 year follow-up showed a reduction in progression with either ACE inhibition (65%, enalapril) or AT1R blockade (70%, losartan) [241]. A further study generated from RASS indicated that enalapril and losartan reduced diabetic retinopathy progression only in patients with glycaemic levels $\geq$7.5% [242].

Whether Ang II blockade is suitable for the clinical treatment of diabetic retinopathy is not resolved. The Appropriate Blood Pressure Control in Diabetes (ABCD) trial reported no difference in the progression of diabetic retinopathy in hypertensive type 2 diabetic people who had intensive or moderate blood pressure control [243]. Furthermore, the Action in Diabetes and Vascular Disease Controlled Evaluation (ADVANCE) trial reported that administration of a fixed combination of an ACE inhibitor (perindopril) and a diuretic (indapamide), reduced cardiovascular mortality but had no effect on retinopathy risk [244]. In summary, there appears to be some benefit of RAS blockade in diabetic retinopathy, which will require further exploration.

6. Perspective

Although hypertension is a known risk factor for AMD and DR, there are indeed a large number of normotensive patients with AMD or DR who have the potential risk of hypotension caused by the use of antihypertensive agents including AT1-R blockers and ACE inhibitors. In contrast, since PRR is present in the major organs but not in the circulation, PRRB does not affect circulatory RAS or systemic blood pressure. Interestingly, PRRB treatment to mice with CNV or diabetes-induced retinal inflammation was shown to cause not only tissue RAS deactivation but also additional suppression of PRR signaling-mediated expression of MCP-1 and VEGF, the major factor responsible for the development of these angiogenic and inflammatory disorders. Consequently, inhibition of RAPS with PRRB may prove more useful as a novel therapeutic strategy for vision-threatening diseases including AMD and DR than RAS suppression with conventional AT1-R blockers or ACE inhibitors.

References

[1] Paul, M; Mehr, AP; Kreutz, R. Physiology of local renin-angiotensin systems. *Physiological Reviews,* 2006;86(3):747-803.

[2] Mukoyama, M. Expression cloning of type 2 angiotensin II receptor reveals a unique class of seven-transmembrane receptors. *J Biol Chem,* 1993; 268(33):24539-24542.

[3] Murphy, TJ; Wayne Alexander, R; Criendling, KK; Runge, MS; Bernstein, KE. Isolation of a cDNA encoding the vascular type-1 angiotensin II receptor. *Nature,* 1991; 351(6323):233-236.

[4] de Gasparo, M; Levens, NR. Pharmacology of Angiotensin II receptors in the kidney. *Kidney. Int,* 1994;46:1486-1491.

[5] Douglas, JG; Hopfer U. Novel aspect of angiotensin receptors and signal transduction in kidney. *Annu. Rev. Physiol,* 1994;56:649-669.

[6] Fyhrquist, F; Metsärinne, K; Tikkanen, I. Role of angiotensin II in blood pressureregulation and in the pathophysiology of cardiovascular disorders. *J Hum Hypertens,* 1995;5:19-24.

[7] Beevers, G; Lip, GY; O'Brien, E. ABC of hypertension: The pathophysiology of hypertension. *BMJ,* 2001;322:912-916.

[8] Metsärinne, KP; Helin, KH; Saijonmaa, O; Stewen, P; Sirviö, ML; Fyhrquist, FY. Tissuespecific regulation of angiotensin-converting enzyme by angiotensin II and losartan in the rat. *Blood Press,* 1996;5:363-370.

[9] Bader, M; Peters, J; Baltatu, O; Müller, DN; Luft, FC; Ganten, D. Tissue renin-angiotensin systems: new insights from experimental animal models in hypertension research. *J Mol Med,* 2001;79:76-102.

[10] Kramkowski, K; Mogielnicki, A; Buczko, W. The physiological significance of the alternative pathways of angiotensin II production. *J Physiol Pharmacol,* 2006;57:529-539.

[11] Tikellis, C; Bernardi, S; Burns, WC. Angiotensin-converting enzyme 2 is a key modulator of the renin-angiotensin system in cardiovascular and renal disease. *Curr Opin Nephrol Hypertens,* 2011;20:62-68.

[12] Santos, RA; Simoes, E; Silva, AC; Maric, C; Silva, DM; Machado, RP; de Buhr, I. Angiotensin (1-7) is an endogenous ligand for the G-protein-coupled receptor Mas. *Proc Natl Acad Sci USA*, 2003;8:825882-63.

[13] Kostenis, E; Milligan, G; Christopoulos, A; Sanchez-Ferrer, CF; Heringer-Walther, S; Sexton, PM. G-protein-coupled receptor Mas is a physiological antagonist of the angiotensin II type I receptor. *Circulation*, 2005;111:1806-1813.

[14] Nguyen G. Renin, (pro)renin and receptor: an update. *Clin Sci (Lond)*, 2011;120:169-78.

[15] Wilkinson-Berka, JL; Miller, AG; Fletcher, EL. Prorenin and the (pro)renin receptor: do they have a pathogenic role in the retina? *Front Biosci (Elite Ed)*, 2010;2:1054-1064.

[16] Burckle, CA; Jan Danser, AH; Muller, DN; Garrelds, IM; Gasc, JM; Popova, E; Plehm, R; Peters, J; Bader, M; Nguyen, G. Elevated blood pressure and heart rate in human renin receptor transgenic rats. *Hypertension*, 2006;47:552-556.

[17] Ichihara, A; Suzuki, F; Nakagawa, T; Kaneshiro, Y; Takemitsu, T; Sakoda, M; Nabi, AH, Nishiyama, A; Sugaya, T; Hayashi, M; Inagami, T. Prorenin receptor blockade inhibits development of glomerulosclerosis in diabetic angiotensin II type 1a receptor-deficient mice. *J Am Soc Nephrol,* 2006;17:1950-1961.

[18] Ichihara, A; Kaneshiro, Y; Takemitsu, T; Sakoda, M; Suzuki, F; Nakagawa, A; Nishiyama, A; Inagami, T; Hayashi, M. Nonproteolytic activation of prorenin contributes to development of cardiac fibrosis in genetic hypertension. *Hypertension,* 2006;47:894-900.

[19] Kaneshiro, Y; Ichihara, A; Sakoda, M; Takemitsu, T; Nabi, AH; Uddin, MN; Nakagawa, T; Nishiyama, A; Suzuki, F; Inagami, T;Itoh, H. Slowly Progressive, Angiotensin II-Independent Glomerulosclerosis in Human(Pro)renin Receptor-Transgenic Rats. *J Am Soc Nephrol*, 2007;18, 1789-1795.

[20] Nguyen, G; Delarue, F; Berrou, J; Rondeau, E; Sraer, JD. Specific receptor binding of renin on human mesangial cells in culture increases plasminogen activator inhibitor-1 antigen. *Kidney Int*, 1996;50:1897-1903.

[21] Danser, AH; van den Dorpel, MA; Deinum, J; Derkx, FH; Peperkamp, E; de Jong, PT; Schalekamp, MA. Prorenin in vitreous and subretinal fluid of the human eye. *Clin. Exp. Hypertens*, 1988;A10:1297-1299.

[22] Nguyen, GF; Delarue, C; Burckle, L; Bouzhir, T; Sraer, JD. Pivotal role of the renin/prorenin receptor in angiotensin II production and cellular responses to renin. *J Clin Invest*, 2002;109:1417-1427.

[23] Danser, AH; Deinum, J. Renin, prorenin and the putative (pro)renin receptor. *Hypertension*, 2005;46:1069-1076.

[24] Batenburg, WW; Krop, M; Garrelds, IM; de Vries, R; de Bruin, RJ; Burckle, CA; Muller, DN; Bader, M; Nguyen, G; Danser, AH. Prorenin is the endogenous agonist of the (pro)renin receptor. Binding kinetics of renin and prorenin in rat vascular smooth muscle cells overexpressing the human (pro)renin receptor. *J. Hypertens*, 2007;25:2441-2453.

[25] Satofuka, S., A. Ichihara, N. Nagai, K. Yamashiro, T.Koto, H. Shinoda, K. Noda, Y. Ozawa, M. Inoue, K.Tsubota, F. Suzuki, Y. Oike & S. Ishida: Suppression of ocular inflammation in endotoxin-induced uveitis byinhibiting nonproteolytic activation of prorenin. *InvestOphthalmol Vis Sci* 47, 2686-2692(2006)

[26] Satofuka, S; Ichihara, A; Nagai, N; Koto, T; Shinoda, H; Noda, K; Ozawa, Y; Inoue, M; Tsubota, H; Itoh, H; Oike, Y; Ishida, S. Role of nonproteolytically activated prorenin in pathologic, but not physiologic, retinal neovascularization. *Invest Ophthalmol Vis Sci,* 2007;48:422-429.

[27] Cruciat, CM; Ohkawara, B; Acebron, SP; Karaulanov, E; Reinhard, C; Ingelfinger, D; Boutros, M; Niehrs, C. Requirement of prorenin receptor and vacuolar H+-ATPase-mediated acidification for Wnt signaling. *Science,* 2010;327:459-463.

[28] Huang, Y; Noble, NA; Zhang, J; Xu, C; Border, WA. Renin-stimulated TGF-beta1 expression is regulated by a mitogen-activated protein kinase in mesangial cells. *Kidney Int*, 2007;72:45-52.

[29] Ichihara, A; Kaneshiro, Y; Takemitsu, Y; Sakoda, T; Nakagawa, M; Nishiyama, T; Kawachi, H; Shimizu, F; Inagami, T. Contribution of nonproteolytically activated prorenin in glomeruli to hypertensive renal damage. *J AmSoc Nephrol,* 2006;7:2495-2503.

[30] Kaneshiro, Y; Ichihara, A; Sakoda, M; Takemitsu, T; Nabi, AH; Uddin, MN; Nakagawa, T; Nishiyama, A; Suzuki, F; Inagami, T;Itoh, H. Slowly Progressive, Angiotensin II-Independent Glomerulosclerosis in Human(Pro)renin Receptor-Transgenic Rats. *J Am Soc Nephrol*, 2007;18, 1789-1795.

[31] Satofuka, S; Kanda, A; Ishida, S.Receptor-associated prorenin system in the pathogenesis of retinal diseases. *Frontiers in Bioscience*, 2012;S4:1449-1460.

[32] Ichihara, A; Suzuki, F; Nakagawa, T; Kaneshiro, Y; Takemitsu, T; Sakoda, M; Nabi, AH, Nishiyama, A; Sugaya, T; Hayashi, M; Inagami, T. Prorenin receptor blockade inhibits development of glomerulosclerosis in diabetic angiotensin II type 1a receptor-deficient mice. *J Am Soc Nephrol,* 2006;17:1950-1961.

[33] Ichihara, A; Hayashi, M; Kaneshiro, Y; Suzuki, F; Nakagawa, T; Tada, Y; Koura, Y; Nishiyama, A; Okada, H; Uddin, MN; Nabi, AH; Ishida, Y; Inagami, T; Saruta, T. Inhibition of diabetic nephropathy by a decoypeptide corresponding to the "handle" region fornonproteolytic activation of prorenin. *J Clin Invest,* 2004;114: 1128-1135.

[34] Takahashi, H; Ichihara, A; Kaneshiro, Y; Inomata, K; Sakoda, M; Takemitsu, T; Nishiyama, A; Itoh, H. Regression of Nephropathy Developed in Diabetes by (Pro)renin Receptor Blockade. *J Am Soc Nephrol,* 2007;18:2054-2061.

[35] Suzuki, F; Hayakawa, M; Nakagawa, T; Nasir, UM; Ebihara, A; Iwasawa, A; Ishida, Y; Nakamura, Y;Murakami, K. Human prorenin has "gate and handle" regions for its non-proteolytic activation. *J Biol Chem,* 2003;278:22217-22222.

[36] Satofuka, S; Ichihara, A; Nagai, N; Noda, K; Ozawa, Y; Fukamizu, A; Tsubota, K; Itoh, H; Oike, Y; Ishida, S. (Pro)reninreceptor-mediated signal transduction and tissue reninangiotensinsystem contribute to diabetes-induced retinalinflammation. *Diabetes,* 2009;58:1625-1633.

[37] Nurun, NA; Uddin, NM; Nakagawa, T; Iwata, H; Ichihara, A; Inagami, T; Suzuki, F. Role of "handle"region of prorenin prosegment in the non-proteolytic activation of prorenin by binding to membrane anchored(pro)renin receptor. *Front Biosci,* 2007;12:4810-4817.

[38] Satofuka, S; Ichihara, A; Nagai, N; Noda, K; Ozawa, Y; Fukamizu, A; Tsubota, K; Itoh, H; Oike, I; Ishida, S. (Pro)renin receptor promotes choroidal neovascularization by activating its signal transduction and tissue renin-angiotensinsystem. *Am J Pathol,* 2008;173:1911-1918.

[39] Ichihara, A; Kaneshiro, Y; Takemitsu, T; Sakoda, M; Suzuki, F; Nakagawa, A; Nishiyama, A; Inagami, T; Hayashi, M. Nonproteolytic activation of prorenin contributes to development of cardiac fibrosis in genetic hypertension. *Hypertension,* 2006;47:894-900.

[40] Rong, P; Wilkinson-Berka, JL; Skinner, SL. Control of renin secretion from adrenal gland in transgenic Ren-2 and normal rats. *Mol Cell Endocrinol*, 2001;173:203-212.

[41] Wilkinson-Berka, JL; Kelly, DJ; Rong, P; Campbell, DJ; Skinner, SL. Characterisation of a thymic renin-angiotensin system in the transgenic m(Ren-2)27 rat. *Mol Cell Endocrinol* , 2002;194: 201-209.

[42] Berka, JL; Stubbs, AJ; Wang, DZ; DiNicolantonio, R; Alcorn, D; Campbell, DJ; Skinner, SL. Renin-containing Muller cells of the retina display endocrine features. *Invest Ophthalmol Vis Sci*, 1995;36:1450-1458.

[43] Sarlos, S; Rizkalla, B; Moravski, CJ; Cao, Z; Cooper, ME; Wilkinson-Berka, JL. Retinal angiogenesis is mediated by an interaction between the angiotensin type 2 receptor, VEGF, and angiopoietin. *Am J Pathol*, 2003;163: 879-887.

[44] Igić, R; Robinson, CJ; Milosević, Z; Wilson, CM; Erdös, EG. Activity of renin and angiotensin I converting enzyme in retina and ciliary body. *Lijec Vjesn*, 1977;99(8):482-484.

[45] Wheeler-Schilling, TH; Kohler, K; Sautter, M; Guenther, E. Angiotensin II receptor subtype gene expression and cellular localization in the retina and non-neuronal ocular tissues of the rat. *Eur J Neurosci*, 1999. 11;3387-3394

[46] Savaskan, E; Loffler, KU; Meier, F; Muller-Spahn, F; Flammer, J; Meyer, P. Immunohistochemical localization of angiotensin-converting enzyme, angiotensin II and AT1 receptor in human ocular tissues. *Ophthalmic Res*, 2004. 36;312-320

[47] Senanayake, P; Drazba, J; Shadrach, K; Milsted, A; Rungger-Brandle, E; Nishiyama, K; Miura, S; Karnik, S; Sears, JE; Hollyfield, JG. Angiotensin II and its receptor subtypes in the human retina. *Invest Ophthalmol Vis Sci*, 2007;48: 3301-3311

[48] Striker, GE; Praddaude, F; Alcazar, O; Cousins, SW; Marin-Castano, ME. Regulation of angiotensin II receptors and extracellular matrix turnover in human retinal pigment epithelium: role of angiotensin II. *Am J Physiol Cell Physiol*, 2008;295:C1633-1646

[49] Wagner, J; Jan Danser, AH; Derkx, FH; de Jong, TV; Paul, M; Mullins, JJ; Schalekamp, MA; Ganten, D. Demonstration of renin mRNA, angiotensinogen mRNA, and angiotensin converting enzyme mRNA expression in the human eye: evidence for an intraocular renin-angiotensin system. *Br J Ophthalmol*, 1996; 80:159-163.

[50] Cunha-Vaz, J. The blood-ocular barriers. *Surv Ophthalmol*, 1979;23:279-296.

[51] Danser, AHJ; Derkx, FHM; Admiraal, PJJ; Deinum, J; de Jong, PTVM; Schalekamp, MADH. Angiotensin levels in the eye. *Invest Ophthalmol Vis Sci*, 1994;35:1008-1018

[52] Otani, A; Takagi, H; Suzuma, K; Honda, Y. Angiotensin II potentiates endothelial growth factor-induced angiogenic activity in retinal microcapillary endothelial cells. *Circ Res,*1998;82:619-628.

[53] Strauss, O. The retinal pigment epithelium in visual function. *Physiol Rev*, 2005; 85:845-881.

[54] Milenkovic, VM; Brockmann, M; Meyer, C; Desch, M; Schweda, F; Kurtz, A; Todorov, V; Strauss, O. Regulation of the renin expression in the retinal pigment epithelium by systemic stimuli. *Am J Physiol Renal Physiol*, 2010;299:F396-F403.

[55] Fletcher, EL; Phipps, JA; Ward, MM; Vessey, KA; Wilkinson-Berka, JL. The renin-angiotensin system in retinal health and disease: Its influence on neurons, glia and the vasculature. *Prog Retin Eye Res*, 2010;29:284-311.

[56] Jacobi, PC; Osswald, H; Jurklies, B; Zrenner, E. Neuromodulatory effects of the reninangiotensin system on the cat electroretinogram. *Invest Ophthalmol Vis Sci*, 1994; 35: 973-980.

[57] Jurklies, B; Eckstein, A; Jacobi, P; Kohler, K; Risler, T; Zrenner, E. The renin-angiotensin system-a possible neuromodulator in the human retina? *Ger J Ophthalmol*, 1995;4:144-150.

[58] Klein, R; Peto, T; Bird, A; Vannewkirk, MR.The epidemiology of age-related macular degeneration. *Am J Ophthalmol*, 2004;137:486-495.

[59] Young, RW. Pathophysiology of age-related macular degeneration. *Surv Ophthalmol*, 1987;31: 291-306.

[60] Bressler, SB; Maguire, MG; Bressler, NM; Fine. SL. Relationship of drusen and abnormalities of the retinal pigment epithelium to the prognosis of neovascular macular degeneration. The Macular Photocoagulation Study Group. *Arch Ophthalmol*, 1990;108: 1442-1447.

[61] Sarks, SH; Van Driel, D; Maxwell, L; Killingsworth, M. Softening of drusen and subretinal neovascularization. *Trans Ophthalmol Soc U K,* 1980;100:414-422.

[62] Vinding, T. Occurrence of drusen, pigmentary changes and exudative changes in the macula with reference to age-related macular degeneration. An epidemiological study of 1000 aged individuals. *Acta Ophthalmol* (Copenh), 1999;68:410-414.

[63] Clemons, TE; Milton, RC; Klein, R; Seddon, JM; Ferris 3rd, FL. Risk factors for the incidence of advanced age-related macular degeneration in the Age-Related Eye Disease Study (AREDS). AREDS Report No. 19. *Ophthalmology*, 2005;112:533-539.

[64] Evans, JR. 2001. Risk factors for age-related macular degeneration. *Prog. Retin. Eye Res*, 2001;20:227-253.

[65] Khan, JC; Thurlby, DA; Shahid, H; Clayton, DG; Yates, JR; Bradley, M; Moore, AT, Bird, AC. Smoking and age related macular degeneration: the number of pack years of cigarette smoking is amajor determinant of risk for both geographic atrophy and choroidal neovascularisation. *Br. J. Ophthalmol*, 2006;90,:75-80.

[66] Sepp, T; Khan, JC; Thurlby, DA, Shahid, H, Clayton, DG; Moore, AT; Bird, AC; Yates, JR. Complement factor H variant Y402H is a major risk determinant for geographic atrophy and choroidal neovascularization in smokers and nonsmokers. *Invest. Ophthalmol. Vis. Sci*, 2006;47;536-540.

[67] Smith, W; Assink, J; Klein, R; Mitchell, P; Klaver, CC; Klein, BE; Hofman, A; Jensen, S; Wang, JJ; de Jong, PT. Risk factors for age-related macular degeneration: pooled findings from three continents. Ophthalmology, 2001;108:697-704.

[68] Praddaude, F; Cousins, SW; Pêcher, C; Marin-Castaño, ME. Angiotensin II-induced hypertension regulates AT1 receptor subtypes and extracellular matrix turnover in mouse retinal pigment epithelium.*Exp Eye Res*, 2009;89(1):109-118.

[69] Aumailley, M; Gayraud, B. Structure and biological activity of the extracellular matrix. *J Mol Med,*1998;76:253-265.

[70] Kugler, A. Matrix metalloproteinases and their inhibitors. *Anticancer Res,* 1999;19:1589-1592.

[71] Jacot, TA; Striker, GE; Stetler-Stevenson, M. Mesangial cells from transgenic mice with progressive glomerulosclerosis exhibit stable, phenotypic changes including undetectable MMP-9 and increased type IV collagen. *Lab Invest,* 1996;75:791-799.

[72] Peten, EP; Garcia-Perez, A; Terada, Y. Age-related changes in alpha 1- and alpha 2-chain type IV collagen mRNAs in adult mouse glomeruli: competitive PCR. *Am J Physiol,* 1992;263:F951-F957.

[73] Belkhiri, A; Richards, C; Whaley, M. Increased expression of activated matrix metalloproteinase-2 by human endothelial cells after sublethal H2O2 exposure. *Lab Invest,* 1997;77:533-539.

[74] Green, WR. Histopathology of age-related macular degeneration. *Mol Vis,* 1999, 5:27.

[75] Ishibashi, T; Patterson, R; Ohnishi, Y; Inomata, H; Ryan, S. Formation of drusen in the human eye. *Am. J. Ophthalmol*, 1986;101:342–353.

[76] Burns, R; Feeney Burns, L. Clinico-morphologic correlations of drusen of Bruch's membrane. *Trans Am Ophthalmol Soc*, 1980;78:206–225.

[77] Zhu, ZR; Goodnight, R; Nishimura, T; Sorgente, N; Ogden, TE; Ryan, SJ. Experimental changes resembling the pathology of drusen in Bruch's membrane in the rabbit. *Curr Eye Res,*1988;7:581-592.

[78] Sarks, S; Cherepanoff, S; Killingsworth, M; Sarks, J. Relationship of basal laminar deposit and membranous debris to the clinical presentation of early Age-related macular degeneration. *Invest Ophthalmol Vis Sci*, 2007; 48:968-977.

[79] Marin-Castaño, ME; Csaky, KG; Cousins, SW. Nonlethal oxidant injury to human retinal pigment epithelium cells causes cell membrane blebbing but decreased MMP-2 activity. *Invest Ophthalmol Vis Sci*, 2005;46(9):3331-3340.

[80] Marin-Castaño, ME; Striker, GE; Alcazar, O; Catanuto, P; Espinosa-Heidmann, DG; Cousins, SW. Repetitive nonlethal oxidant injury to retinal pigment epithelium decreased extracellular matrix turnover in vitro and induced sub-RPE deposits in vivo. *Invest Ophthalmol Vis Sci*, 2006;47(9):4098-4112.

[81] Alcazar, O; Cousins, SW; Marin-Castaño, ME. MMP-14 and TIMP-2 overexpression protects against hydroquinone-induced oxidant injury in RPE: implications for extracellular matrix turnover. *Invest Ophthalmol Vis Sci*, 2007;48(12):5662-70.

[82] Alcazar, O; Hawkridge, AM; Collier, TS; Cousins, SW; Bhattacharya, SK; Muddiman, DC; Marin-Castano, ME. Proteomics characterization of cell membrane blebs in human retinal pigment epithelium cells. *Mol Cell Proteomics*, 2009;8(10):2201-2211.

[83] Wiesner, C; Faix, J; Himmel, M; Bentzien, F; Linder, S. KIF5B and KIF3A/KIF3B kinesins drive MT1-MMP surface exposure, CD44 shedding, and extracellular matrix degradation in primary macrophages. *Blood*, 2010;116(9):1559-69.

[84] Deryugina, EI; Bourdon, MA; Reisfeld, RA; Strongin, A. Remodeling of collagen matrix by human tumor cells requires activation and cell surface association of matrix metalloproteinase-2. *Cancer Res,* 1989; 58:3743-3750.

[85] Atkison, SJ; Petterson, ML; Butler, MJ; Murphy, G. Membrane type 1 matrix metalloproteinase and gelatinase A synergistically degrade type I collagen in a cell model. *FEBS Lett,* 2001; 491:222-226.

[86] Spagnoli, LG; Sambuy, Y; Palmieri, G. Age-related modulation of vascular smooth muscle cells proliferation following arterial wall damage. *Artery*, 1985;13:187-198.

[87] Jonas, JB; Hayreh, SS; Martus, P. Influence of arterial hypertension and diet-induced atherosclerosis on macular drusen. *Graefes Arch Clin Exp Ophthalmol*, 2003;24(2):125-134.

[88] Hayreh, SS; Servais, GE; Virdi, PS. Macular lesions in malignant arterial hypertension. *Ophthalmologica*, 1989;198:230-246.

[89] Hyman, L; Schachat, AP; He, Q; Leske, MC. Hypertension, cardiovascular disease, and age-related macular degeneration. Age-Related Macular Degeneration Risk Factors Study Group. *Arch Ophthalmol*, 2000;118:351-358.

[90] Taylor, WR. Hypertensive vascular disease and inflammation: mechanical and humoral mechanisms. *Curr Hypertens.Rep*, 1999;1:96-101.

[91] Lee, MA; Bohm, M; Paul, M; Ganten, D. Tissue renin-angiotensin systems. Their role in cardiovascular disease. *Circulation*, 1993;87:IV7-13.

[92] Berka, JL; Stubbs; AJ; Wang, DZ; DiNicolantonio, R; Alcorn, D; Campbell, DJ; Skinner, SL. Renin-containing Muller cells of the retina display endocrine features. *Invest Ophthalmol Vis Sci*, 1995; 36:1450-1458.

[93] Kohler, K; Wheeler-Schilling, T; Jurklies, B; Guenther, E. Angiotensin II in the rabbit retina. *Vis Neurosci*, 1997;14:63-71.

[94] Wagner, J; Jan Danser, AH; Derkx, FH; de Jong, TV; Paul, M; Mullins, JJ; Schalekamp, MA; Ganten, D. Demonstration of renin mRNA, angiotensinogen mRNA, and angiotensin converting enzyme mRNA expression in the human eye: evidence for an intraocular renin-angiotensin system. *Br J Ophthalmol*, 1996;80: 159-163.

[95] Castoldi, G; Di Gioia, CR; Pieruzzi, F; d'Orlando, C; Van de Greef, WM; Busca, G; Sperti, G; Stella, A. ANG II increases TIMP-1 expression in rat aortic smooth muscle cells in vivo. *Am J Physiol Heart Circ Physiol,* 2003;284:H635-643.

[96] Eagleton, MJ; Ballard, N; Lynch, E; Srivastava, SD; Upchurch, GR Jr; Stanley, JC. Early increased MT1-MMP expression and late MMP-2 and MMP-9 activity during Angiotensin II induced aneurysm formation. *J Surg Res,* 2006;135:345-51.

[97] Huang, W; Yu, LF; Zhong, J; Qizo, MM; Jiang, FX; Du, F; Tian, XL; Wu, YL. Angiotensin II Type 1 Receptor Expression in Human Gastric Cancer and Induces MMP2 and MMP9 Expression in MKN-28 Cells. *Dig Dis Sci*, 2008; 53(1):163-168.

[98] Seeger, H; Lippert, C; Wallwiener, D; Mueck, AO. Valsartan and candesartan can inhibit deteriorating effects of angiotensin II on coronary endothelial function. *J Renin Angiotensin Aldosterone Syst*, 2001;2:141-143.

[99] Uchiyama-Tanaka, Y; Matsubara, H; Nozawa, Y; Murasawa, S; Mori, Y; Kosaki, A; Maruyama, K; Masaki, H; Shibasaki, Y; Fujiyama, S; Nose, A; Iba, O; Hasagawa, T; Tateishi, E; Higashiyama, S; Iwasaka, I. Angiotensin II signaling and HB-EGF shedding via metalloproteinase in glomerular mesangial cells. *Kidney Int*, 2001;60:2153-2163.

[100] Wang, M; Zhang, J; Spinetti, G; Jiang, LQ; Monticone, R; Zhao, D; Cheng, L; Krawczyk, M; Talan, M; Pintu, SG; Lakatta, EG. Angiotensin II activates matrix metalloproteinase type II and mimics age-associated carotid arterial remodeling in young rats. *Am J Pathol*, 2005;167:1429-1442.

[101] Weiss, RH; Ramirez, A.TGF-beta- and angiotensin-II-induced mesangial matrix protein secretion is mediated by protein kinase C. *Nephrol Dial Transplant*, 1998;13:2804-2813.

[102] Wolf, G; Ziyadeh, NF. Renal tubular hypertrophy induced by angitensin II. *Semin Nephrol,* 1997;17:448-454.
[103] Sarlos, S; Rizkalla, B; Moravski, CJ; Cao, Z; Cooper, ME; Wilkinson-Berka, JL. Retinal angiogenesis is mediated by an interaction between the angiotensin type 2 receptor, VEGF and angiopoietin. *Am J Pathol*, 2003;879-887.
[104] Han SY, Jee YH, Han KH, Kang YS, Kim HK, Han JY, Kim YS, Cha DR. An imbalance between MMP-2 and tissue inhibitor of matrix metalloproteinase-2 contributes to the development of early nephropathy. *Nephrol Dal Transplant*, 2006;21:2406-2416.
[105] Arenas, IA; xu, Y; Lopez-Jaramillo, P; Davidge, ST. Angiotensin II-induced MMP-2 release from endothelial cells is mediated by TNF-alpha. *Am J Physiol Cell Physio,* 2004; 286:779-7784.
[106] Lijnen, P; Papparella, I; Petrov, V; Semplicini, A; Fagard, R. Angiotensin II-stimulated collagen production in cardiac fibroblasts is mediated by reactive oxygen species. *J Hypertens,* 2006;24:757-766.
[107] Flamant, M; Placier, S; Dubroca, C; Esposito, B; Lopes, I; Chatziantoniou, C; tedgui, A; Dussaule, JC; Lehoux, S. Role of Matrix Metalloproteinases in early hypertensive vascular remodeling. *Hypertension*, 2007;50:213-218.
[108] Wolf, G. Angiotensin II and tubular development. *Nephol Dial Transplant*, 2002;17:48-51.
[109] Cui, XL; Ding, Y; Alexander, LD; Bao, C; Al-Khalili, OK; Simonson, M; Eaton, DC; Douglas, JG. Oxidative signaling in renal epithelium: Critical role of cytosolic phospholipase A2 and p38(SAPK). *Free Radical Biology and Medicine*, 2006;41:190-192.
[110] Pons, M; Cousins, SW; Alcazar, O; Striker, GE; Marin-Castaño, ME. Angiotensin II-induced MMP-2 activity and MMP-14 and basigin protein expression are mediated via the angiotensin II receptor type 1-mitogen-activated protein kinase 1 pathway in retinal pigment epithelium implications for age-related macular degeneration. *Am J Pathol*, 2011 ;178(6):2665-81.
[111] Ichijo, H; Nishida, E; Irie, K; ten Dijke, P; Saitoh, M; Moriguchi, T; Takagi, M; Matsumoto, K; Miyazono, G; Gotoh, Y. Induction of apoptosis by ASK1, a mammalian MAPKKK that activates SAPK/JNK and p38 signaling pathways. *Science*, 1997, 275:90-94.
[112] Sugden, PH; Clerk, A. Regulation of the ERK subgroup of MAP kinase cascades through G protein-coupled receptors. *Cell Signal*, 1997;9: 337-351.
[113] Taniyama, Y; Ushio-Fukai, M; Hitomi, H; Rocic, P; Kingsley, MJ; Pfahnl, C; Weber, DS; Alexander, RW; Griendling, KK. Role of p38 MAPK and MAPKAPK-2 in angiotensin II-induced Akt activation in vascular smooth muscle cells. Am J Physiol Cell Physiol, 2004, 287:C494-499.
[114] Chen, Z; Gibson, TB; Robinson, F; Silvestro, L; Pearson, G; Xu, B; Wright, A; Vanderbilt, C; Cobb, MH. MAP kinases. *Chem Rev*, 2001;101:2449-2476.
[115] Lewis, TS; Shapiro, PS; Ahn, NG. Signal transduction through MAP kinase cascades. *Adv Cancer Res*, 1998;74:49-139.
[116] Pearson, G; Robinson, F; Beers-Gibson, T; Xu, BE; Karandikar, M; Berman, K; Cobb, MH. Mitogen-activated protein (MAP) kinase pathways: regulation and physiological functions. *Endocr Rev*, 2001;22:153-183.

[117] Alcazar, O; Cousins, SW; Striker, GE; Marin-Castano, ME. (Pro)renin receptor is expressed in human retinal pigment epithelium and participates in extracellular matrix remodeling. *Exp Eye Res*, 2009;89(5):638-47.
[118] Rodrigues, EB. Inflammation in dry age-related macular degeneration. *Ophthalmologica*, 2007;221;143-152.
[119] Chisolm, GM III; Hazen, SL; Fox, PL; Cathcart, MK. The oxidation of lipoproteins by monocytes-macrophages. Biochemical and biological mechanisms. *J Biol Chem*, 1999; 274(37):25959-25962.
[120] Grossniklaus, HE; Ling, JX; Wallace, TM; Dithmar, S; Lawson, DH; Cohen, C et al. Macrophage and retinal pigment epithelium expression of angiogenic cytokines in choroidal neovascularization. *Mol Vis*, 2002; 8:119-126.
[121] Cousins, SW; Espinosa-Heidmann, DG; Csaky, KG. Monocyte activation in patients with age-related macular degeneration: a biomarker of risk for choroidal neovascularization? *Arch Ophthalmo*l, 2004; 122(7):1013-1018.
[122] Espinosa-Heidmann, DG; Suner, IJ; Hernandez, EP; Monroy, D; Csaky, KG; Cousins, SW. Macrophage depletion diminishes lesion size and severity in experimental choroidal neovascularization. *Invest Ophthalmol Vis Sci*, 2003; 44(8):3586-3592.
[123] Patel, M; Chan, CC. Immunopathological aspects of age-related macular degeneration. *Semin Immunopathol*, 2008;30: 97-110
[124] Victor Chong, NH; Johnson, LV; Anderson, DH. An integrated hypothesis that considers drusen as biomarkers of immune-mediated processes at the RPE-Bruch's membrane interface in aging and age-related macular degeneration. *Prog Retin Eye Res*, 2001; 20: 705-732.
[125] Donoso, LA; Kim, D; Frost, A; Callahan, A; Hageman, G. The role of inflammation in the pathogenesis of age-related macular degeneration. *Surv Ophthalmol*, 2006; 51: 137-152.
[126] Haines, JL; Hauser, MA; Schmidt, S; Scott, WK; Olson, LM. Complement factor H variant increases the risk of age-related macular degeneration. *Science*, 2005; 308: 419-421.
[127] Lommatzsch, A; Hermans, P; Muller, KD; Bornfeld, N; Bird, AC. Are low inflammatory reactions involved in exudative age-related macular degeneration? Morphological and immunhistochemical analysis of AMD associated with basal deposits. *Graefes Arch Clin Exp Ophthalmol*, 2008; 246: 803-810.
[128] Penfold, PL; Madigan, MC; Gillies, MC; Provis, JM. Immunological and aetiological aspects of macular degeneration. *Prog Retin Eye Res*, 2001; 20: 385-414.
[129] 129.Killingsworth, MC; Sarks, JP; Sarks, SH. Macrophages related to Bruch's membrane in age-related macular degeneration. *Eye (Lond)*, 1999; 4 (Pt 4): 613-621.
[130] Dastgheib, K; Green WR. Granulomatous reaction to Bruch's membrane in age-related macular degeneration. *Arch Ophthalmol*, 1994; 112: 813-818.
[131] Grossniklaus, HE; Ling, JX; Wallace, TM; Dithmar, S; Lawson, DH.Macrophage and retinal pigment epithelium expression of angiogenic cytokines in choroidal neovascularization. *Mol Vis*, 2002; 8: 119-126.
[132] Lopez, PF; Grossniklaus, HE; Lambert, HM; Aaberg, TM; Capone, A. Pathologic features of surgically excised subretinal neovascular membranes in age-related macular degeneration. *Am J Ophthalmol*, 1991; 112: 647-656.

[133] Oh, H; Takagi, H; Takagi, C; Suzuma, K; Otani, A. The potential angiogenic role of macrophages in the formation of choroidal neovascular membranes. *Invest Ophthalmol Vis Sci*, 1999; 40: 1891-1898.

[134] Yi, X; Takahashi, K; Ogata, N; Uyama, M. Immunohistochemical proof of origin of macrophages in laser photocoagulation lesion in the retina. *Jpn J Ophthalmol*, 1996; 40: 192-201.

[135] Ding, X; Patel, M; Chan, CC. Molecular pathology of age-related macular degeneration. *Prog Retin Eye Res,* 2009; 28: 1-18.

[136] Luft FC, Mervaala E, Muller DN, Gross V, Schmidt F, Joon KP, et al. Hypertension-induced end-organ damage: a new transgenic approach to an old problem. *Hypertension.* 1999;33:212–218.

[137] Alexander RW. Hypertension and the pathogenesis of atherosclerosis: oxidative stress and the mediation of arterial inflammatory response, a new perspective. *Hypertension.* 1995;25:155–161.

[138] Yla-Herttuala, S; Lipton, BA; Rosenfeld, ME; Srakioja, T; Yoshimura, T; Leonard, EJ. Expression of monocyte chemoattractant protein-1 in macrophage-rich areas of human and rabbit atherosclerotic lesions. *Proc Natl Acad Sci USA,* 1991;88:5252–5256.

[139] Yu, X; Dluz, S; Graves, DT; Zhang, L; Antoniades, HN; Hollander, W. Elevated expression of monocyte chemoattractant protein-1 by vascular smooth muscle cells in hypercholesterolemic primates. *Proc Natl Acad Sci USA, 1*992;89:6953–6957.

[140] Capers, Q; Alexander, RW; Lou, P; De Leon, H; Wilcox, JN; Ishizaka, N. Monocyte chemoattractant protein-1 expression in aortic tissues of hypertensive rats. *Hypertension, 1*997;30:1397-1402.

[141] Behr, TM; Wang, XK; Aijar, N; Coatney, RW; Li, X; Koster, P. Monocyte chemoattractant protein-1 is upregulated in rats with volume overloaded congestive heart failure. *Circulation,* 2000;102:1315-1322.

[142] Hilgers, KF; Hartner, A; Porst, M; Mai, M; Wittmann, M; Hugo, C. Monocyte chemoattractant protein-1 and macrophage infiltration in hypertensive kidney injury. *Kidney Int,* 2000;58:2408-2419.

[143] Hernandez-Presa, M; Bustos, C; Ortego, M; Tunon, J; Renedo, G; Ruiz-Ortega, M; Egido, J. Angiotensin-converting enzyme inhibition prevents arterial nuclear factor-kappa B activation, monocyte chemoattractant protein-1 expression, and macrophage infiltration in a rabbit model of early accelerated atherosclerosis. *Circulation, 1*997;95:1532–1541.

[144] *Ruiz*-Ortega, M; Ruperez, M; Lorenzo, O; Esteban, V; Blanco, J; Mezzano, S. Angiotensin II regulates the synthesis of proinflammatory cytokines and chemokines in the kidney. *Kidney Int,* 2002;62(suppl 82):12–22.

[145] Tham, DM; Martin-McNulty, B; Wang, YX; Wilson, DW; Vergona, R; Sullivan, ME. Angiotensin II is associated with activation of NF-kappa B-mediated genes and downregulation of PPARs. *Physiol Genom,* 2002;11:21–31.

[146] Yoshimura, T; Leonard, EJ. Identification of high affinity receptors for human monocyte chemoattractant protein-1 on human monocytes. *J Immunol,* 1990;145:292–297.

[147] Charo, IF; Myers, SJ; Herman, A; Franci, C; Connolly, AJ; Coughlin, SR. Molecular cloning and functional expression of two monocyte chemoattractant protein-1 receptors reveals alternative splicing of the carboxyl-terminal trails. *Proc Natl Acad Sci USA,* 1994;91:2752–2756.

[148] Uetama, T; Ohno-Matsui, K; Nakahama, K; Morita, I; Mochizuki, M. Phenotypic change regulates monocyte chemoattractant protein-1 (MCP-1) gene expression in human retinal pigment epithelial cells. *J Cell Physiol,* 2003; 197: 77-85.

[149] Higgins, GT; Wang, JH; Dockery, P; Cleary, PE; Redmond, HP. Induction of angiogenic cytokine expression in cultured RPE by ingestion of oxidized photoreceptor outer segments. *Invest Ophthalmol Vis Sci,* 2003; 44: 1775-1782.

[150] Ambati, J; Anand, A; Fernandez, S; Sakurai, E; Lynn, BC. An animal model of age-related macular degeneration in senescent Ccl-2- or Ccr-2-deficient mice. *Nat Med,* 2003; 9: 1390-1397.

[151] Tuo, J; Bojanowski, CM; Zhou, M; Shen, D; Ross, RJ. Murine ccl2/cx3cr1 deficiency results in retinal lesions mimicking human age-related macular degeneration. *Invest Ophthalmol Vis Sci*, 2007; 48: 3827-3836.

[152] Penfold, PL; Madigan, MC; Gillies, MC; Provis, JM. Immunological and aetiological aspects of macular degeneration. *Prog Retin Eye Res*, 2001; 20(3):385-414.

[153] Basso, N; Paglia N, Stella I, de Cavanagh, EM; Ferder, L; Arnaiz, M; Inserra, F. Protective effect of the inhibition of the renin-angiotensis system on aging. *Regul Pept*, 2005;128:247-252.

[154] Diz, D; Lewis, K. Dahl memorial lecture: the renin-angiotensisn system and aging. *Hypertension*, 2008;52:37-43.

[155] Cushman, WC. Are there benefits to specific antihypertensive drug therapy? *Am J Hypertens,* 2003;16:31–35.

[156] Timmermans, PB; Wong, PC; Chiu, AT; Herblin, WF; Benfield, P; Carini, DJ. Angiotensin II receptors and angiotensin II receptor antagonists. *Pharmacol Rev,* 1993;45:205–251.

[157] Heart Outcomes Prevention Evaluation Study Investigators. Effects of an angiotensin-converting enzyme inhibitor, ramipril, on cardiovascular events in high-risk patients. *N Engl J Med.* 2000;342:145–153.

[158] Dahlof, B; Devereux, RB; Kjeldsen, SE; Julius, S; Beevers, G; Faire, U. for the LIFE Study Group. Cardiovascular morbidity and mortality in the Losartan Intervention For Endpoint reduction in hypertension study (LIFE): a randomised trial against atenolol. *Lancet,* 2002;359:995–1003.

[159] Hisada, Y; Sygaya, T; Yamanouchi, M; Uchida, H; Fujimura, H; Sakurai, H. Angiotensin II plays a pathologic role in immune-mediated renal injury in mice. *J Clin Invest,* 1999;103:627–635.

[160] Behr, TM; Willette, RN; Coatney, RW; Berova, M; Angermann, CE; Anderson, K. Eprosartan improves cardiac performance, reduces cardiac hypertrophy and mortality and downregulates myocardial MCP-1 and inflammation in hypertensive heart disease. *J Hypertens,* 2004;22:583–592

[161] Funakoshi, Y; Ichiki, T; Shimokawa, H; Egashira, K; Takeda, K; Kaibuchi, K. Rho-kinase mediates angiotensin II-induced monocyte chemoattractant protein-1 expression in rat vascular smooth muscle cells. *Hypertension,* 2001;38:100-104.

[162] Wu, L; Iwai, M; Nakagami, H; Li, Z; Chen, R; Suzuki, J. Roles of angiotensin II type 2 receptor stimulation associated with selective angiotensin II type 1 receptor blockade with valsartan in the improvement of inflammation-induced vascular injury. *Circulation,* 2001;104:2716-2721.

[163] Sozzani, S; Luini, W; Molino, M; Jilek, P; Bottazzi, B; Cerletti, C. The signaling transduction pathway involved in the migration induced by a monocyte chemotactic cytokine. *J Immunol,* 1991;147:2215–2221.

[164] Chen, XL; Tummala, PE; Olbrych, MT; Alexander, RW; Medford, RM. Angiotensin II induces monocyte chemoattractant protein-1 gene expression in rat vascular smooth muscle cells. *Circ Res,* 1998;83:952–959.

[165] Locati, M; Zhou, D; Luini, W; Evangelista, V; Mantovani, A; Sozzani, S. Rapid induction of arachidonic acid release by monocyte chemotactic protein-1 and related chemokines: role of Ca^{2+} influx, synergism with platelet-activating factor and significance for chemotaxis. *J Biol Chem,* 1994;269:4746-4753.

[166] Yu, BP; Chung, HY. Adaptive mechanisms to oxidative stress during aging. *Mech Ageing Dev*, 2006; 127:436–443.

[167] Kim, HJ; Jung, KJ; Yu, BP; Cho, CG; Choi, JS; Chung, HY. Modulation of redox-sensitive transcription factors by calorie restriction during aging. *Mech Ageing Dev*, 2002; 123:1589–1595.

[168] Chung, HY; Kim, HJ; Kim, KW; Choi, JS; Yu, BP. Molecular inflammation hypothesis of aging based on the anti-aging mechanism of calorie restriction. *Microsc Res Tech*, 2002; 59:264–272.

[169] Chung, HY; Cesari, M; Anton, S; Marzetti, E; Giovannini, S; Seo, AY; Carter, C; Yu, BP; Leeuwenburgh, C. Molecular inflammation: underpinnings of aging and age-related diseases. *Ageing Res Rev*, 2009; 8:18–30.

[170] Miyata, N; Yamakoshi, Y; Nakanishi, I. Reactive species responsible for biological actions of photo excited fullerenes. *Yakugaku Zasshi*, 2002; 120:1007–1016.

[171] Murkies, A. Phytoestrogens what is the current knowledge? *Aust Fam Physician*, 1998; 27:S47–S51.

[172] Ferris, FL; Fine, SL; Hyman, L. Agerelated macular degeneration and blindness due to neovascular maculopathy. *Arch Ophthalmol*, 1984;102:1640-1642.

[173] Klein, RQ; Wang, BE; Klein, S; Moss, E; Meuer SM.The relationship of age-related maculopathy, cataract, and glaucoma to visual acuity. *InvestOphthalmol Vis Sci,* 1995;36, 182-191.

[174] Ishibashi, T; Hata, Y; Yoshikawa, H; Nakagawa, K; Sueishi, K; Inomata H. Expression of vascular endothelial growth factor in experimental choroidal neovascularization. *Graefes Arch Clin Exp Ophthalmol,*1997;235:159-167.

[175] Nagai, N; Oike, Y; Izumi-Nagai, K; Urano, T; Kubota, Y; Noda, K; Ozawa, Y; Inoue, M; Tsubota, K; Suda, T; S, Ishida. Angiotensin II type 1 receptor-mediated inflammation is required for choroidal neovascularization.*Arterioscler Thromb Vasc Biol* ,2006;26, 2252-2259(2006)

[176] Sakurai, E; Taguchi, H; Anand, A; Ambati, BK; Gragoudas, ES; Miller, JW; Adamis, AP; Ambati, J.Targeted disruption of the CD18 or ICAM-1 gene inhibits choroidal neovascularization. *Invest Ophthalmol Vis Sci*, 2003;44:2743-2749.

[177] Yeh, DC; Bula, DV; Miller, JW; Gragoudas, ES; Arroyo, JG. Expression of leukocyte adhesion moleculesin human subfoveal choroidal neovascular membranes treated with and without photodynamic therapy. *InvestOphthalmol Vis Sci,* 2004;45: 2368-2373.
[178] Sakurai, E; Anand, A; Ambati, BK; van Rooijen, N; Ambati, J. Macrophage depletion inhibits experimentalchoroidal neovascularization. *Invest Ophthalmol Vis Sci*, 2003;44:3578-3585.
[179] Tsutsumi, C; Sonoda,KH; Egashira, K; Qiao, H; Hisatomi, T; Nakao, S; Ishibashi, M; Charo, IF; Sakamoto, T; Murata, T; Ishibashi, T. The critical role of ocular-infiltrating macrophages in the development ofchoroidal neovascularization. *J Leukoc Biol,* 2003;74:25-32.
[180] Yau, JW; Rogers, SL; Kawasaki, R; Lamoureux, EL; Kowalski, JW; Bek T et al. Global prevalence and major risk factors of diabetic retinopathy. *Diabetes Care*, 2012;35:556-564.
[181] Fong, DS; Aiello, L; Gardner, TW; King, GL; Blankenship, G; Cavallerano, JD et al. Retinopathy in diabetes. *Diabetes Care*, 2004;27(Suppl 1):S84-87.
[182] Wilkinson, CP; Ferris, FL; Klein, RE; Lee, PP; Agardh, CD; Davis, M et al. Proposed international clinical diabetic retinopathy and diabetic macular edema disease severity scales. *Ophthalmology*, 2003;110:1677-1682.
[183] 183. Downie, LE; Vessey, K; Miller, A; Ward, MM; Pianta, MJ; Vingrys, AJ, et al. Neuronal and glial cell expression of angiotensin II type 1 (AT1) and type 2 (AT2) receptors in the rat retina. *Neuroscience*, 2009;161:195-213.
[184] Ishizaki, E; Takai, S; Ueki, M; Maeno, T; Maruichi, M; Sugiyama, T et al. Correlation between angiotensin-converting enzyme, vascular endothelial growth factor, and matrix metalloproteinase-9 in the vitreous of eyes with diabetic retinopathy. *Am J Ophthalmol,* 2006;141:129-134,
[185] Miller, AG; Tan, G; Binger, KJ; Pickering, RJ; Thomas, MC; Nagaraj, RH et al. Candesartan attenuates diabetic retinal vascular pathology by restoring glyoxalase-I function. *Diabetes*, 2010;59:3208-3215.
[186] Otani, A; Takagi, H; Oh, H; Koyama, S; Honda, Y. Angiotensin II induces expression of the Tie2 receptor ligand, angiopoietin-2, in bovine retinal endothelial cells. *Diabetes*, 2001;50:867-875.
[187] Otani, A; Takagi, H; Suzuma, K; Honda, Y. Angiotensin II potentiates vascular endothelial growth factor-induced angiogenic activity in retinal microcapillary endothelial cells. *Circ Res*, 1998;82:619-628.
[188] Yamagishi, S; Imaizumi, T. Pericyte biology and diseases. *Int J Tissue React*, 2005;27:125-135.
[189] Kawamura, H; Kobayashi, M; Li, Q; Yamanishi, S; Katsumura, K; Minami, M et al. Effects of angiotensin II on the pericyte-containing microvasculature of the rat retina. *J Physiol*, 2004;561:671-683.
[190] Zhang, T; Wu, DM; Xu, GZ; Puro, DG. The electrotonic architecture of the retinal microvasculature: modulation by angiotensin II. *J Physiol*, 2011;589:2383-2399.
[191] Nadal, JA; Scicli, GM; Carbini, LA; Nussbaum, JJ; Scicli, AG. Angiotensin II and retinal pericytes migration. *Biochem Biophys Res Commun*, 1999;266: 382-385.
[192] Nadal, JA; Scicli, GM; Carbini, LA; Scicli, AG. Angiotensin II stimulates migration of retinal microvascular pericytes: involvement of TGF-beta and PDGF-BB. *Am J Physiol Heart Circ Physiol*, 2002;282:H739-748.

[193] Yamagishi, S; Takeuchi, M; Matsui, T; Nakamura, K; Imaizumi, T; Inoue, H. Angiotensin II augments advanced glycation end product-induced pericyte apoptosis through RAGE overexpression. *FEBS Lett*, 2005;579:4265-4270.

[194] Danser, AH; van den Dorpel, MA; Deinum, J; Derkx, FH; Franken, AA; Peperkamp, E et al. Renin, prorenin, and immunoreactive renin in vitreous fluid from eyes with and without diabetic retinopathy. *J Clin Endocrinol Metab*, 1989;68:160-167.

[195] Okada, Y; Yamanaka, I; Sakamoto, T; Hata, Y; Sassa, Y; Yoshikawa, H et al. Increased expression of angiotensin-converting enzyme in retinas of diabetic rats. *Jpn J Ophthalmol*, 2001;45:585-591.

[196] Verma, A; Shan, Z; Lei, B; Yuan, L; Liu, X; Nakagawa, T et al. ACE2 and Ang-(1–7) confer protection against development of diabetic retinopathy. *Mol Ther*, 2012;20:28-36.

[197] Wakisaka, M; Yoshinari, M; Nakamura, S; Asano, T; Sonoki, K; Shi, A et al. Suppression of sodium-dependent glucose uptake by captopril improves high-glucose-induced morphological and functional changes of cultured bovine retinal pericytes. *Microvasc Res*, 1999;58:215-23.

[198] Zhang, JZ; Gao, L; Widness, M; Xi, X; Kern, TS. Captopril inhibits glucose accumulation in retinal cells in diabetes. *Invest Ophthalmol Vis Sci*, 2003;44:4001-4005.

[199] Gilbert, RE; Kelly, DJ; Cox, AJ; Wilkinson-Berka, JL; Rumble, JR; Osicka, T et al. Angiotensin converting enzyme inhibition reduces retinal overexpression of vascular endothelial growth factor and hyperpermeability in experimental diabetes. *Diabetologia*, 2000;43:1360-1367.

[200] Moravski, CJ; Skinner, SL; Stubbs, AJ; Sarlos, S; Kelly, DJ; Cooper, ME et al. The renin–angiotensin system influences ocular endothelial cell proliferation in diabetes: transgenic and interventional studies. *Am J Pathol*, 2003;162:151-160.

[201] Wilkinson-Berka, JL; Tan, G; Jaworski, K; Ninkovic, S. Valsartan but not atenolol improves vascular pathology in diabetic Ren-2 rat retina. *Am J Hypertens*, 2007;20:423-430.

[202] Zhang, JZ; Xi, X; Gao, L; Kern, TS. Captopril inhibits capillary degeneration in the early stages of diabetic retinopathy. *Curr Eye Res*, 2007;32:883-889.

[203] 203. Chen, P; Scicli, GM; Guo, M; Fenstermacher, JD; Dahl, D; Edwards, PA et al. Role of angiotensin II in retinal leukostasis in the diabetic rat. *Exp Eye Res*, 2006;83:1041-1051.

[204] 204. Mori, F; Hikichi, T; Nagaoka, T; Takahashi, J; Kitaya, N; Yoshida, A. Inhibitory effect of losartan, an AT1 angiotensin II receptor antagonist, on increased leucocyte entrapment in retinal microcirculation of diabetic rats. *Br J Ophthalmol*, 2002;86:1172-1124.

[205] 205. Silva, KC; Pinto, CC; Biswas, SK; Souza, DS; de Faria, JB; de Faria, JM. Prevention of hypertension abrogates early inflammatory events in the retina of diabetic hypertensive rats. *Exp Eye Res*, 2007;85:123-129.

[206] Zhang, JZ; Xi, X; Gao, L; Kern, TS. Captopril inhibits capillary degeneration in the early stages of diabetic retinopathy. *Curr Eye Res*, 2007;32:883-889.

[207] Wilkinson-Berka, JL; Tan, G; Binger, KJ; Sutton, L; McMaster, K; Deliyanti, D et al. Aliskiren reduces vascular pathology in diabetic retinopathy and oxygen-induced retinopathy in the transgenic (mRen-2)27 rat. *Diabetologia*, 2011;54:2724-2735.

[208] Rungger-Brandle, E; Dosso, AA; Leuenberger, PM. Glial reactivity, an early feature of diabetic retinopathy. *Invest Ophthalmol Vis Sci*, 2000;41:1971-1980.

[209] Krady, JK; Basu, A; Allen, CM; Xu, Y; LaNoue, KF; Gardner, TW et al. Minocycline reduces proinflammatory cytokine expression, microglial activation, and caspase-3 activation in a rodent model of diabetic retinopathy. *Diabetes*, 2005;54:1559-1565.

[210] Gastinger, MJ; Singh, RS; Barber, AJ. Loss of cholinergic and dopaminergic amacrine cells in streptozotocin-diabetic rat and Ins2Akita-diabetic mouse retinas. *Invest Ophthalmol Vis Sci,* 2006;47:3143-150.

[211] Barber, AJ; Lieth, E; Khin, SA; Antonetti, DA; Buchanan, AG; Gardner, TW. Neural apoptosis in the retina during experimental and human diabetes. Early onset and effect of insulin. *J Clin Invest*, 1998;102:783-791.

[212] Lieth, E; Barber, AJ; Xu, B; Dice, C; Ratz, MJ; Tanase, D et al. Glial reactivity and impaired glutamate metabolism in short-term experimental diabetic retinopathy. Penn State Retina Research Group. *Diabetes*, 1998;47:815-820.

[213] Park, SH; Park, JW; Park, SJ; Kim, KY; Chung, JW; Chun, MH et al. Apoptotic death of photoreceptors in the streptozotocin-induced diabetic rat retina. *Diabetologia*, 2003;46:1260-1268.

[214] Bresnick, GH; Korth, K; Groo, A; Palta, M. Electroretinographic oscillatory potentials predict progression of diabetic retinopathy. Preliminary report. *Arch Ophthalmol*, 1984;102:1307-1311.

[215] Bresnick, GH; Palta, M. Predicting progression to severe proliferative diabetic retinopathy. *Arch Ophthalmol*, 1987;105:810-814.

[216] Phipps, JA; Fletcher, EL; Vingrys, AJ. Paired-flash identification of rod and cone dysfunction in the diabetic rat. *Invest Ophthalmol Vis Sci*, 2004;45:4592-4600.

[217] Sokol, S; Moskowitz, A; Skarf, B; Evans, R; Molitch, M; Senior, B. Contrast sensitivity in diabetics with and without background retinopathy. *Arch Ophthalmol*, 1985;103:51-54.

[218] Fletcher, EL; Phipps, JA; Ward, MM; Vessey, KA; Wilkinson-Berka, JL. The renin–angiotensin system in retinal health and disease: its influence on neurons, glia and the vasculature. *Prog Retin Eye Res*, 2010;29:284-311.

[219] Bui, BV; Armitage, JA; Tolcos, M; Cooper, ME; Vingrys, AJ. ACE inhibition salvages the visual loss caused by diabetes. *Diabetologia*, 2003;46:401-408.

[220] . Kurihara, T; Ozawa, Y; Nagai, N; Shinoda, K; Noda, K; Imamura, Y et al. Angiotensin II type 1 receptor signaling contributes to synaptophysin degradation and neuronal dysfunction in the diabetic retina. *Diabetes*, 2008;57:2191-2198.

[221] Nakamura, H; Inoue, T; Arakawa, N; Shimizu, Y; Yoshigae, Y; Fujimori, I et al. Pharmacological and pharmacokinetic study of olmesartan medoxomil in animal diabetic retinopathy models. *Eur J Pharmacol*, 2005;512:239-246.

[222] Phipps, JA; Wilkinson-Berka, JL; Fletcher, EL. Retinal dysfunction in diabetic Ren-2 rats is ameliorated by treatment with valsartan but not atenolol. *Invest Ophthalmol Vis Sci*, 2007;48:927-934.

[223] Sugiyama, T; Okuno, T; Fukuhara, M; Oku, H; Ikeda, T; Obayashi, H et al. Angiotensin II receptor blocker inhibits abnormal accumulation of advanced glycation end products and retinal damage in a rat model of type 2 diabetes. *Exp Eye Res*, 2007;85:406-412.

[224] Garrido, AM; Griendling, KK. NADPH oxidases and angiotensin II receptor signaling. *Mol Cell Endocrinol*, 2009;302:148-158.

[225] . Schramm, A; Matusik, P; Osmenda, G; Guzik, TJ. Targeting NADPH oxidases in vascular pharmacology. *Vascul Pharmacol*, 2012.

[226] Giacco, F; Brownlee, M. Oxidative stress and diabetic complications. *Circ Res*, 2010;107:1058-1070.

[227] Mataftsi, A; Dimitrakos, SA; Adams, GG. Mediators involved in retinopathy of prematurity and emerging therapeutic targets. *Early Hum Dev*, 2011;87:683-690.

[228] Bedard, K; Krause, KH. The NOX family of ROS-generating NADPH oxidases: physiology and pathophysiology. *Physiol Rev*, 2007;87:245-313.

[229] Al-Shabrawey, M; Bartoli, M; El-Remessy, AB; Platt, DH; Matragoon, S; Behzadian, MA et al. Inhibition of NAD(P)H oxidase activity blocks vascular endothelial growth factor overexpression and neovascularization during ischemic retinopathy. *Am J Pathol*, 2005;167:599-607.

[230] Saito, Y; Geisen, P; Uppal, A; Hartnett, ME. Inhibition of NAD(P)H oxidase reduces apoptosis and avascular retina in an animal model of retinopathy of prematurity. *Mol Vis* ,2007;13:840-853.

[231] Al-Shabrawey, M; Rojas, M; Sanders, T; Behzadian, A; El-Remessy, A; Bartoli, Met al. Role of NADPH oxidase in retinal vascular inflammation. *Invest Ophthalmol Vis Sci*, 2008;49:3239-3244.

[232] Li, J; Wang, JJ; Yu, Q; Chen, K; Mahadev, K; Zhang, SX. Inhibition of reactive oxygen species by Lovastatin downregulates vascular endothelial growth factor expression and ameliorates blood-retinal barrier breakdown in db/db mice: role of NADPH oxidase 4. *Diabetes*, 2010;59:1528-1538.

[233] Chen, P; Guo, AM; Edwards, PA; Trick, G; Scicli, AG. Role of NADPH oxidase and ANG II in diabetes-induced retinal leukostasis. Am J Physiol Regul Integr *Comp Physiol*, 2007;293:R1619-1629.

[234] Fukumoto, M; Takai, S; Ishizaki, E; Sugiyama, T; Oku, H; Jin, D et al. Involvement of angiotensin II-dependent vascular endothelial growth factor gene expression via NADPH oxidase in the retina in a type 2 diabetic rat model. *Curr Eye Res*, 2008;33:885-891.

[235] The Diabetes Control and Complications Trial/Epidemiology of Diabetes Interventions and Complications Research Group. Retinopathy and nephropathy in patients with type 1 diabetes four years after a trial of intensive therapy. *N Engl J Med*, 2000;342:381-389.

[236] United Kingdom Prospective Diabetes Study Group. Tight blood pressure control and risk of macrovascular and microvascular complications in type 2 diabetes: UKPDS 38. *Br Med J*, 1998;317:703-713.

[237] Chaturvedi, N; Sjolie, AK; Stephenson, JM; Abrahamian, H; Keipes, M; Castellarin, A,et al. Effect of lisinopril on progression of retinopathy in normotensive people with type 1 diabetes. The EUCLID Study Group. EURODIAB Controlled Trial of Lisinopril in Insulin-Dependent Diabetes Mellitus. *Lancet*, 1998;351:28-31.

[238] Sjolie, AK; Klein, R; Porta, M; Orchard, T; Fuller, J; Parving, HH et al. Effect of candesartan on progression and regression of retinopathy in type 2 diabetes (DIRECT-Protect 2): a randomised placebo-controlled trial. *Lancet*, 2008;372:1385-1393.

[239] Sola, A; Saldeno, YP; Favareto, V. Clinical practices in neonatal oxygenation: where have we failed? What can we do? *J Perinatol*, 2008;28(Suppl 1):S28-34.

[240] Sjolie, AK; Klein, R; Porta, M; Orchard, T; Fuller, J; Parving, HH et al. Retinal microaneurysm count predicts progression and regression of diabetic retinopathy. Post hoc results from the DIRECT Programme. Diabet Med 2011;28:345-351.

[241] Mauer, M; Zinman, B; Gardiner, R; Suissa, S; Sinaiko, A; Strand, T et al. Renal and retinal effects of enalapril and losartan in type 1 diabetes. *N Engl J Med*, 2009;361:40-51.

[242] Harindhanavudhi, T; Mauer, M; Klein, R; Zinman, B; Sinaiko, A; Caramori, ML. Benefits of renin–angiotensin blockade on retinopathy in type 1 diabetes vary with glycemic control. *Diabetes Care*, 2011;34:1838-1842.

[243] Estacio, RO; Jeffers, BW; Gifford, N; Schrier, RW. Effect of blood pressure control on diabetic microvascular complications in patients with hypertension and type 2 diabetes. *Diabetes Care*, 2000;23(Suppl 2):B54-64.

[244] Patel, A; MacMahon, S; Chalmers, J; Neal, B; Woodward, M; Billot, L et al. Effects of a fixed combination of perindopril and indapamide on macrovascular and microvascular outcomes in patients with type 2 diabetes mellitus (the ADVANCE trial): a randomised controlled trial. *Lancet,* 2007;370:829-840.

In: Renin-Angiotensin System
Editors: Ayako Himura and Takeshi Sato

ISBN: 978-1-62417-788-0

Chapter III

Implication of the Renin-Angiotensin System in Obesity and Diabetes

Paul Tan[1,2]***, Mark F. Germano***[1,5]***, Jolanta Gutkowska***[1,3]
and Julie L. Lavoie[1,4,*]

[1]Research Center of the University of Montreal Hospital Center (CRCHUM) and
[2]Biochemistry, [3]Medicine and [4]Kinesiology Department of the University of Montreal, Montreal, Quebec, Canada
[5]Faculty of Medical Sciences, Universidade Nova de Lisboa, Lisbon, Portugal

Abstract

For a few decades now, the renin-angiotensin system (RAS) has been well known for its implication in the regulation of blood pressure and fluid homeostasis. Furthermore, dysregulation of the RAS has been implicated in many pathological states including obesity, hypertension, diabetes and chronic kidney disease. Due to the elevated consumption of foods that are rich in fat, salt and glucose, typical of a Western diet, obesity and diabetes are two of the greatest causes of morbidity and consumption of health care resources in North America. Interestingly, inhibition of the RAS has been shown to induce weight loss, and increased activation of the RAS in obesity suggests a potential link between the RAS and obesity-related hypertension. Indeed, increased adipose tissue cell size has been associated with a stimulation of the local RAS activity in this tissue which then spills over into the circulation. This in turn contributes to an increase in the circulating levels of angiotensin II and may thus produce a vasoconstrictive state. Moreover, constant fat accumulation eventually causes adipose tissue inflammation, oxidative and nitritive stress which can promote the development of insulin resistance and, with time, type 2 diabetes which are also consequences of local RAS overactivation in the pancreas. Clinically, RAS inhibitors are by far the preferred anti-hypertensive treatment in patients at risk of developing diabetes as they do not impact negatively glucose homeostasis regulation. This chapter will detail the implication of the RAS in the pathology of obesity and diabetes.

* Address of correspondence: Julie L. Lavoie, PhD, Centre de Recherche du CHUM (CRCHUM), Technopole Angus, 2901 Rachel E., bureau 310, Montréal, Québec, H1W 4A4, Tel: (514) 890-8000 ext. 23612; Fax: (514) 412-7655; Email: julie.lavoie.3@umontreal.ca.

Introduction

Insight into the renin-angiotensin system (RAS) can be traced back to 1898 when Tigerstedt and Bergman first described renin [1]. In the classical pathway, renin secreted from the juxtaglomerular cells of the kidney cleaves angiotensinogen (AGT) from the liver to produce the decapeptide angiotensin I (Ang-I). The angiotensin-converting enzyme (ACE) in the vascular endothelium of the lungs then cleaves this decapeptide to produce the octapeptide Ang-II (Figure 1). Conversely, the systemic RAS has now been expanded into novel pathways which include vascular and other tissues that have local RAS activity [2, 3] as well as enzymes, such as cathepsins and chymase, that have been found to be able to produce Ang-I and Ang-II respectively (Figure 1) [4, 5]. Moreover, discovery of other effector angiotensin peptides and characterization of their production has increased the complexity of our current understanding of the RAS. For example, ACE2 can lead to the production of Ang (1-7) either by direct cleavage of Ang-II or by producing Ang (1-9) from Ang-I followed by ACE cleavage (Figure 1) [6]. Aminopeptidases convert Ang-II to Ang-III which can then be converted into Ang-IV (Figure 1) [5]. Once produced, each of these angiotensin peptides' effects are mediated through its own specific cell surface receptor (Figure 1).

Effects most commonly associated with the RAS are produced by Ang-II through its stimulation of the Ang-II type 1 receptor (AT1R) which includes vasoconstriction, stimulation of aldosterone release and sympathetic nerve activity, promotion of cell growth and inflammation. Ang-III is also a ligand of this receptor although its affinity for the AT1R is much lower than that of the Ang-II [7, 8]. Conversely, opposite effects are produced by the Ang-II stimulation of the AT2R, which in addition also promotes apoptosis [7, 9], protects neural tissue [10] and possibly synergistically promotes AT1R inflammation [11]. Interestingly, although the AT2R is expressed at significant levels during fetal life, these levels quickly drop after birth, and it has been suggested that the predominant effect of Ang-II by the AT1R is due to a paucity of AT2R [12]. Opposite effects of the AT1R and AT2R have also been shown on blood pressure and glucose metabolism [13]. Indeed, hyperglycemia has been demonstrated to increase RAS components resulting in a rise in Ang-II synthesis [14]. This increase can cause insulin resistance in several tissues by decreasing glucose uptake and utilization probably via the stimulation of the AT1R since an AT1R inhibitor has been shown to redirect glucose uptake into utilization [14].

The more recent Ang-IV and Ang (1-7) peptides also have their own receptors, the AT4R and the Mas receptor (MasR) respectively. The implication of the AT4R in metabolic disorders has not been established although it should be noted that the AT4R is itself a transmembrane insulin-regulated aminopeptidase (IRAP) which may have a role in glucose homeostasis [15]. On the other hand, Ang (1-7) seems to mainly have opposite effects to those observed with the stimulation of the AT1R as it has an antidiuretic effect and inhibits cell growth [16, 17]. It has yet to be elucidated however if all of these effects are mediated only by the MasR since it has been shown that Ang (1-7) can also stimulate AT2R. Indeed, it has been reported that Ang (1-7) can exert a vasodepressor effect through the stimulation of AT2R in hypertensive rats [18]. Although Ang (1-7)'s affinity for AT2R is lower than Ang-II, it has considerable selectivity for AT2R compared to AT1R [19].

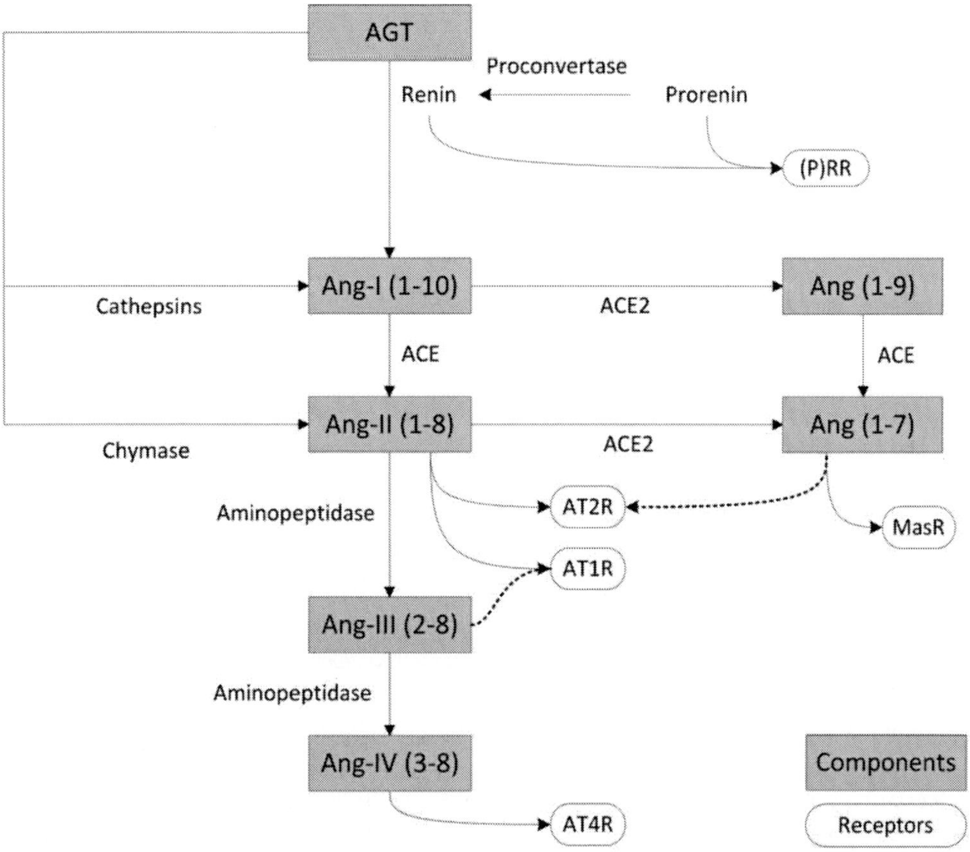

Figure 1. RAS cascade of reaction on effector receptors.
Angiotensinogen (AGT) is cleaved by renin to produce the decapeptide angiotensin I (Ang-I). Angiotensin converting enzyme (ACE) then catalyses the removal of two carboxyterminal amino acids from Ang-I to produce Ang-II. Ang-I and Ang-II can be produced independently of the classical RAS cascade via cathepsins and chymase. ACE2 cleaves the carboxyterminal amino acid of either Ang-I or Ang-II leading to the production of Ang (1-7). Aminopeptidases further break down Ang-II producing Ang-III and Ang-IV.
Grey boxes = Component peptides. White Boxes(rounded edges) = Receptors. Dotted line indicates minor binding relevance.

Important Facts on the Renin-Angiotensin System Components

Renin

Renin is produced by a proconvertase which cleaves 43 amino acids from the N-terminal prosegment of the inactive precursor prorenin [20]. Renin is highly species specific which means, for example, that mouse renin cannot cleave human AGT [21]. Since AGT conversion to Ang-I is considered to be the rate-limiting step of the RAS, renin KO mice have been generated to study the effects on blood pressure. As expected, these mice have decreased blood pressure and undetectable circulating levels of renin, Ang-I and Ang-II [22]. Blood pressure can be restored in these mice by infusing Ang-II. The same group later demonstrated that these KO mice also had lower body weight, fat mass, adipocyte size and were resistant to diet-induced obesity as a result of their higher metabolic rate and fat excretion. They also had lower plasma insulin levels. Most of these changes were reversed with Ang-II administration [23]. These studies thus showed the importance of Ang-II in controlling blood pressure, weight gain and insulin sensitivity.

(Pro)renin Receptor

Plasma prorenin concentrations are several folds higher than those of renin which suggests that this pro-enzyme may have a physiological role [24]. Prorenin's enzymatic cleft is hidden by its prosegment restricting access to AGT. This pro-enzyme is almost exclusively secreted by the kidney although other tissues have been shown to also contribute such as the adrenal glands, eyes, mast cells, reproductive system and placenta [25]. It has been demonstrated that prorenin and renin, collectively referred to as (pro)renin, bind to the mannose-6-phosphate receptor in cardiac cells followed by an intracellular internalization of the enzyme [26]. They can also bind to the renin binding protein (RnBP) in human adipose tissue [27] although the effects of this are unclear. It has been proposed that the RnBP could inhibit renin activity and vice versa [28]. Indeed, it has been proposed that RnBP exists as a homodimer which dissociates to form a heterodimer when binding with renin which would result in auto-inhibition of their activity.

Recently, a new receptor for (pro)renin has been discovered by Nguyen's group called the (pro)renin receptor [(P)RR] [29]. When renin binds to the (P)RR, the catalytic efficiency of the conversion of AGT into Ang-I is increased by 4-fold [29]. However, the (P)RR has a higher affinity for prorenin than renin [30]. By binding to the (P)RR, prorenin can be activated in a reversible non-proteolytic manner which involves a conformational change of the enzyme [31]. As such, (pro)renin binding to the (P)RR has been shown to lead to an increased Ang-I formation [32]. Moreover, (pro)renin binding to the (P)RR can lead to the phosphorylation of its tyrosine and serine residues which produces an activation of the extracellular regulated kinase 1/2 (ERK1/2) [29] as well as to the stimulation of other signaling pathways[32]. Thus, (pro)renin binding to the (P)RR can activate both Ang-II dependent and independent pathways.

In recent studies in humans, it has been found that polymorphisms of the (P)RR gene were correlated with blood pressure [33, 34]. When the human (P)RR gene is targeted to rat vascular smooth muscle cells, blood pressure and heart rate increased after 6 months of age [35]. When ubiquitously overexpressed, human (P)RR transgenic rats presented with proteinuria and glomerulosclerosis [36]. Furthermore, the receptor was also proposed to be implicated in fetal development since complete (P)RR deletion in a mouse model was proven to be lethal [37]. (P)RR gene mutation in humans has also been reported to produce X-linked mental retardation and epilepsy [38].

As such, the involvement of the (P)RR in different pathologies has been evaluated using a (P)RR inhibitor. This antagonist, also referred to as the handle region peptide (HRP), is a segment of the prorenin prosegment which binds to the (P)RR in a competitive manner [39].

Using the HRP in diabetic rats, it was shown that Ang-I and Ang-II content could be decreased in the kidney and that diabetic nephropathy was prevented without any effect on hyperglycemia.

Angiotensin-converting Enzymes

In normal conditions, Ang-II can regulate ACE activity as was shown in a study where Ang-II infusion decreased ACE expression and activity in the lung and testis of rats [40]. Conversely, in a pathological state such as hypertension, it is known that Ang-II executes the opposite effect by increasing ACE expression and decreasing ACE2 expression through AT1R stimulation of ERK1/2 and p38 mitogen-activated protein kinase (MAPK) signaling pathways [41]. In another study in obese Zucker rats, ACE expression was upregulated whereas ACE2 was downregulated, although they didn't show that these modulations were due to Ang-II even if the latter increased compared to lean rats [42]. This suggests that the ACE/ACE2 ratio might be important when considering any pathology since both enzymes produce different peptides which have opposing effects.

Angiotensin II Receptors

As mentioned above, Ang-II mediates its physiological effects through the AT1R and AT2R, two seven transmembrane domains receptors which are G-protein coupled receptors [43]. Binding of Ang-II to AT1R leads to intracellular signaling in which the G_q protein activates phospholipase C (PLC). The latter, using phospholipids from plasma membranes, generates second messengers, such as diacylglycerol. In turn, this activates protein kinase C and inositol triphosphate which stimulate the release of intracellular calcium. This pathway leads to the regulation of many cardiovascular and renal processes. Another pathway activated by the AT1R is the MAPK which regulates cellular proliferation [44]. This signaling pathway can either be activated directly by binding of Ang-II to its receptor or by downstream tyrosine transactivation of growth factor receptors such as epidermal growth factor receptor or platelet-derived growth factor receptor.

AT2R signaling is slightly different than that of the AT1R. Indeed, binding of Ang-II to the AT2R activates a phosphotyrosine phosphatase through Giα2 and Giα3 proteins which then deactivate MAPK by dephosphorylation [45]. Prolonged activation of AT2R has also been shown to induce apoptosis [46].

Renin-Angiotensin System and Obesity

The RAS is regulated by energy intake and it becomes overactivated systemically and locally in the case of obesity in humans [47]. Moreover, obesity has been associated with an increase in circulating levels of AGT, renin, aldosterone and ACE compared to lean subjects [48-55]. Increased sympathetic tone from the nervous system in obesity [56] may in part be responsible for elevated plasma renin levels as beta-adrenergic stimulation causes a rise in systemic renin levels and activity [57]. Human adipose tissue seems to mirror the circulating levels of the RAS as increased local levels of renin, ACE and AT1R expression can be observed in obesity [58] although AGT concentrations seem to vary [47]. This increased local production of Ang-II may spillover into the circulation and thus contribute to the increased circulating Ang-II associated with obesity.

Plasma aldosterone concentrations have also been found to be elevated in obesity and have been shown to correlate with the body mass index [59]. In obese hypertensive subjects, weight loss has been associated with a reduction in aldosterone levels [60]. Indeed, adipose tissue secretes factors that have aldosterone stimulating effects, such as Ang-II [61], complement-C1q tumor necrosis factor (TNF)-related protein 1 [62] and oxidized derivatives of linoleic acid [63, 64]. In hypertensive rats, treatment with both aldosterone synthase and aldosterone inhibitors produced a decrease in aldosterone levels and body weight [65]. Eplerenone or spironolactone, both aldosterone antagonists, can also attenuate glomerular hyperfiltration, sodium retention and hypertension associated with diet-induced obesity in dogs [66], humans [67, 68] and mice [69].

AT1R blockers (ARB) have also been shown to reduce weight gain, fat mass and adipocyte cell size in rodents [70-74] and humans [75-78]. ACE-deficient mice have been shown to have decreased body weight and abdominal fat mass [79] whereas ACE inhibitors in rats produced a decrease in adipocyte cell size and fat mass [70, 80, 81]. RAS inhibitors effects on body weight may be as a result of a decrease in food intake [82-84] potentially by having central effects as certain ARBs have been demonstrated to be able to penetrate the blood-brain barrier in rats [85]. Moreover, it has been suggested that an intact leptin signaling is required to decrease body weight and food intake since no changes could be observed in *fa/fa* Zucker rats treated with an ARB [83]. It has also been shown that ARB treatments lead to increased adiponectin concentrations [86, 87], which has been reported to increase glucose utilization and fatty acid oxidation in muscle [88].

Therefore, obesity is related to an activation of both systemic and local RAS from different tissues. The experimental evidence highlights the complexity of the interactions between the RAS and obesity and illustrates the care that must be taken in choosing animal models when studying the RAS.

Local RAS

All components of the RAS have been shown to be expressed and functional in several organs such as the heart, brain, kidney, pancreas and adipose tissue [2]. As such, local RAS may contribute to the many functions that were attributed originally to its systemic components.

Adipose Tissue

Studies in high-caloric diet overfed men showed that in response to weight gain there was an enhanced expression of many RAS components, such as AGT and ACE, and possibly increased Ang-II production in subcutaneous abdominal adipose tissue [89]. Similar data has been obtained in other human studies [57, 58, 90] as well as in animal models [91-93]. In addition, in 3T3-L1 (mouse adipocyte cell line) and human adipocytes, Ang-II has been shown to increase lipogenesis by increasing triglyceride content and lipogenic enzymes such as fatty acid synthase and glycerol-3-phosphate dehydrogenase through its stimulation of the AT2R [94]. In line with these results, systemic AT2R KO mice on a high-fat diet had reduced adipocyte size which produced a decrease in fat mass and fat cell mass [95, 96]. As such, the local RAS in adipose tissue has been proposed to be implicated in the pathogenesis of obesity as well as its related diseases [97].

Renin

Discrepancy exists concerning the detection of renin in adipose tissue. Indeed, although some studies were able to detect its presence in human subcutaneous adipose tissue [4], human preadipocytes [98] and adipocytes [4, 99], others have failed to detect any trace [27, 100, 101].What is known thus far is that renin mRNA is detected reproducibly in human preadipocytes and adipocytes but remains mostly undetectable in whole adipose tissue with the exception of one study [4]. Indeed, Karlsson *et al* (1998), measured renin mRNA in human subcutaneous abdominal adipose tissue, adipocytes and stroma [4]. They found renin mRNA to be more abundant in adipocytes than in whole adipose tissue without any presence in stroma. However, in contrast to the other studies which found renin to be undetectable, this study investigated subcutaneous adipose tissue whereas other studies had looked at visceral adipose tissue. This suggests that there may be variability in the expression of renin depending on the adipose tissue depot studied. In line with this hypothesis, one study didn't detect renin mRNA in human mammary adipocytes, which is contrast to all the other studies which had investigated adipocytes isolated from subcutaneous adipose tissue [27]. Hence, even though renin has been studied for more than five decades, not much light has been shed on the ability to reproducibly detect renin production in adipose tissue. Some have suggested that renin can be taken up from the circulation into local tissues [100, 101]. If this is the case in adipose tissue, renin levels may be too low to be detectable but could still produce significant amounts of Ang-I due to its interaction with the (P)RR which has been found to increase renin's catalytic activity to convert AGT to Ang-I by 4 fold, as mentioned above [29]. Adipose tissue is a heterogeneous tissue which is composed of different cell types such as connective tissues, nerves, stromovacular cells and immune cells [102]. Depending on whether obesity is present or not, if renin is produced in adipocytes or other cells present in adipose tissue, then it may be diluted by other types of cells present in whole adipose tissue. Studies using sensitive technology focusing on specific cell types such as real-time PCR should be considered when trying to confirm renin's presence in adipose tissue.

Angiotensinogen

Although adipose tissue AGT mRNA and circulating AGT levels generally increase with obesity in mice and humans, hepatic AGT mRNA levels in diet-induced obesity [103] and in genetically obese Zucker rats [104] have been reported to be unchanged, suggesting a tissue specific regulation of AGT. Thus, increased circulating AGT levels may be as a result of increased production in other tissues, such as adipose tissue which may contribute up to 30% of the plasma AGT concentrations measured in obesity [105].

However, a controversy exists regarding the modulation of AGT expression in adipose tissue by obesity. Indeed, its expression has been shown to be either upregulated [91, 106] [91, 103] or downregulated [50, 107, 108] in humans and rodents. Differences in species, genetic models and posttranscriptional modifications could possibly explain the discrepancy in RAS component expression. In studies where AGT expression was measured in adipose tissue, circulating levels were always significantly higher in obese subjects. Although diet-induced obesity in rodents mirrors what is seen in humans [91, 106] since both systemic and adipose RAS have been observed to be increased, genetic obesity models can either have increased levels of adipose tissue AGT, for example, as is the case with *ob/ob* mice, *db/db* mice and *fa/fa* Zucker rat or decreased levels, such as in the viable yellow mice [47]. Both *ob/ob* and *db/db* mice are obesity models where mice are either leptin-deficient or leptin receptor-deficient, respectively. Similarly to the *db/db* mice, the *fa/fa* Zucker rat is leptin receptor-deficient and the viable yellow mouse has a mutation in the agouti gene which increases the storage and decreases the utilization of fat. The *ob/ob* and *db/db* mice and the *fa/fa* Zucker rats are more susceptible to gain weight since they lack the leptin-mediated effect on appetite compared to viable yellow mouse which has a functional leptin system. As a result, the discrepancy observed in adipose AGT between these different rodent models might highlight the importance of leptin resistance and leptin effects such as reduced food intake and increased energy expenditure on RAS regulation.

In contrast, a study also using *db/db* mice found a decrease in AGT mRNA in adipose tissue [107]. Interestingly, these authors observed that AGT mRNA in adipose tissue could be increased by treating the mice with an anti-oxidant suggesting that oxidative stress can also regulate AGT expression. Because *db/db* mice have a deficiency in the leptin receptor, increases in leptin production may be present to compensate. Moreover, leptin has been shown to increase oxidative stress by upregulating nicotinamide adenine dinucleotide phosphate (NADPH) oxidase which is an enzyme that generates superoxide and by facilitating endothelin-1 generation [109]. Thus, the potential increase in leptin levels in *db/db* mice might promote oxidative stress in this genetic model of obesity and may thus be an added factor which contributes to the discrepancy observed in AGT expression.

Of note, regional differences seem to exist regarding AGT expression in adipose tissue. In studies using human adipose tissue, AGT mRNA upregulation was found in visceral adipose tissue [110] whereas downregulation was observed in subcutaneous adipose tissue [50]. Similarly, in a rodent study, no change in mouse and transgenic human AGT expression was detected in subcutaneous adipose tissue with obesity whereas visceral adipose tissue displayed an increase in AGT expression [103]. Differences in gene expression in these two adipose tissue site have already been reported in obese humans where expression of inflammatory and oxidative stress pathway genes were higher in visceral adipose tissue while expression of insulin homeostasis and growth factor genes were higher in subcutaneous adipose tissue [111]. Also, in rodents, expression of lipogenesis and lipolysis genes has been reported to be higher in subcutaneous fat whereas fatty acid oxidation genes were more expressed in visceral fat [112].

Interestingly, acute refeeding and chronic energy influx have both been shown to increase AGT expression in adipose tissue while fasting decreases mRNA levels suggesting that AGT is in part regulated by food intake [93]. Thus, tissues collected in fasting animals might possibly mask the effects of chronic energy excess on AGT expression.

In any case, the true physiological significance of AGT production by adipose or other tissues is debatable as it is believed that renal renin release is the rate-limiting step of RAS activation. However, it should be noted that other enzymes are able to cleave AGT and produce Ang-II independently of the classic RAS pathway, namely cathepsins and chymase, and that these enzymes have been found to be increased with obesity [93, 101], although physiological significance of these enzymes is unclear [4, 5]. Nonetheless, in a highly elaborate study, Massiera *et al.* (2001) generated 3 different mouse models where AGT was either overexpressed specifically in adipose tissue, KO systemically or expressed only in adipose tissue [105]. In mice overexpressing AGT in adipose tissue, a significant increase in plasma AGT, body weight, fat mass, fat cell size, fatty acid synthase activity in epididymal adipose tissue was detected. Moreover, hyperinsulinemia and hypertension were also present whereas fat cell number and locomotor activity was decreased. In AGT KO mice, all of the above mentioned parameters were reversed, that is mice had undetectable levels of plasma AGT as well as decreased body weight, fat mass, fat cell size, fatty acid synthase activity and systolic blood pressure. When AGT was expressed only in adipose tissue, the phenotype observed in mice which overexpressed AGT in adipose tissue was reproduced demonstrating that local AGT was critical in this phenotype. Thereafter, several groups generated similar mouse models by overexpressing AGT in adipose tissue, systemic AGT KO or expressing AGT only in adipose tissue and reproduced the same results [96, 113-115]. Taken together, these studies demonstrate that spillover of adipose tissue AGT into the circulation can contribute to increase blood pressure. Moreover, they establish that AGT overexpression in adipose tissue can lead to adipocyte hypertrophy and hypoplasia and as such, may contribute significantly to the development of obesity.

Angiotensin II Receptor

In rodents, AT1R exists in two isoforms AT1aR and AT1bR which mainly differ by their tissue localization and regulation [7]. In mammalians, no isoforms had been found until recently when the existence of four functionally distinct human AT1R splice variants with different affinity for Ang-II was reported [116]. Each variant has a different expression level in different tissues suggesting that they may have different functions. Ang-II effects through AT1R variants depend on Ang-II concentration and on AT1R density on each cell type. Using AT1aR KO mice on a high-fat diet, Kouyama *et al.* (2005) observed that these mice gained less body weight when placed on a high-fat diet compared to wild-type (WT) mice and this was associated with a significant decrease in adipocyte cell size[117]. Conversely, no changes in body weight or adipocyte size could be observed between the WT and AT1aR KO mice when they were fed a normal diet. Hence, these data suggested that although AT1aR may not have any effects on adipocyte cell size at baseline, these receptors may be implicated in fat accumulation in pathological conditions such as obesity. In contrast, Putnam *et al.* (2012) recently reported an increase in adipocyte cell size and a decrease in cell number in AT1aR KO mice compared to WT mice on a normal diet. These authors proposed that this may be as a consequence of an increased lipid accumulation in adipocytes despite the similar fat mass observed in the two groups. [118]. However, this controversy might be due to the age difference of the mice at the end of the study and to difference in the normal diet composition. Indeed, in Kouyama's study, the diet used contained 5,4% fat and mice were 18 weeks of age at sacrifice whereas in Putnam's study, fat content in the chow was 10% and mice were 24-26 weeks of age. As such, double the amount of fat in the diet coupled with the advancing age of the animals might explain why Putnam's AT1R KO mice had increased adipocyte size due to lipid accumulation compared to WT mice on normal diet, similarly to what was observed by Kouyama's group in their obese animals. This is even more likely since Putnam *et al.*'s AT1R KO mice on high-fat diet seemed to have reached their maximum adipocyte size and/or limit capacity to stock lipids compared to WT mice as suggested by that group.

(Pro)renin Receptor

In adipose tissue from obese women, (P)RR expression has been detected, although no differences were observed when comparing to lean women and after weight loss [50]. In another human study, the authors showed that the (P)RR was produced in the stromal portion of human adipose tissue in preadipocyte and non-preadipocyte cells [119]. Furthermore, it is expressed in the periphery of cells suggesting that (P)RR is a membrane receptor as has been shown by others in other tissues [119]. Again, no differences in (P)RR were detected between lean and obese women. However, both studies had relatively small number of subjects and both were done exclusively in women. Hence, since the (P)RR has been shown to be present on the X chromosome [29] and that gender differences have been observed in regards to the expression of other RAS components [120, 121], we cannot rule out that a gender effect could be implicated in the lack of differences in (P)RR observed between lean and obese subjects. A part from this, not much is known about the (P)RR's implication in obesity. What is known is that adipose tissue is a major source of circulating AGT and Ang-II [122]. It has also been demonstrated that ERK1/2 signaling enhances adipogenesis [123]. Since renin binding to (P)RR improves Ang-I production by several folds and that (P)RR has more affinity for prorenin, both Ang-II dependent and independent pathway might play a role in obesity although additional studies are needed to evaluate the implication of the (P)RR in adipose tissue.

Put together these studies strongly support a role for the local adipose tissue RAS in the pathogenesis of obesity. Indeed, mice systemically deficient in AGT, renin, ACE, AT1R or AT2R have been shown to be protected from high-fat diet-induced obesity and present with adipose tissue hypotrophy [79, 95, 113, 117, 124]. On the other hand, mice deficient in MasR have increased abdominal fat mass and higher adipose AGT expression probably due to increased proliferation since transforming growth factor-β (TGF-β) expression was found to be upregulated [125]. Interestingly, in all of these studies, there was no association between the RAS knockout (KO) and food consumption, suggesting that the effects of adipose tissue RAS on body weight and composition are not through the modulation of energy intake in this case. On the other hand, renin-deficient mice have increased gastrointestinal loss of dietary fat which could contribute to the weight gain resistance associated with the deficiency in the RAS [124], although AGT and ACE KO mice have been reported to have no changes in lipid absorption [79, 113]. This may be as a result of renin's Ang-II independent pathway through binding to the (P)RR which could have an effect on intestinal fat absorption [126]. Renin deficiency might have dampened this effect of the (P)RR leading to dietary fat loss whereas AGT and ACE deficiency still has functional renin. Taken together, these studies provide evidence that Ang-II has a role in the progression of obesity and could be counter-regulated via the ACE2/Ang (1-7)/MasR axis.

Pancreas

A local pancreatic RAS has been reported to be present in rats and humans [127, 128]. In rodents, renin has been detected in islet beta cells which secrete insulin [129], AGT was found in alpha cells which secrete glucagon [130] and ACE is expressed in islet periphery [131]. As such, all components required to produce Ang-II locally seem to be in place. Moreover, both AT1R and AT2R are localized in beta cells [132, 133] but AT2R has also been found in delta cells which secrete somatostatin [134]. In addition, AT1R was not only found in the plasma membrane of beta cells but also in the cytoplasm which suggests that it may be internalized after it binds to Ang-II or retained in the cytosol after synthesis [135].

Interestingly, AGT and AT1R expression have been found to be increased in the pancreas of type 2 diabetic animal models [131, 136]. In addition, in humans, Ang-II infusion has been reported to reduce glucose-induced insulin secretion and to increase plasma glucose after an oral glucose tolerance test suggesting that the pancreatic RAS may alter glucose homeostasis deleteriously [137]. In line with these results, in isolated mice islets of Langerhans, Ang-II caused a dose-dependent decrease in insulin secretion and in (pro)insulin synthesis which was reversed by the administration of an AT1R inhibitor [138]. This suggests that the Ang-II-induced decrease in insulin secretion might be partially due to an altered (pro)insulin synthesis in the pancreas. In the same study, they also showed that an AT2R blocker had no effect on insulin secretion supporting the premise that the effects of Ang-II are exclusively through the AT1R. Conversely, in another study, short term exposure of beta cells to Ang-II caused a rapid and short stimulation of insulin secretion [133]. The authors proposed that insulin secretion might be regulated by increased intracellular calcium levels since it is known that Ang-II via AT1R signaling can increase the latter through PLC stimulation [43] and/or L-type voltage dependent calcium channels [139]. Blocking L-type calcium channels or PLC in human islet moderately decreased Ang-II-induced calcium elevation suggesting that this Ang-II effect is through the stimulation of calcium channel and the release of calcium from intracellular stores. These studies thus highlight a discrepancy regarding the Ang-II effects on insulin secretion which suggests that it may have both short and long-term effects. As such, short-term effects would increase insulin secretion by increasing intracellular calcium content whereas long-term effects would decrease insulin secretion probably by reducing (pro)insulin synthesis.

Insulin secretion has been reported to be improved in mice by AT1R inhibitors [136, 140]. As such, given that hypertensive patients treated with beta-blockers or thiazides have been reported to have higher risk of developing diabetes [141], RAS inhibitors are typically the preferred treatment for hypertensive diabetic patients. This is supported by the data generated by many clinical trials which have demonstrated that ACE inhibitors [142, 143] and AT1R blockers [144, 145] lower the risk of developing diabetes.

Moreover, AT1R seems to be implicated in beta cell mass. Indeed, AT1R blockers have been reported to increase beta cell mass probably through Ang-II mechanisms that control proliferation, apoptosis, inflammation and oxidative stress [146]. For instance, it was reported that ACE inhibitors and AT1R blockers could reduce apoptosis and oxidative stress in islets of diabetic Zucker rats [131]. In line with these results, in isolated rat pancreatic stellate cells, which are implicated in pancreatitis, high glucose increased Ang-II levels, TGF-β and cell proliferation [147]. All of these effects were lessened by treating the cells with ACE inhibitors and AT1R antagonists. Moreover, when rats are fed with a high-fat diet for a prolonged period of time, nuclear factor kappa-light-chain-enhancer of activated B cells (NF-κβ), interleukin-1β (IL-1β), uncoupling protein-2 (UCP-2), caspase-3 content, AT1R expression and the number of apoptotic cells are increased in the pancreas but can be reduced by the administration of an ACE inhibitor or an AT1R blocker [148]. In *db/db* mice, it was reported that AT1R blocker downregulated NADPH oxidase resulting in a suppression of oxidative stress and UCP2 expression in islets of the pancreas [149].This suggests that the RAS contributes to increase inflammation, oxidative stress and apoptosis in the pancreas in pathological states.

Brain

In contrast, central Ang-II infusion has already been shown to reduce weight gain, food intake and to raise energy expenditure [150]. Indeed, mice overexpressing human renin and human AGT in the brain had increased thermogenesis in brown and white adipose tissue as well as elevated energy expenditure through a beta-adrenergic dependant stimulation of cAMP signaling [151]. Moreover, others have demonstrated that centrally administered Ang-II results in an increased expression of beta-3-adrenergic receptor in white adipose tissue (WAT) and brown adipose tissue (BAT) as well as an elevation in UCP1 in BAT [150]. In addition, high RAS activity in the brain has been shown to decrease food intake [152]. Conversely, ARBs have been proposed to centrally decrease food intake [85]. Since ARBs block AT1R and Ang-II has been shown to decrease food intake in the brain, we could speculate that this effect might be through the AT2R. Indeed, Ohinata *et al.* have reported that central infusion of Ang-II reduced food intake and this was inhibited by the administration of an AT2R blocker and was absent in a whole body AT2R KO mice compared to wild type and AT1R KO mice [153].

Conversely, energy expenditure is consistently increased in all RAS component KO mice as well as in studies investigating ARB treated mice [79, 95, 113, 117, 124, 154]. These studies have suggested the implication of increased hepatic fatty acid oxidation, BAT UCP1, locomotor activity and β-oxidation in muscle as potential mechanisms that may contribute to the observed effects.

Taken together, these data suggest that local RAS in the brain may act to counterbalance other peripheral local RAS systems when systemic RAS activity is elevated. This may be through a negative feedback loop where high levels of Ang-II from adipose tissue or pancreas may reach the brain to trigger negative energy balance [152].

Renin-angiotensin System and Inflammation

In a chronic overfed state, there is an increase in adipose tissue expansion associated with adipocyte hypertrophy. This could contribute to produce endoplasmic reticulum stress that would bring about a proinflammatory state in adipose tissue which eventually leads to pathologies such as chronic inflammation, insulin resistance or hepatic injury [155, 156].

Adipose tissue is known to secrete different molecules known as adipokines. Proinflammatory markers, a family of adipokines, are secreted by adipose tissue macrophages (ATM). For example, monocyte chemoattractant protein-1 (MCP-1) are produced and secreted by adipose tissue, the major source of this marker, to increase the recruitment of macrophages [157]. In turn, these newly recruited macrophages further contribute to increase the secretion of proinflammatory markers. As such, a vicious circle is established between MCP-1 secretion and macrophage recruitment which further promotes inflammation resulting in damaged and inflamed adipose tissue [158]. Since Ang-II has been reported to induce the release of proinflammatory markers by adipose tissue, the RAS may be implicated in this inflammatory process [97].

Angiotensin II Induces Inflammation

Ang-II has been shown to induce the expression of several proinflammatory markers and chemokines such as MCP-1, IL-6 and IL-8 in rat preadipocytes and adipose tissue [159], murine 3T3-L1 preadipocytes cell line [160] and human adipocytes [161]. In line with this data, treatment with ARBs has been shown to decrease macrophages and inflammatory markers in rat epididymal adipose tissue and adipocytes [71, 73, 74]. It has been suggested that Ang-II might be involved in the stimulation of MCP-1 expression through the activation of NF-κB. Indeed, in a study using rats, Ang-II increased MCP-1 expression in a time and dose dependent manner in adipose tissue which was decreased by the administration of either an AT1R blocker or a NF-κB blocker [159]. This suggests that Ang-II regulation of MCP-1 is via the AT1R through the stimulation of the NF-κB signaling pathway. Similarly, it was shown that an ARB and NF-κB blocker prevented Ang-II stimulation of IL-6 and IL-8 gene and protein expression in cultured human adipocytes whereas AT2R blocker partially attenuated this stimulation [161]. Moreover, NF-κB activation by Ang-II via AT2R has been shown in PC12 cells, a rat adrenal pheochromocytoma cell line that only expresses AT2R, COS7, a kidney cell line that doesn't normally express ATR, and rat glomerular endothelial cells that express both AT1R and AT2R [11]. These authors then overexpressed either the AT1R or AT2R in COS7 cells. Ang-II activated NF-κB in COS7 cells expressing AT1R or AT2R, in PC12 cells via AT2R and via AT1R and AT2R in rat glomerular endothelial cells. The administration of an AT2R blocker reduced NF-κB activation in COS7 transfected with AT2R and PC12 cells while AT1R blocker had no effect on COS7 cells transfected with AT1R. Finally, both AT1R and AT2R blockers decreased NF-κB activation in rat glomerular endothelial cells. This thus suggests that Ang-II stimulation of NF-κB is through mainly AT2R although an interaction between both AT1R and AT2R may also be implicated.

An interaction between AT1R and AT2R in terms of their counter-regulatory effects has been shown in spontaneously hypertensive rats and fructose-induced insulin resistance of hypertensive rats [13, 162], as an AT1R blocker reduced blood pressure in both studies and AT2R antagonist had no effect in Otsuka's study [162] or increased blood pressure in the Hsieh's study [13]. However, in Otsuka's study, blood pressure was measured by the tail-cuff method while Hsieh measured it using a pressure transducer. As such, methodological differences may have contributed to the results reported in these studies. In rat brain neurons, Ang-II was shown to cause a decrease in potassium current via AT1R which was later increased through AT2R and vice versa [163] This suggests that interaction between AT1R and AT2R is crucial. Changes in the expression and protein of either ATRs might explain why the previous study found that NF-κB activation by Ang-II is via AT2R while they also observed NF-κB activation through both type of receptors in rat glomerular endothelial cells where they were normally expressed [11].

It has also been shown in adipocytes that Ang-II raises the phosphorylation of p65, a subunit of NF-κB, which promotes the translocation of NF-κB into the nucleus where it will act as a transcription factor to increase proinflammatory gene transcription [161].

It should be mentioned that ACE2 overexpression in macrophages also inhibits MCP-1 expression by Ang-II suggesting that Ang (1-7)/MasR axis antagonizes these Ang-II effects by increasing Ang (1-7) levels and reducing local Ang-II concentrations [164].

In contrast, there is a study showing that Ang-II alone couldn't increase the expression of MCP-1 in 3T3-L1 preadipocyte cell line. They rather observed that the stimulation of the TNF-α increased MCP-1 mRNA expression and protein and that Ang-II could enhance the expression of MCP-1 [160]. Both Ang-II and TNF-α stimulation increased phosphorylation of ERK and p38 MAPK. This increase was abolished by ERK, p38 MAPK or NF-κB inhibitors. Also, IκBα phosphorylation was increased by TNF-α alone but not by Ang-II. These data suggest that Ang-II could act as a facilitator of the TNF-α-induced MCP-1 expression via ERK and p38 MAPK.

Chemotaxis is the property of a cell to migrate towards a chemoattractant molecule. As such, monocytes are attracted to the site of inflammation by chemoattractants such as MCP-1. It has been shown that Ang-II could enhance chemotaxis in human T and NK cells where all components of the RAS are present and functional [165]. Also, Ang-II has been found to increase monocyte adhesion in aortic endothelial cells in essential hypertensive patients compared to normotensive patients. Treatment with an AT1R inhibitor decreased circulating monocytes adhesion although the expression of adhesion molecules such as CD11b, CD54 and CCR5 was increased [166]. The mechanisms involved in these effects are still however unclear.

Taken together, these studies suggest that Ang-II can enhance the expression and synthesis of inflammatory markers by an NF-κB pathway in synergy with other chemokines. This may thus contribute to increase inflammation in any tissue. Indeed, by enhancing MCP-1 expression, Ang-II can promote macrophage infiltration by increasing their chemotaxis and adhesion near the target tissue.

Renin-angiotensin System and Oxidative Stress

Oxidative stress happens when the balance between reactive oxygen species (ROS) production and antioxidant defences is compromised. ROS are produced from oxygen into superoxide, hydrogen peroxide (H_2O_2), peroxynitrate and hypochlorous acid (HOCl), and are well-known for their potentially deleterious effects. Superoxide production, for instance by NADPH oxidase, can damage lipids, proteins or DNA. Superoxide can then be processed by superoxide dismutase (SOD) into H_2O_2 which is the key molecule which can generate other ROSs such as HOCl or the hydroxyl radical. Hydrogen peroxide can however be processed by antioxidant enzymes, such as catalase or glutathione peroxidase, to produce water [167]. It has been reported that oxidative stress associated with obesity is as a result of decreased antioxidant capacity with and increasing amount of body fat [168]. In parallel, increasing ROS and decreasing anti-oxidant can promote oxidative stress which in turn could contribute to the development and progression of diabetes by increasing ROS and decreasing anti-oxidant [169]. With obesity, increased oxidative stress could, for example, damage key enzymes implicated in the lipogenesis or lipolysis pathways which would result in less fat uptake or less lipid oxidation respectively. Reduced lipogenesis could in turn increase circulating free fatty acids which would contribute to ectopic fat deposition in tissues triggering inflammation and insulin resistance whereas decreased lipolysis would increase fat storage further promoting obesity.

It has been shown in adipose tissue that both ROS production and NADPH oxidase expression are increased and that antioxidant enzyme expressions, such as SOD, glutathione peroxidase and catalase, are decreased in obese mice [170]. Moreover, in obese patients, it has been shown that adipose tissue mass correlates positively with plasma ROS concentration and that weight loss can reduce this, suggesting that increased oxidative stress in obesity is as a result of an increased fat mass [171].

In addition, ROS can also increase the production of plasminogen activator inhibitor-1 (PAI-1), IL-6 and MCP-1 [170] and as such, could contribute to the inflammatory state present in obesity.

Angiotensin II Induces Oxidative Stress

It has been proposed that Ang-II might be implicated in the obesity-related increase in oxidative stress since it has been shown that ARBs can decrease ROS and NADPH oxidase expression in adipose tissue of obese mice without any effect on body weight [172]. In addition, Ang-II has been shown to activate NADPH oxidase in different cell types by stimulating its subunits such as Nox1, p47phox, p67phox and p22phox [167], thus suggesting a direct effect on oxidative stress production. Also, given that the Ang (1-7)/MasR axis antagonizes the effects of the AT1R [173], it has been shown that Ang (1-7) could suppress ROS production and NADPH oxidase subunits expression such as p22phox, gp91phox, Nox4, p47phox, p67phox through the stimulation of the MasR in 3T3-L1 adipocyte. Furthermore, MasR blocker reversed these effects on oxidative stress [174] further supporting the contribution of Ang-II in the increased oxidative stress associated with obesity.

Moreover, Ang-II infusion, which produces hypertension in rats, increased vascular superoxide formation [175]. Many studies have also demonstrated that different RAS inhibitors can decrease fat mass [73, 74, 80], as mentioned previously, which could thus reduce ROS and NADPH oxidase expression levels.

In mice, direct inhibition of NADPH oxidase or NF-κB could reverse the increased MCP-1 expression in adipose tissue produced by Ang-II [176]. In a similar study in rat glomerular endothelial cells, Pan *et al.* (2009) also found that Ang-II increased the protein levels of NADPH oxidase subunit p47phox, MCP-1 synthesis and ROS generation which were abolished by the administration of an AT1R and NADPH oxidase inhibitors [177]. As such, these two studies suggest that Ang-II induces MCP-1 through a NADPH oxidase-dependent NF-κB pathway.

In addition, Ang-II can not only regulate NADPH oxidase but it can also increase lipoxygenase activity, another enzyme capable of producing superoxide anions in mice macrophages [178]. Indeed, Ang-II administration has been shown to increase lipoxygenase activity and expression in human aortic smooth muscle cells, aortic endothelial cells and monocytes [179].As such, increased Ang-II associated with obesity may also stimulate this pathway to increase the production of ROS.

Finally, in rats, Ang-II has been shown to upregulate endothelial nitric oxide synthase (eNOS) expression which could increase NO production [180]. This may thus be one of the mechanisms by which Ang-II regulates the bioavailability of NO. Since Ang-II also leads to the formation of ROS, it can interact with NO to form peroxynitrate which causes nitration of tyrosine residues [167] Thus, increased oxidative stress in obesity can impair pathways such as insulin signaling implicated in glucose uptake by impairing proper protein folding or damaging them which would alter their functions.

Renin Angiotensin System and Hypertension

Obesity is often associated with an increase in blood pressure in rodents [91, 181, 182] and in humans [183, 184]. In addition, the western style diet which is characterized by a high-fat and high-salt content, certainly contributes to obesity-related hypertension in North America. Moreover, weight loss has been shown to have beneficial effects on blood pressure [185, 186]. Of particular interest, obesity is often associated with an increase in circulating Ang-II [91] and dysregulation of the RAS is a well-known culprit for the development of hypertension. Indeed, Ang-II can not only induce vasoconstriction, through the stimulation of the AT1R, but it can also act on the adrenal cortex to promote the release of aldosterone which in turn will increase renal sodium and water reabsorption as well as potassium excretion which can lead to an increase in blood pressure [187].

In support of this hypothesis, weight loss of as little as 5% produced a reduction of 7 mmHg in systolic blood pressure in menopausal women [50] and was associated with a reduction in circulating levels of AGT, ACE, renin and aldosterone which were found to be increased in these obese women. Several other studies have demonstrated this relation between weight loss and blood pressure [188, 189]

Many have proposed the role of local RAS in adipose tissue in obesity-related hypertension [190]. Indeed, adipose tissue AGT overexpression in mice resulted in an increase in fat mass and blood pressure while adipose tissue AGT deficiency had the opposite effect, lowering blood pressure and fat mass [105].

Aldosterone

Ang-II's stimulation of aldosterone release is probably through the regulation of aldosterone synthase enzyme which converts 11-deoxycorticosterone to aldosterone [191]. Ang-II infusion in obese rats caused elevated blood pressure but also stimulated growth in the zona glomerula, increased adrenal AT1R density and aldosterone synthase which might explain their higher circulating aldosterone levels when compared to lean rats [192].

Leptin

Leptin is an adipokine secreted into the circulation exclusively by adipose tissue and proportionally to the amount of fat mass. Circulating leptin can then act on the brain to reduce appetite and stimulate energy expenditure by increasing sympathetic stimulation to peripheral tissues [193]. It has been suggested that leptin expression and secretion in obesity are upregulated directly by hyperinsulinemia and glucocorticoids synergistically in human adipose tissue [194]. As such, circulating leptin has been shown to be increased with obesity to try and counter the associated overfeeding condition and increase energy expenditure to decrease fat accumulation [103].

Interestingly, Ang-II has been shown to stimulate the production of leptin via the AT1R by an ERK1/2 signaling pathway which is dose and time dependent [195]. Recently, it was reported that the metabolic effects of leptin on food intake and body weight were reduced in obese mice compared to normal mice suggesting that obesity is related to a state of leptin resistance although leptin stimulation of renal sympathetic activity and increased blood pressure are preserved [196].

Indeed, it has been shown in *ob/ob* mice that blood pressure decreased despite severe obesity [197]. This suggests that leptin may modulate blood pressure probably through sympathetic excitation of the kidney.

Renin-angiotensin System and Insulin Resistance

Insulin resistance occurs when cells are unable to respond to circulating levels of insulin either due to a mutation in the insulin receptor or any downstream molecules present in the insulin signaling pathway such as the insulin receptor substrate (IRS), PI3K and Akt [43]. As a consequence, cellular nutrient uptake is altered thus resulting in high plasma glucose and triglyceride content which leads to glucose intolerance and dyslipidemia. In this condition, insulin levels also rise as a compensatory mechanism.

In obesity, high circulating free fatty acids (FFA) levels [198] can cause insulin resistance [199], while decreasing circulating FFA can ameliorate the latter [200]. In addition, obesity is associated with a decrease in the activation of Akt and in the translocation of glucose transporter 4 (GLUT4) to the plasma membrane which both contribute to the development of insulin resistance [201].

Angiotensin II Induces Insulin Resistance

Implication of the RAS in the development of insulin resistance has been demonstrated using RAS KO models [79, 114, 115, 117, 124], RAS inhibitors [70, 71, 73, 87] and RAS overexpression models [115, 176]. Globally, these studies have shows that RAS deficiency in mice improves glucose tolerance and insulin sensitivity by increasing plasma adiponectin and decreasing plasma glucose and insulin.

Ang-II has been shown to impair insulin signaling by decreasing Akt activation and GLUT 4 translocation in rat skeletal muscle as well as by increasing NF-κB and oxidative stress. As such, treatments with AT1R, NADPH oxidase or NF-κB inhibitors, improve insulin signaling and reduce NF-κB and oxidative stress [202]. Similar data were also obtained in rats overexpressing renin in the pancreas where Ang-II decreased total IRS1, IRS2, Akt and increased NADPH oxidase activity [203] and treatment with a renin inhibitor reversed all these effects. Finally, it was reported in adipose tissue that AT1R blocker could increase activation of insulin signaling and decrease MCP-1 and TNF-α [71]. A recent study in rat skeletal muscle cells also suggests that nitrative stress is also implicated in insulin resistance as they showed that incubation with Ang-II could induce tyrosine nitration of ERK1/2, which inhibits IRS-1/2, and Akt [204]. A study in diabetic rats showed that losartan, an AT1R inhibitor, lowered the production of ROS and NO by decreasing eNOS in the kidney [205]. This suggests that Ang-II can modulate both ROS and NO synthesis which can in turn impair the insulin signaling pathway leading to insulin resistance.

Adiponectin

Adiponectin is an adipokine specifically secreted from adipose tissue which is known to have insulin-sensitizing and anti-inflammatory effects [206]. Indeed, adiponectin KO mice present with insulin resistance [207]. Moreover, when adiponectin is administrated to mice, their glucose levels decrease and their insulin sensitivity is improved [208]. In humans, it has been shown that obesity leads to decreased adiponectin circulating levels and adipose tissue expression [209, 210]. Exercise and diet intervention have been shown to increase adiponectin concentrations and insulin sensitivity in obese teenagers [211]. Adiponectin binds to the adiponectin receptor 1 (AdipoR1) and AdipoR2 in order to mediate its physiological effects. These receptors are present in the liver, muscle, heart, adipose tissue, osteoblast, pancreas, leukocytes and brain. They have been shown in the brain, for example, to modulate food intake and energy expenditure [212]. AdipoR1 deficiency in mice produces glucose intolerance whereas AdipoR2 KO mice are lean, resistant to obesity and have improved glucose tolerance [213]. This suggests that AdipoR1 is more implicated in the beneficial effects of adiponectin such as improving glucose tolerance whereas AdipoR2 has opposing effects. With high-fat feeding, both hepatic AdipoR1 and AdipoR2 and muscle AdipoR1 were shown to be upregulated. This suggests that advancing age and obesity can increase both AdipoRs [214]. In streptozotocin diabetic mice, AdipoR1 expression was higher in muscle but was brought back to normal levels with insulin treatment, suggesting a negative feed-back effect on the receptor with the normalization of glycemia or increased insulinemia [215]. In insulin-resistant *db/db* mice, AdipoR1 expression was reduced in skeletal muscle cells probably due to the hyperinsulinemia present in this mice model whereas hepatic AdipoR2 expression was unchanged [215]. The authors proposed that the AdipoR1 rather than the AdipoR2 seemed to be more implicated in glucose and fat metabolism suggesting that in an insulin resistant state, high insulin levels might ultimately decrease the availability of AdipoR1 which has beneficial effects on insulin sensitivity. Interestingly, Ang-II infusion leads to a decrease in adiponectin circulating levels in high-fructose fed rats, an effect which is thought to be through the AT1R since an AT1R antagonist brought adiponectin back to normal level [216]. Moreover, RAS inhibitors, such as renin inhibitors, ARBs and ACE inhibitors, have been shown to increase plasma adiponectin levels in diabetic and diet-induced obesity rodents as well as in humans with impaired glucose tolerance or essential hypertension [73, 74, 87, 217-219]. It seems that the AT2R could counterbalance the AT1R effects on adiponectin as its inhibition attenuated adiponectin protein expression in 3T3-L1 cells [86]. The effect of the RAS on adiponectin might be through the activation of the peroxisome proliferator-activated receptor gamma (PPARγ) since its blocker could inhibit irbesartan-induced adiponectin protein expression [86]. The same group has previously found that irbesartan could increase adipocyte differentiation by PPARγ [220]. However, this increase was also preserved in AT1R KO cells suggesting that irbesartan's effect on adipocyte differentiation was mainly through the stimulation of PPARγ not by antagonizing the AT1R. As such, these studies demonstrate a link between the RAS and adiponectin production which may contribute to the RAS effects on insulin sensitivity.

ACE2/Angiotensin (1-7)/Mas Receptor

In rat muscles, it has been shown that Ang (1-7) improves by 30% the insulin resistance produced by Ang-II with an associated increase in Akt Ser (473) phosphorylation [221]. They further demonstrated in this study that this effect was through the stimulation of the MasR since an inhibitor of this receptor abolished the insulin-mediated glucose transport activity and Akt phosphorylation [221]. The beneficial effects of the Ang (1-7)/MasR axis on insulin resistance seems to extend beyond muscle as similar results have been found in liver and adipose tissue of fructose-fed rats [222]. In addition, MasR deficiency in mice causes an increase in fasting circulating concentrations of glucose and insulin. This is also associated with a decrease in insulin sensitivity as well as a reduced adipocyte glucose uptake due to a reduction in adipose tissue GLUT4 protein with no change in serum adiponectin [125]. This suggests that the MasR is implicated in glucose homeostasis and fat metabolism.

In streptozotocin-induced diabetic rats, ACE2 activity was reduced in renal glomeruli and normalized after insulin treatment whereas ACE activity was unchanged which resulted in an increase in Ang-II levels in kidney glomeruli [223]. In obese mice, ACE2 expression, protein and activity were upregulated in epididymal and subcutaneous adipose tissues after 1 week of high-fat feeding [224]. At 4 months of high-fat feeding, ACE2 mRNA remained elevated in adipose tissues whereas the protein and activity were no longer increased. At this age, these mice also had increased blood pressure and plasma glucose. Interestingly, they found that in 3T3-L1 adipocyte cell line that an increase in ADAM17 expression, a metallopeptidase that cleaves TNF-α from cell membranes, was associated with a decrease in ACE2 activity at membrane and that an ADAM17 inhibitor decreased ACE2 activity in the media. Moreover, a similar upregulation in ADAM17 mRNA was found in adipose tissue from the high-fat fed mice with a parallel increase in plasma ACE2 activity. Therefore, this may be as a result of ACE2 shedding from cell membrane produced by ADAM17 [225]. As such, by cleaving ACE2 from the membrane, ADAM17 may decrease the availability of membrane-bound ACE2 and thus increase plasma ACE2 activity. Based on this study, it seems that the ADAM17 effects on ACE2 protein occurs only after prolonged high-fat feeding. As a consequence, there may be an increase in local Ang-II production with an associated decrease in Ang (1-7) which would promote insulin resistance.

Conclusion

The implication of the RAS in pathology is very broad and complex. After many decades, we are just starting to understand how the RAS is involved in the development of obesity and diabetes as well as its many associated diseases. Indeed, obesity and diabetes can promote hypertension, cancer, macrovascular diseases and insulin resistance just to name a few. Because all these processes are somehow connected by the RAS, drugs targeting this system may be beneficial for the treatment of obese and diabetic patients. Animal models have been of great use to improve our understanding of the RAS since it is not always possible to collect the needed materials in patients. But animal models have their limitations and results obtained from these studies will need to be carefully validated in humans since different animal models have led to conflicting results. Therapeutic future challenges will be to design drugs with high specificity and affinity for blocking the local tissue RAS at doses sufficient to have significant impact on the targeted tissues.

References

[1] Basso N, Terragno NA: History about the discovery of the renin-angiotensin system. *Hypertension* 2001, 38:1246-1249.

[2] Paul M, Poyan MA, Kreutz R: Physiology of local renin-angiotensin systems. *Physiol Rev.* 2006, 86:747-803.

[3] Admiraal PJ, Derkx FH, Danser AH, Pieterman H, Schalekamp MA: Metabolism and production of angiotensin I in different vascular beds in subjects with hypertension. *Hypertension* 1990, 15:44-55.

[4] Karlsson C, Lindell K, Ottosson M, Sjostrom L, Carlsson B, Carlsson LM: Human adipose tissue expresses angiotensinogen and enzymes required for its conversion to angiotensin II. *J.Clin.Endocrinol.Metab* 1998, 83:3925-3929.

[5] Schmieder RE, Hilgers KF, Schlaich MP, Schmidt BM: Renin-angiotensin system and cardiovascular risk. *Lancet* 2007, 369:1208-1219.

[6] Donoghue M, Hsieh F, Baronas E, Godbout K, Gosselin M, Stagliano N, Donovan M, Woolf B, Robison K, Jeyaseelan R, Breitbart RE, Acton S: A novel angiotensin-converting enzyme-related carboxypeptidase (ACE2) converts angiotensin I to angiotensin 1-9. *Circ.Res.* 2000, 87:E1-E9.

[7] De Gasparo M, Catt KJ, Inagami T, Wright JW, Unger T: International union of pharmacology. XXIII. The angiotensin II receptors. *Pharmacol Rev* 2000, 52:415-472.

[8] Rowe BP, Dixon B: Angiotensin III depressor action in the conscious rabbit is blocked by losartan but not PD 123319. *Hypertension* 2000, 35:130-134.

[9] Carey RM: Cardiovascular and renal regulation by the angiotensin type 2 receptor: the AT2 receptor comes of age. *Hypertension* 2005, 45:840-844.

[10] Imai Y, Kuba K, Rao S, Huan Y, Guo F, Guan B, Yang P, Sarao R, Wada T, Leong-Poi H, Crackower MA, Fukamizu A, Hui CC, Hein L, Uhlig S, Slutsky AS, Jiang C, Penninger JM: Angiotensin-converting enzyme 2 protects from severe acute lung failure. *Nature* 2005, 436:112-116.

[11] Wolf G, Wenzel U, Burns KD, Harris RC, Stahl RA, Thaiss F: Angiotensin II activates nuclear transcription factor-kappaB through AT1 and AT2 receptors. *Kidney Int.* 2002, 61:1986-1995.

[12] Kalupahana NS, Moustaid-Moussa N: The adipose tissue renin-angiotensin system and metabolic disorders: a review of molecular mechanisms. *Crit Rev.Biochem.Mol.Biol.* 2012, 47:379-390.

[13] Hsieh PS, Tai YH, Loh CH, Shih KC, Cheng WT, Chu CH: Functional interaction of AT1 and AT2 receptors in fructose-induced insulin resistance and hypertension in rats. *Metabolism* 2005, 54:157-164.

[14] Putnam K, Shoemaker R, Yiannikouris F, Cassis LA: The renin-angiotensin system: a target of and contributor to dyslipidemias, altered glucose homeostasis, and hypertension of the metabolic syndrome. *Am.J.Physiol Heart Circ.Physiol* 2012, 302:H1219-H1230.

[15] Demaegdt H, Gard P, De Backer JP, Lukaszuk A, Szemenyei E, Toth G, Tourwe D, Vauquelin G: Binding of "AT4 receptor" ligands to insulin regulated aminopeptidase (IRAP) in intact Chinese hamster ovary cells. *Mol.Cell Endocrinol.* 2011, 339:34-44.

[16] Kostenis E, Milligan G, Christopoulos A, Sanchez-Ferrer CF, Heringer-Walther S, Sexton PM, Gembardt F, Kellett E, Martini L, Vanderheyden P, Schultheiss HP, Walther T: G-protein-coupled receptor Mas is a physiological antagonist of the angiotensin II type 1 receptor. *Circulation* 2005, 111:1806-1813.

[17] Tallant EA, Ferrario CM, Gallagher PE: Angiotensin-(1-7) inhibits growth of cardiac myocytes through activation of the mas receptor. *Am.J.Physiol Heart Circ.Physiol* 2005, 289:H1560-H1566.

[18] Walters PE, Gaspari TA, Widdop RE: Angiotensin-(1-7) acts as a vasodepressor agent via angiotensin II type 2 receptors in conscious rats. *Hypertension* 2005, 45:960-966.

[19] Bosnyak S, Jones ES, Christopoulos A, Aguilar MI, Thomas WG, Widdop RE: Relative affinity of angiotensin peptides and novel ligands at AT1 and AT2 receptors. *Clin.Sci.(Lond)* 2011, 121:297-303.

[20] Batenburg WW, Danser AH: (Pro)renin and its receptors: pathophysiological implications. *Clin.Sci.(Lond)* 2012, 123:121-133.

[21] Takahashi S, Fukamizu A, Hatae T, Yamada Y, Sugiyama F, Kajiwara N, Yagami K, Murakami K: Species-specific kinetics of mouse renin contribute to maintenance of normal blood pressure in transgenic mice with overexpressed human angiotensinogen. *J.Vet.Med.Sci.* 1992, 54:1191-1193.

[22] Takahashi N, Lopez ML, Cowhig JE, Jr., Taylor MA, Hatada T, Riggs E, Lee G, Gomez RA, Kim HS, Smithies O: Ren1c homozygous null mice are hypotensive and polyuric, but heterozygotes are indistinguishable from wild-type. *J.Am.Soc.Nephrol.* 2005, 16:125-132.

[23] Takahashi N, Li F, Hua K, Deng J, Wang CH, Bowers RR, Bartness TJ, Kim HS, Harp JB: Increased energy expenditure, dietary fat wasting, and resistance to diet-induced obesity in mice lacking renin. *Cell Metab* 2007, 6:506-512.

[24] Danser AH, Derkx FH, Schalekamp MA, Hense HW, Riegger GA, Schunkert H: Determinants of interindividual variation of renin and prorenin concentrations: evidence for a sexual dimorphism of (pro)renin levels in humans. *J.Hypertens.* 1998, 16:853-862.

[25] Krop M, Danser AH: Circulating versus tissue renin-angiotensin system: on the origin of (pro)renin. *Curr.Hypertens.Rep.* 2008, 10:112-118.

[26] van Kesteren CA, Danser AH, Derkx FH, Dekkers DH, Lamers JM, Saxena PR, Schalekamp MA: Mannose 6-phosphate receptor-mediated internalization and activation of prorenin by cardiac cells. *Hypertension* 1997, 30:1389-1396.

[27] Engeli S, Gorzelniak K, Kreutz R, Runkel N, Distler A, Sharma AM: Co-expression of renin-angiotensin system genes in human adipose tissue. *J.Hypertens.* 1999, 17:555-560.

[28] Takahashi S, Kumagai M, Shindo S, Saito K, Kawamura Y: Renin inhibits N-acetyl-D-glucosamine 2-epimerase (renin-binding protein). *J.Biochem.* 2000, 128:951-956.

[29] Nguyen G, Delarue F, Burckle C, Bouzhir L, Giller T, Sraer JD: Pivotal role of the renin/prorenin receptor in angiotensin II production and cellular responses to renin. *J.Clin.Invest.* 2002, 109:1417-1427.

[30] Lu X, Danser AH, Meima ME: HRP and prorenin: focus on the (pro)renin receptor and vacuolar H+-ATPase. *Front Biosci.(Schol.Ed)* 2011, 3:1205-1215.

[31] Jan Danser AH, Batenburg WW, van Esch JH: Prorenin and the (pro)renin receptor--an update. *Nephrol.Dial.Transplant.* 2007, 22:1288-1292.

[32] Ahmed B, Lavoie J: Renin receptor as a new drug target. *Current Drug Target* 2010.

[33] Hirose T, Hashimoto M, Totsune K, Metoki H, Asayama K, Kikuya M, Sugimoto K, Katsuya T, Ohkubo T, Hashimoto J, Rakugi H, Takahashi K, Imai Y: Association of (pro)renin receptor gene polymorphism with blood pressure in Japanese men: the Ohasama study. *Am.J.Hypertens.* 2009, 22:294-299.

[34] Ott C, Schneider MP, Delles C, Schlaich MP, Hilgers KF, Schmieder RE: Association of (pro)renin receptor gene polymorphism withblood pressure in Caucasian men. *Pharmacogenet.Genomics* 2011.

[35] Burckle CA, Jan Danser AH, Muller DN, Garrelds IM, Gasc JM, Popova E, Plehm R, Peters J, Bader M, Nguyen G: Elevated blood pressure and heart rate in human renin receptor transgenic rats. *Hypertension* 2006, 47:552-556.

[36] Kaneshiro Y, Ichihara A, Takemitsu T, Sakoda M, Suzuki F, Nakagawa T, Hayashi M, Inagami T: Increased expression of cyclooxygenase-2 in the renal cortex of human prorenin receptor gene-transgenic rats. *Kidney Int.* 2006, 70:641-646.

[37] Burckle C, Bader M: Prorenin and its ancient receptor. *Hypertension* 2006, 48:549-551.

[38] Ramser J, Abidi FE, Burckle CA, Lenski C, Toriello H, Wen G, Lubs HA, Engert S, Stevenson RE, Meindl A, Schwartz CE, Nguyen G: A unique exonic splice enhancer mutation in a family with X-linked mental retardation and epilepsy points to a novel role of the renin receptor. *Hum.Mol.Genet.* 2005, 14:1019-1027.

[39] Ichihara A, Hayashi M, Kaneshiro Y, Suzuki F, Nakagawa T, Tada Y, Koura Y, Nishiyama A, Okada H, Uddin MN, Nabi AH, Ishida Y, Inagami T, Saruta T: Inhibition of diabetic nephropathy by a decoy peptide corresponding to the "handle" region for nonproteolytic activation of prorenin. *J.Clin.Invest* 2004, 114:1128-1135.

[40] Schunkert H, Ingelfinger JR, Hirsch AT, Pinto Y, Remme WJ, Jacob H, Dzau VJ: Feedback regulation of angiotensin converting enzyme activity and mRNA levels by angiotensin II. *Circ.Res.* 1993, 72:312-318.

[41] Koka V, Huang XR, Chung AC, Wang W, Truong LD, Lan HY: Angiotensin II up-regulates angiotensin I-converting enzyme (ACE), but down-regulates ACE2 via the AT1-ERK/p38 MAP kinase pathway. *Am.J.Pathol.* 2008, 172:1174-1183.

[42] Samuel P, Ali Q, Sabuhi R, Wu Y, Hussain T: High Na intake increases renal angiotensin II levels and reduces expression of the ACE2-AT(2)R-MasR axis in obese Zucker rats. *Am.J.Physiol Renal Physiol* 2012, 303:F412-F419.

[43] Olivares-Reyes JA, Arellano-Plancarte A, Castillo-Hernandez JR: Angiotensin II and the development of insulin resistance: implications for diabetes. *Mol.Cell Endocrinol.* 2009, 302:128-139.

[44] Hunyady L, Catt KJ: Pleiotropic AT1 receptor signaling pathways mediating physiological and pathogenic actions of angiotensin II. *Mol.Endocrinol.* 2006, 20:953-970.

[45] Padia SH, Carey RM: AT(2) receptors: beneficial counter-regulatory role in cardiovascular and renal function. *Pflugers Arch.* 2012.

[46] Jones ES, Vinh A, McCarthy CA, Gaspari TA, Widdop RE: AT2 receptors: functional relevance in cardiovascular disease. *Pharmacol.Ther.* 2008, 120:292-316.

[47] Kalupahana NS, Moustaid-Moussa N: The renin-angiotensin system: a link between obesity, inflammation and insulin resistance. *Obes.Rev.* 2012, 13:136-149.

[48] Cooper R, McFarlane-Anderson N, Bennett FI, Wilks R, Puras A, Tewksbury D, Ward R, Forrester T: ACE, angiotensinogen and obesity: a potential pathway leading to hypertension. *J.Hum.Hypertens.* 1997, 11:107-111.

[49] Licata G, Scaglione R, Ganguzza A, Corrao S, Donatelli M, Parrinello G, Dichiara MA, Merlino G, Cecala MG: Central obesity and hypertension. Relationship between fasting serum insulin, plasma renin activity, and diastolic blood pressure in young obese subjects. *Am.J.Hypertens.* 1994, 7:314-320.

[50] Engeli S, Bohnke J, Gorzelniak K, Janke J, Schling P, Bader M, Luft FC, Sharma AM: Weight loss and the renin-angiotensin-aldosterone system. *Hypertension* 2005, 45:356-362.

[51] Uckaya G, Ozata M, Sonmez A, Kinalp C, Eyileten T, Bingol N, Koc B, Kocabalkan F, Ozdemir IC: Plasma leptin levels strongly correlate with plasma renin activity in patients with essential hypertension. *Horm.Metab Res.* 1999, 31:435-438.

[52] Bloem LJ, Manatunga AK, Tewksbury DA, Pratt JH: The serum angiotensinogen concentration and variants of the angiotensinogen gene in white and black children. *J.Clin.Invest.* 1995, 95:948-953.

[53] Umemura S, Nyui N, Tamura K, Hibi K, Yamaguchi S, Nakamaru M, Ishigami T, Yabana M, Kihara M, Inoue S, Ishii M: Plasma angiotensinogen concentrations in obese patients. *Am.J.Hypertens.* 1997, 10:629-633.

[54] Cooper R, Forrester T, Ogunbiyi O, Muffinda J: Angiotensinogen levels and obesity in four black populations. ICSHIB Investigators. *J Hypertens.* 1998, 16:571-575.

[55] Schorr U, Blaschke K, Turan S, Distler A, Sharma AM: Relationship between angiotensinogen, leptin and blood pressure levels in young normotensive men. *J.Hypertens.* 1998, 16:1475-1480.

[56] Troisi RJ, Weiss ST, Parker DR, Sparrow D, Young JB, Landsberg L: Relation of obesity and diet to sympathetic nervous system activity. *Hypertension* 1991, 17:669-677.

[57] Goossens GH, Jocken JW, Blaak EE, Schiffers PM, Saris WH, van Baak MA: Endocrine role of the renin-angiotensin system in human adipose tissue and muscle: effect of beta-adrenergic stimulation. *Hypertension* 2007, 49:542-547.

[58] Gorzelniak K, Engeli S, Janke J, Luft FC, Sharma AM: Hormonal regulation of the human adipose-tissue renin-angiotensin system: relationship to obesity and hypertension. *J.Hypertens.* 2002, 20:965-973.

[59] Goodfriend TL, Egan B, Stepniakowski K, Ball DL: Relationships among plasma aldosterone, high-density lipoprotein cholesterol, and insulin in humans. *Hypertension* 1995, 25:30-36.

[60] Dall'Asta C, Vedani P, Manunta P, Pizzocri P, Marchi M, Paganelli M, Folli F, Pontiroli AE: Effect of weight loss through laparoscopic gastric banding on blood pressure, plasma renin activity and aldosterone levels in morbid obesity. *Nutr.Metab Cardiovasc.Dis.* 2009, 19:110-114.

[61] Spat A, Hunyady L: Control of aldosterone secretion: a model for convergence in cellular signaling pathways. *Physiol Rev.* 2004, 84:489-539.

[62] Jeon JH, Kim KY, Kim JH, Baek A, Cho H, Lee YH, Kim JW, Kim D, Han SH, Lim JS, Kim KI, Yoon dY, Kim SH, Oh GT, Kim E, Yang Y: A novel adipokine CTRP1 stimulates aldosterone production. *FASEB J.* 2008, 22:1502-1511.

[63] Ehrhart-Bornstein M, Lamounier-Zepter V, Schraven A, Langenbach J, Willenberg HS, Barthel A, Hauner H, McCann SM, Scherbaum WA, Bornstein SR: Human adipocytes secrete mineralocorticoid-releasing factors. *Proc.Natl.Acad.Sci.U.S.A* 2003, 100:14211-14216.

[64] Goodfriend TL, Ball DL, Egan BM, Campbell WB, Nithipatikom K: Epoxy-keto derivative of linoleic acid stimulates aldosterone secretion. *Hypertension* 2004, 43:358-363.

[65] Menard J, Gonzalez MF, Guyene TT, Bissery A: Investigation of aldosterone-synthase inhibition in rats. *J.Hypertens.* 2006, 24:1147-1155.

[66] de Paula RB, da Silva AA, Hall JE: Aldosterone antagonism attenuates obesity-induced hypertension and glomerular hyperfiltration. *Hypertension* 2004, 43:41-47.

[67] White WB, Carr AA, Krause S, Jordan R, Roniker B, Oigman W: Assessment of the novel selective aldosterone blocker eplerenone using ambulatory and clinical blood pressure in patients with systemic hypertension. *Am.J.Cardiol.* 2003, 92:38-42.

[68] Brown NJ, Nakamura S, Ma L, Nakamura I, Donnert E, Freeman M, Vaughan DE, Fogo AB: Aldosterone modulates plasminogen activator inhibitor-1 and glomerulosclerosis in vivo. *Kidney Int.* 2000, 58:1219-1227.

[69] Keidar S, Hayek T, Kaplan M, Pavlotzky E, Hamoud S, Coleman R, Aviram M: Effect of eplerenone, a selective aldosterone blocker, on blood pressure, serum and macrophage oxidative stress, and atherosclerosis in apolipoprotein E-deficient mice. *J.Cardiovasc.Pharmacol.* 2003, 41:955-963.

[70] Furuhashi M, Ura N, Takizawa H, Yoshida D, Moniwa N, Murakami H, Higashiura K, Shimamoto K: Blockade of the renin-angiotensin system decreases adipocyte size with improvement in insulin sensitivity. *J.Hypertens.* 2004, 22:1977-1982.

[71] Munoz MC, Giani JF, Dominici FP, Turyn D, Toblli JE: Long-term treatment with an angiotensin II receptor blocker decreases adipocyte size and improves insulin signaling in obese Zucker rats. *J.Hypertens.* 2009, 27:2409-2420.

[72] Mori Y, Itoh Y, Tajima N: Angiotensin II receptor blockers downsize adipocytes in spontaneously type 2 diabetic rats with visceral fat obesity. *Am.J.Hypertens.* 2007, 20:431-436.

[73] Lee MH, Song HK, Ko GJ, Kang YS, Han SY, Han KH, Kim HK, Han JY, Cha DR: Angiotensin receptor blockers improve insulin resistance in type 2 diabetic rats by modulating adipose tissue. *Kidney Int.* 2008, 74:890-900.

[74] Zorad S, Dou JT, Benicky J, Hutanu D, Tybitanclova K, Zhou J, Saavedra JM: Long-term angiotensin II AT1 receptor inhibition produces adipose tissue hypotrophy accompanied by increased expression of adiponectin and PPARgamma. *Eur.J.Pharmacol.* 2006, 552:112-122.

[75] Goossens GH, Moors CC, van der Zijl NJ, Venteclef N, Alili R, Jocken JW, Essers Y, Cleutjens JP, Clement K, Diamant M, Blaak EE: Valsartan improves adipose tissue function in humans with impaired glucose metabolism: a randomized placebo-controlled double-blind trial. *PLoS.One.* 2012, 7:e39930.

[76] Makita S, Abiko A, Naganuma Y, Moriai Y, Nakamura M: Effects of telmisartan on adiponectin levels and body weight in hypertensive patients with glucose intolerance. *Metabolism* 2008, 57:1473-1478.

[77] Chujo D, Yagi K, Asano A, Muramoto H, Sakai S, Ohnishi A, Shintaku-Kubota M, Mabuchi H, Yamagishi M, Kobayashi J: Telmisartan treatment decreases visceral fat accumulation and improves serum levels of adiponectin and vascular inflammation markers in Japanese hypertensive patients. *Hypertens.Res.* 2007, 30:1205-1210.

[78] Shimabukuro M, Tanaka H, Shimabukuro T: Effects of telmisartan on fat distribution in individuals with the metabolic syndrome. *J.Hypertens.* 2007, 25:841-848.

[79] Jayasooriya AP, Mathai ML, Walker LL, Begg DP, Denton DA, Cameron-Smith D, Egan GF, McKinley MJ, Rodger PD, Sinclair AJ, Wark JD, Weisinger HS, Jois M, Weisinger RS: Mice lacking angiotensin-converting enzyme have increased energy expenditure, with reduced fat mass and improved glucose clearance. *Proc.Natl.Acad.Sci.U.S.A* 2008, 105:6531-6536.

[80] Mathai ML, Naik S, Sinclair AJ, Weisinger HS, Weisinger RS: Selective reduction in body fat mass and plasma leptin induced by angiotensin-converting enzyme inhibition in rats. *Int.J.Obes.(Lond)* 2008, 32:1576-1584.

[81] Weisinger RS, Stanley TK, Begg DP, Weisinger HS, Spark KJ, Jois M: Angiotensin converting enzyme inhibition lowers body weight and improves glucose tolerance in C57BL/6J mice maintained on a high fat diet. *Physiol Behav.* 2009, 98:192-197.

[82] Voigt JP, Bramlage P, Fink H: Hypophagic effect of the angiotensin AT1 receptor antagonist irbesartan in rats. *Eur.J.Pharmacol.* 2007, 564:131-137.

[83] Muller-Fielitz H, Markert A, Wittmershaus C, Pahlke F, Johren O, Raasch W: Weight loss and hypophagia after high-dose AT1-blockade is only observed after high dosing and depends on regular leptin signalling but not blood pressure. *Naunyn Schmiedebergs Arch.Pharmacol.* 2011, 383:373-384.

[84] Telmisartan suppresses food intake in mice via the melanocortin pathway. *Obesity Research & Clinical Practice* 2011, 5:e93-e100.

[85] Gohlke P, Weiss S, Jansen A, Wienen W, Stangier J, Rascher W, Culman J, Unger T: AT1 receptor antagonist telmisartan administered peripherally inhibits central responses to angiotensin II in conscious rats. *J.Pharmacol.Exp.Ther.* 2001, 298:62-70.

[86] Clasen R, Schupp M, Foryst-Ludwig A, Sprang C, Clemenz M, Krikov M, Thone-Reineke C, Unger T, Kintscher U: PPARgamma-activating angiotensin type-1 receptor blockers induce adiponectin. *Hypertension* 2005, 46:137-143.

[87] Furuhashi M, Ura N, Higashiura K, Murakami H, Tanaka M, Moniwa N, Yoshida D, Shimamoto K: Blockade of the renin-angiotensin system increases adiponectin concentrations in patients with essential hypertension. *Hypertension* 2003, 42:76-81.

[88] Yamauchi T, Kamon J, Minokoshi Y, Ito Y, Waki H, Uchida S, Yamashita S, Noda M, Kita S, Ueki K, Eto K, Akanuma Y, Froguel P, Foufelle F, Ferre P, Carling D, Kimura S, Nagai R, Kahn BB, Kadowaki T: Adiponectin stimulates glucose utilization and fatty-acid oxidation by activating AMP-activated protein kinase. *Nat.Med.* 2002, 8:1288-1295.

[89] Alligier M, Meugnier E, Debard C, Lambert-Porcheron S, Chanseaume E, Sothier M, Loizon E, Hssain AA, Brozek J, Scoazec JY, Morio B, Vidal H, Laville M: Subcutaneous adipose tissue remodeling during the initial phase of weight gain induced by overfeeding in humans. *J.Clin.Endocrinol.Metab* 2012, 97:E183-E192.

[90] Faloia E, Gatti C, Camilloni MA, Mariniello B, Sardu C, Garrapa GG, Mantero F, Giacchetti G: Comparison of circulating and local adipose tissue renin-angiotensin system in normotensive and hypertensive obese subjects. *J.Endocrinol.Invest* 2002, 25:309-314.

[91] Boustany CM, Bharadwaj K, Daugherty A, Brown DR, Randall DC, Cassis LA: Activation of the systemic and adipose renin-angiotensin system in rats with diet-induced obesity and hypertension. *Am.J.Physiol Regul.Integr.Comp Physiol* 2004, 287:R943-R949.

[92] Giacchetti G, Sechi LA, Griffin CA, Don BR, Mantero F, Schambelan M: The tissue renin-angiotensin system in rats with fructose-induced hypertension: overexpression of type 1 angiotensin II receptor in adipose tissue. *J.Hypertens.* 2000, 18:695-702.

[93] Frederich RC, Jr., Kahn BB, Peach MJ, Flier JS: Tissue-specific nutritional regulation of angiotensinogen in adipose tissue. *Hypertension* 1992, 19:339-344.

[94] Jones BH, Standridge MK, Moustaid N: Angiotensin II increases lipogenesis in 3T3-L1 and human adipose cells. *Endocrinology* 1997, 138:1512-1519.

[95] Yvan-Charvet L, Even P, Bloch-Faure M, Guerre-Millo M, Moustaid-Moussa N, Ferre P, Quignard-Boulange A: Deletion of the angiotensin type 2 receptor (AT2R) reduces adipose cell size and protects from diet-induced obesity and insulin resistance. *Diabetes* 2005, 54:991-999.

[96] Yvan-Charvet L, Massiera F, Lamande N, Ailhaud G, Teboul M, Moustaid-Moussa N, Gasc JM, Quignard-Boulange A: Deficiency of angiotensin type 2 receptor rescues obesity but not hypertension induced by overexpression of angiotensinogen in adipose tissue. *Endocrinology* 2009, 150:1421-1428.

[97] Yvan-Charvet L, Quignard-Boulange A: Role of adipose tissue renin-angiotensin system in metabolic and inflammatory diseases associated with obesity. *Kidney Int.* 2011, 79:162-168.

[98] Schling P, Mallow H, Trindl A, Loffler G: Evidence for a local renin angiotensin system in primary cultured human preadipocytes. *Int.J.Obes.Relat Metab Disord.* 1999, 23:336-341.

[99] Fowler JD, Johnson ND, Haroldson TA, Brintnall JA, Herrera JE, Katz SA, Bernlohr DA: Regulated renin release from 3T3-L1 adipocytes. *Am.J.Physiol Endocrinol.Metab* 2009, 296:E1383-E1391.

[100] Galvez-Prieto B, Bolbrinker J, Stucchi P, de Las Heras AI, Merino B, Arribas S, Ruiz-Gayo M, Huber M, Wehland M, Kreutz R, Fernandez-Alfonso MS: Comparative expression analysis of the renin-angiotensin system components between white and brown perivascular adipose tissue. *J.Endocrinol.* 2008, 197:55-64.

[101] Giacchetti G, Faloia E, Mariniello B, Sardu C, Gatti C, Camilloni MA, Guerrieri M, Mantero F: Overexpression of the renin-angiotensin system in human visceral adipose tissue in normal and overweight subjects. *Am.J.Hypertens.* 2002, 15:381-388.

[102] Kershaw EE, Flier JS: Adipose tissue as an endocrine organ. *J.Clin.Endocrinol.Metab* 2004, 89:2548-2556.

[103] Rahmouni K, Mark AL, Haynes WG, Sigmund CD: Adipose depot-specific modulation of angiotensinogen gene expression in diet-induced obesity. *Am.J.Physiol Endocrinol.Metab* 2004, 286:E891-E895.

[104] Hainault I, Nebout G, Turban S, Ardouin B, Ferre P, Quignard-Boulange A: Adipose tissue-specific increase in angiotensinogen expression and secretion in the obese (fa/fa) Zucker rat. *Am.J.Physiol Endocrinol.Metab* 2002, 282:E59-E66.

[105] Massiera F, Bloch-Faure M, Ceiler D, Murakami K, Fukamizu A, Gasc JM, Quignard-Boulange A, Negrel R, Ailhaud G, Seydoux J, Meneton P, Teboul M: Adipose angiotensinogen is involved in adipose tissue growth and blood pressure regulation. *FASEB J.* 2001, 15:2727-2729.

[106] Yasue S, Masuzaki H, Okada S, Ishii T, Kozuka C, Tanaka T, Fujikura J, Ebihara K, Hosoda K, Katsurada A, Ohashi N, Urushihara M, Kobori H, Morimoto N, Kawazoe T, Naitoh M, Okada M, Sakaue H, Suzuki S, Nakao K: Adipose tissue-specific regulation of angiotensinogen in obese humans and mice: impact of nutritional status and adipocyte hypertrophy. *Am.J.Hypertens.* 2010, 23:425-431.

[107] Okada S, Kozuka C, Masuzaki H, Yasue S, Ishii-Yonemoto T, Tanaka T, Yamamoto Y, Noguchi M, Kusakabe T, Tomita T, Fujikura J, Ebihara K, Hosoda K, Sakaue H, Kobori H, Ham M, Lee YS, Kim JB, Saito Y, Nakao K: Adipose tissue-specific dysregulation of angiotensinogen by oxidative stress in obesity. *Metabolism* 2010, 59:1241-1251.

[108] Davis D, Liyou N, Lockwood D, Johnson A: Angiotensinogen genotype, plasma protein and mRNA concentration in isolated systolic hypertension. *Clin.Genet.* 2002, 61:363-368.

[109] Dong F, Zhang X, Ren J: Leptin regulates cardiomyocyte contractile function through endothelin-1 receptor-NADPH oxidase pathway. *Hypertension* 2006, 47:222-229.

[110] Dusserre E, Moulin P, Vidal H: Differences in mRNA expression of the proteins secreted by the adipocytes in human subcutaneous and visceral adipose tissues. *Biochim.Biophys.Acta* 2000, 1500:88-96.

[111] Korsic M, Gotovac K, Nikolac M, Dusek T, Skegro M, Muck-Seler D, Borovecki F, Pivac N: Gene expression in visceral and subcutaneous adipose tissue in overweight women. *Front Biosci.(Elite.Ed)* 2012, 4:2834-2844.

[112] Palou M, Priego T, Sanchez J, Rodriguez AM, Palou A, Pico C: Gene expression patterns in visceral and subcutaneous adipose depots in rats are linked to their morphologic features. *Cell Physiol Biochem.* 2009, 24:547-556.

[113] Massiera F, Seydoux J, Geloen A, Quignard-Boulange A, Turban S, Saint-Marc P, Fukamizu A, Negrel R, Ailhaud G, Teboul M: Angiotensinogen-deficient mice exhibit impairment of diet-induced weight gain with alteration in adipose tissue development and increased locomotor activity. *Endocrinology* 2001, 142:5220-5225.

[114] Kim S, Urs S, Massiera F, Wortmann P, Joshi R, Heo YR, Andersen B, Kobayashi H, Teboul M, Ailhaud G, Quignard-Boulange A, Fukamizu A, Jones BH, Kim JH, Moustaid-Moussa N: Effects of high-fat diet, angiotensinogen (agt) gene inactivation, and targeted expression to adipose tissue on lipid metabolism and renal gene expression. *Horm.Metab Res.* 2002, 34:721-725.

[115] Kim S, Soltani-Bejnood M, Quignard-Boulange A, Massiera F, Teboul M, Ailhaud G, Kim JH, Moustaid-Moussa N, Voy BH: The adipose renin-angiotensin system modulates systemic markers of insulin sensitivity and activates the intrarenal renin-angiotensin system. *J.Biomed.Biotechnol.* 2006, 2006:27012.

[116] Martin MM, Willardson BM, Burton GF, White CR, McLaughlin JN, Bray SM, Ogilvie JW, Jr., Elton TS: Human angiotensin II type 1 receptor isoforms encoded by messenger RNA splice variants are functionally distinct. *Mol.Endocrinol.* 2001, 15:281-293.

[117] Kouyama R, Suganami T, Nishida J, Tanaka M, Toyoda T, Kiso M, Chiwata T, Miyamoto Y, Yoshimasa Y, Fukamizu A, Horiuchi M, Hirata Y, Ogawa Y: Attenuation of diet-induced weight gain and adiposity through increased energy expenditure in mice lacking angiotensin II type 1a receptor. *Endocrinology* 2005, 146:3481-3489.

[118] Putnam K, Batifoulier-Yiannikouris F, Bharadwaj KG, Lewis E, Karounos M, Daugherty A, Cassis LA: Deficiency of Angiotensin type 1a receptors in adipocytes reduces differentiation and promotes hypertrophy of adipocytes in lean mice. *Endocrinology* 2012, 153:4677-4686.

[119] Achard V, Boullu-Ciocca S, Desbriere R, Nguyen G, Grino M: Renin receptor expression in human adipose tissue. *Am.J.Physiol Regul.Integr.Comp Physiol* 2007, 292:R274-R282.

[120] Silva-Antonialli MM, Tostes RC, Fernandes L, Fior-Chadi DR, Akamine EH, Carvalho MH, Fortes ZB, Nigro D: A lower ratio of AT1/AT2 receptors of angiotensin II is found in female than in male spontaneously hypertensive rats. *Cardiovasc.Res.* 2004, 62:587-593.

[121] Fischer M, Baessler A, Schunkert H: Renin angiotensin system and gender differences in the cardiovascular system. *Cardiovasc.Res.* 2002, 53:672-677.

[122] Harte A, McTernan P, Chetty R, Coppack S, Katz J, Smith S, Kumar S: Insulin-mediated upregulation of the renin angiotensin system in human subcutaneous adipocytes is reduced by rosiglitazone. *Circulation* 2005, 111:1954-1961.

[123] Prusty D, Park BH, Davis KE, Farmer SR: Activation of MEK/ERK signaling promotes adipogenesis by enhancing peroxisome proliferator-activated receptor gamma (PPARgamma) and C/EBPalpha gene expression during the differentiation of 3T3-L1 preadipocytes. *J.Biol.Chem.* 2002, 277:46226-46232.

[124] Takahashi N, Li F, Hua K, Deng J, Wang CH, Bowers RR, Bartness TJ, Kim HS, Harp JB: Increased energy expenditure, dietary fat wasting, and resistance to diet-induced obesity in mice lacking renin. *Cell Metab* 2007, 6:506-512.

[125] Santos SH, Fernandes LR, Mario EG, Ferreira AV, Porto LC, Alvarez-Leite JI, Botion LM, Bader M, Alenina N, Santos RA: Mas deficiency in FVB/N mice produces marked changes in lipid and glycemic metabolism. *Diabetes* 2008, 57:340-347.

[126] Nguyen G: Renin/prorenin receptors. *Kidney Int.* 2006, 69:1503-1506.

[127] Leung PS, Chan WP, Wong TP, Sernia C: Expression and localization of the renin-angiotensin system in the rat pancreas. *J.Endocrinol.* 1999, 160:13-19.

[128] Tahmasebi M, Puddefoot JR, Inwang ER, Vinson GP: The tissue renin-angiotensin system in human pancreas. *J.Endocrinol.* 1999, 161:317-322.

[129] Leung PS, Chappell MC: A local pancreatic renin-angiotensin system: endocrine and exocrine roles. *Int.J.Biochem.Cell Biol.* 2003, 35:838-846.

[130] Regoli M, Bendayan M, Fonzi L, Sernia C, Bertelli E: Angiotensinogen localization and secretion in the rat pancreas. *J.Endocrinol.* 2003, 179:81-89.

[131] Tikellis C, Wookey PJ, Candido R, Andrikopoulos S, Thomas MC, Cooper ME: Improved islet morphology after blockade of the renin- angiotensin system in the ZDF rat. *Diabetes* 2004, 53:989-997.

[132] Chu KY, Cheng Q, Chen C, Au LS, Seto SW, Tuo Y, Motin L, Kwan YW, Leung PS: Angiotensin II exerts glucose-dependent effects on Kv currents in mouse pancreatic beta-cells via angiotensin II type 2 receptors. *Am.J.Physiol Cell Physiol* 2010, 298:C313-C323.

[133] Ramracheya RD, Muller DS, Wu Y, Whitehouse BJ, Huang GC, Amiel SA, Karalliedde J, Viberti G, Jones PM, Persaud SJ: Direct regulation of insulin secretion by angiotensin II in human islets of Langerhans. *Diabetologia* 2006, 49:321-331.

[134] Wong PF, Lee SS, Cheung WT: Immunohistochemical colocalization of type II angiotensin receptors with somatostatin in rat pancreas. *Regul.Pept.* 2004, 117:195-205.

[135] Re RN: Implications of intracrine hormone action for physiology and medicine. *Am.J.Physiol Heart Circ.Physiol* 2003, 284:H751-H757.

[136] Chu KY, Lau T, Carlsson PO, Leung PS: Angiotensin II type 1 receptor blockade improves beta-cell function and glucose tolerance in a mouse model of type 2 diabetes. *Diabetes* 2006, 55:367-374.

[137] Fliser D, Schaefer F, Schmid D, Veldhuis JD, Ritz E: Angiotensin II affects basal, pulsatile, and glucose-stimulated insulin secretion in humans. *Hypertension* 1997, 30:1156-1161.

[138] Lau T, Carlsson PO, Leung PS: Evidence for a local angiotensin-generating system and dose-dependent inhibition of glucose-stimulated insulin release by angiotensin II in isolated pancreatic islets. *Diabetologia* 2004, 47:240-248.

[139] Suarez C, Tornadu IG, Cristina C, Vela J, Iglesias AG, Libertun C, Diaz-Torga G, Becu-Villalobos D: Angiotensin and calcium signaling in the pituitary and hypothalamus. *Cell Mol.Neurobiol.* 2002, 22:315-333.

[140] Kampf C, Lau T, Olsson R, Leung PS, Carlsson PO: Angiotensin II type 1 receptor inhibition markedly improves the blood perfusion, oxygen tension and first phase of glucose-stimulated insulin secretion in revascularised syngeneic mouse islet grafts. *Diabetologia* 2005, 48:1159-1167.

[141] Mason JM, Dickinson HO, Nicolson DJ, Campbell F, Ford GA, Williams B: The diabetogenic potential of thiazide-type diuretic and beta-blocker combinations in patients with hypertension. *J.Hypertens.* 2005, 23:1777-1781.

[142] Major outcomes in high-risk hypertensive patients randomized to angiotensin-converting enzyme inhibitor or calcium channel blocker vs diuretic: The Antihypertensive and Lipid-Lowering Treatment to Prevent Heart Attack Trial (ALLHAT). *JAMA* 2002, 288:2981-2997.

[143] Hansson L, Lindholm LH, Niskanen L, Lanke J, Hedner T, Niklason A, Luomanmaki K, Dahlof B, de FU, Morlin C, Karlberg BE, Wester PO, Bjorck JE: Effect of angiotensin-converting-enzyme inhibition compared with conventional therapy on cardiovascular morbidity and mortality in hypertension: the Captopril Prevention Project (CAPPP) randomised trial. *Lancet* 1999, 353:611-616.

[144] Pfeffer MA, Swedberg K, Granger CB, Held P, McMurray JJ, Michelson EL, Olofsson B, Ostergren J, Yusuf S, Pocock S: Effects of candesartan on mortality and morbidity in patients with chronic heart failure: the CHARM-Overall programme. *Lancet* 2003, 362:759-766.

[145] Julius S, Weber MA, Kjeldsen SE, McInnes GT, Zanchetti A, Brunner HR, Laragh J, Schork MA, Hua TA, Amerena J, Balazovjech I, Cassel G, Herczeg B, Koylan N, Magometschnigg D, Majahalme S, Martinez F, Oigman W, Seabra GR, Zhu JR: The Valsartan Antihypertensive Long-Term Use Evaluation (VALUE) trial: outcomes in patients receiving monotherapy. *Hypertension* 2006, 48:385-391.

[146] Cheng Q, Law PK, de GM, Leung PS: Combination of the dipeptidyl peptidase IV inhibitor LAF237 [(S)-1-[(3-hydroxy-1-adamantyl)ammo]acetyl-2-cyanopyrrolidine] with the angiotensin II type 1 receptor antagonist valsartan [N-(1-oxopentyl)-N-[[2'-(1H-tetrazol-5-yl)-[1,1'-biphenyl]-4-yl]methyl]-L-valine] enhances pancreatic islet morphology and function in a mouse model of type 2 diabetes. *J.Pharmacol.Exp.Ther.* 2008, 327:683-691.

[147] Ko SH, Hong OK, Kim JW, Ahn YB, Song KH, Cha BY, Son HY, Kim MJ, Jeong IK, Yoon KH: High glucose increases extracellular matrix production in pancreatic stellate cells by activating the renin-angiotensin system. *J.Cell Biochem.* 2006, 98:343-355.

[148] Yuan L, Li X, Li J, Li HL, Cheng SS: Effects of renin-angiotensin system blockade on the islet morphology and function in rats with long-term high-fat diet. *Acta Diabetol.* 2010.

[149] Chu KY, Leung PS: Angiotensin II Type 1 receptor antagonism mediates uncoupling protein 2-driven oxidative stress and ameliorates pancreatic islet beta-cell function in young Type 2 diabetic mice. *Antioxid.Redox.Signal.* 2007, 9:869-878.

[150] de Kloet AD, Krause EG, Scott KA, Foster MT, Herman JP, Sakai RR, Seeley RJ, Woods SC: Central angiotensin II has catabolic action at white and brown adipose tissue. *Am.J.Physiol Endocrinol.Metab* 2011, 301:E1081-E1091.

[151] Grobe JL, Grobe CL, Beltz TG, Westphal SG, Morgan DA, Xu D, de Lange WJ, Li H, Sakai K, Thedens DR, Cassis LA, Rahmouni K, Mark AL, Johnson AK, Sigmund CD: The brain Renin-angiotensin system controls divergent efferent mechanisms to regulate fluid and energy balance. *Cell Metab* 2010, 12:431-442.

[152] Porter JP, Potratz KR: Effect of intracerebroventricular angiotensin II on body weight and food intake in adult rats. *Am.J.Physiol Regul.Integr.Comp Physiol* 2004, 287:R422-R428.

[153] Ohinata K, Fujiwara Y, Fukumoto S, Iwai M, Horiuchi M, Yoshikawa M: Angiotensin II and III suppress food intake via angiotensin AT(2) receptor and prostaglandin EP(4) receptor in mice. *FEBS Lett.* 2008, 582:773-777.

[154] Araki K, Masaki T, Katsuragi I, Tanaka K, Kakuma T, Yoshimatsu H: Telmisartan prevents obesity and increases the expression of uncoupling protein 1 in diet-induced obese mice. *Hypertension* 2006, 48:51-57.

[155] Lionetti L, Mollica MP, Lombardi A, Cavaliere G, Gifuni G, Barletta A: From chronic overnutrition to insulin resistance: the role of fat-storing capacity and inflammation. *Nutr.Metab Cardiovasc.Dis.* 2009, 19:146-152.

[156] Mollica MP, Lionetti L, Putti R, Cavaliere G, Gaita M, Barletta A: From chronic overfeeding to hepatic injury: role of endoplasmic reticulum stress and inflammation. *Nutr.Metab Cardiovasc.Dis.* 2011, 21:222-230.

[157] Sartipy P, Loskutoff DJ: Monocyte chemoattractant protein 1 in obesity and insulin resistance. *Proc.Natl.Acad.Sci.U.S.A* 2003, 100:7265-7270.

[158] Olefsky JM, Glass CK: Macrophages, inflammation, and insulin resistance. *Annu.Rev.Physiol* 2010, 72:219-246.

[159] Tsuchiya K, Yoshimoto T, Hirono Y, Tateno T, Sugiyama T, Hirata Y: Angiotensin II induces monocyte chemoattractant protein-1 expression via a nuclear factor-kappaB-dependent pathway in rat preadipocytes. *Am.J.Physiol Endocrinol.Metab* 2006, 291:E771-E778.

[160] Asamizu S, Urakaze M, Kobashi C, Ishiki M, Norel Din AK, Fujisaka S, Kanatani Y, Bukahari A, Senda S, Suzuki H, Yamazaki Y, Iwata M, Usui I, Yamazaki K, Ogawa H, Kobayashi M, Tobe K: Angiotensin II enhances the increase in monocyte chemoattractant protein-1 production induced by tumor necrosis factor-{alpha} from 3T3-L1 preadipocytes. *J.Endocrinol.* 2009, 202:199-205.

[161] Skurk T, van H, V, Hauner H: Angiotensin II stimulates the release of interleukin-6 and interleukin-8 from cultured human adipocytes by activation of NF-kappaB. *Arterioscler.Thromb.Vasc.Biol.* 2004, 24:1199-1203.

[162] Otsuka S, Sugano M, Makino N, Sawada S, Hata T, Niho Y: Interaction of mRNAs for angiotensin II type 1 and type 2 receptors to vascular remodeling in spontaneously hypertensive rats. *Hypertension* 1998, 32:467-472.

[163] Gelband CH, Zhu M, Lu D, Reagan LP, Fluharty SJ, Posner P, Raizada MK, Sumners C: Functional interactions between neuronal AT1 and AT2 receptors. *Endocrinology* 1997, 138:2195-2198.

[164] Guo YJ, Li WH, Wu R, Xie Q, Cui LQ: ACE2 overexpression inhibits angiotensin II-induced monocyte chemoattractant protein-1 expression in macrophages. *Arch.Med.Res.* 2008, 39:149-154.

[165] Jurewicz M, McDermott DH, Sechler JM, Tinckam K, Takakura A, Carpenter CB, Milford E, Abdi R: Human T and natural killer cells possess a functional renin-angiotensin system: further mechanisms of angiotensin II-induced inflammation. *J.Am.Soc.Nephrol.* 2007, 18:1093-1102.

[166] Syrbe U, Moebes A, Scholze J, Swidsinski A, Dorffel Y: Effects of the angiotensin II type 1 receptor antagonist telmisartan on monocyte adhesion and activation in patients with essential hypertension. *Hypertens.Res.* 2007, 30:521-528.

[167] Sachse A, Wolf G: Angiotensin II-induced reactive oxygen species and the kidney. *J.Am.Soc.Nephrol.* 2007, 18:2439-2446.

[168] Tang J, Yan H, Zhuang S: Inflammation and oxidative stress in obesity-related glomerulopathy. *Int.J.Nephrol.* 2012, 2012:608397.

[169] Maritim AC, Sanders RA, Watkins JB, III: Diabetes, oxidative stress, and antioxidants: a review. *J.Biochem.Mol.Toxicol.* 2003, 17:24-38.

[170] Furukawa S, Fujita T, Shimabukuro M, Iwaki M, Yamada Y, Nakajima Y, Nakayama O, Makishima M, Matsuda M, Shimomura I: Increased oxidative stress in obesity and its impact on metabolic syndrome. *J.Clin.Invest* 2004, 114:1752-1761.

[171] Gletsu-Miller N, Hansen JM, Jones DP, Go YM, Torres WE, Ziegler TR, Lin E: Loss of total and visceral adipose tissue mass predicts decreases in oxidative stress after weight-loss surgery. *Obesity.(Silver.Spring)* 2009, 17:439-446.

[172] Kurata A, Nishizawa H, Kihara S, Maeda N, Sonoda M, Okada T, Ohashi K, Hibuse T, Fujita K, Yasui A, Hiuge A, Kumada M, Kuriyama H, Shimomura I, Funahashi T: Blockade of Angiotensin II type-1 receptor reduces oxidative stress in adipose tissue and ameliorates adipocytokine dysregulation. *Kidney Int.* 2006, 70:1717-1724.

[173] Iwai M, Horiuchi M: Devil and angel in the renin-angiotensin system: ACE-angiotensin II-AT1 receptor axis vs. ACE2-angiotensin-(1-7)-Mas receptor axis. *Hypertens.Res.* 2009, 32:533-536.

[174] Liu C, Lv XH, Li HX, Cao X, Zhang F, Wang L, Yu M, Yang JK: Angiotensin-(1-7) suppresses oxidative stress and improves glucose uptake via Mas receptor in adipocytes. *Acta Diabetol.* 2012, 49:291-299.

[175] Laursen JB, Rajagopalan S, Galis Z, Tarpey M, Freeman BA, Harrison DG: Role of superoxide in angiotensin II-induced but not catecholamine-induced hypertension. *Circulation* 1997, 95:588-593.

[176] Kalupahana NS, Massiera F, Quignard-Boulange A, Ailhaud G, Voy BH, Wasserman DH, Moustaid-Moussa N: Overproduction of angiotensinogen from adipose tissue induces adipose inflammation, glucose intolerance, and insulin resistance. *Obesity.(Silver.Spring)* 2012, 20:48-56.

[177] Pan Q, Yang XH, Cheng YX: Angiotensin II stimulates MCP-1 production in rat glomerular endothelial cells via NAD(P)H oxidase-dependent nuclear factor-kappa B signaling. *Braz.J.Med.Biol.Res.* 2009, 42:531-536.

[178] Scheidegger KJ, Butler S, Witztum JL: Angiotensin II increases macrophage-mediated modification of low density lipoprotein via a lipoxygenase-dependent pathway. *J.Biol.Chem.* 1997, 272:21609-21615.

[179] Kim JA, Gu JL, Natarajan R, Berliner JA, Nadler JL: A leukocyte type of 12-lipoxygenase is expressed in human vascular and mononuclear cells. Evidence for upregulation by angiotensin II. *Arterioscler.Thromb.Vasc.Biol.* 1995, 15:942-948.

[180] Hennington BS, Zhang H, Miller MT, Granger JP, Reckelhoff JF: Angiotensin II stimulates synthesis of endothelial nitric oxide synthase. *Hypertension* 1998, 31:283-288.

[181] Dobrian AD, Davies MJ, Prewitt RL, Lauterio TJ: Development of hypertension in a rat model of diet-induced obesity. *Hypertension* 2000, 35:1009-1015.

[182] Barnes MJ, Lapanowski K, Conley A, Rafols JA, Jen KL, Dunbar JC: High fat feeding is associated with increased blood pressure, sympathetic nerve activity and hypothalamic mu opioid receptors. *Brain Res.Bull.* 2003, 61:511-519.

[183] Schiel R, Beltschikow W, Kramer G, Stein G: Overweight, obesity and elevated blood pressure in children and adolescents. *Eur.J.Med.Res.* 2006, 11:97-101.

[184] Gryglewska B, Grodzicki T, Kocemba J: Obesity and blood pressure in the elderly free-living population. *J.Hum.Hypertens.* 1998, 12:645-647.

[185] Su HY, Sheu WH, Chin HM, Jeng CY, Chen YD, Reaven GM: Effect of weight loss on blood pressure and insulin resistance in normotensive and hypertensive obese individuals. *Am.J.Hypertens.* 1995, 8:1067-1071.

[186] Schotte DE, Stunkard AJ: The effects of weight reduction on blood pressure in 301 obese patients. *Arch.Intern.Med.* 1990, 150:1701-1704.

[187] Gullapalli N, Bloch MJ, Basile J: Renin-angiotensin-aldosterone system blockade in high-risk hypertensive patients: current approaches and future trends. *Ther.Adv.Cardiovasc.Dis.* 2010, 4:359-373.

[188] Blumenthal JA, Babyak MA, Hinderliter A, Watkins LL, Craighead L, Lin PH, Caccia C, Johnson J, Waugh R, Sherwood A: Effects of the DASH diet alone and in combination with exercise and weight loss on blood pressure and cardiovascular biomarkers in men and women with high blood pressure: the ENCORE study. *Arch.Intern.Med.* 2010, 170:126-135.

[189] Stevens VJ, Obarzanek E, Cook NR, Lee IM, Appel LJ, Smith WD, Milas NC, Mattfeldt-Beman M, Belden L, Bragg C, Millstone M, Raczynski J, Brewer A, Singh B, Cohen J: Long-term weight loss and changes in blood pressure: results of the Trials of Hypertension Prevention, phase II. *Ann.Intern.Med.* 2001, 134:1-11.

[190] Segura J, Ruilope LM: Obesity, essential hypertension and renin-angiotensin system. *Public Health Nutr.* 2007, 10:1151-1155.

[191] Bassett MH, White PC, Rainey WE: The regulation of aldosterone synthase expression. *Mol.Cell Endocrinol.* 2004, 217:67-74.

[192] Muller-Fielitz H, Lau M, Johren O, Stellmacher F, Schwaninger M, Raasch W: Blood pressure response to angiotensin II is enhanced in obese Zucker rats and is attributed to an aldosterone-dependent mechanism. *Br.J.Pharmacol.* 2012, 166:2417-2429.

[193] Francischetti EA, Genelhu VA: Obesity-hypertension: an ongoing pandemic. *Int.J.Clin.Pract.* 2007, 61:269-280.

[194] Fried SK, Ricci MR, Russell CD, Laferrere B: Regulation of leptin production in humans. *J.Nutr.* 2000, 130:3127S-3131S.

[195] Skurk T, van H, V, Blum WF, Hauner H: Angiotensin II promotes leptin production in cultured human fat cells by an ERK1/2-dependent pathway. *Obes.Res.* 2005, 13:969-973.

[196] Rahmouni K, Morgan DA, Morgan GM, Mark AL, Haynes WG: Role of selective leptin resistance in diet-induced obesity hypertension. *Diabetes* 2005, 54:2012-2018.

[197] Mark AL, Shaffer RA, Correia ML, Morgan DA, Sigmund CD, Haynes WG: Contrasting blood pressure effects of obesity in leptin-deficient ob/ob mice and agouti yellow obese mice [In Process Citation]. *J Hypertens.* 1999, 17:1949-1953.
[198] Reaven GM, Hollenbeck C, Jeng CY, Wu MS, Chen YD: Measurement of plasma glucose, free fatty acid, lactate, and insulin for 24 h in patients with NIDDM. *Diabetes* 1988, 37:1020-1024.
[199] Boden G, Chen X, Ruiz J, White JV, Rossetti L: Mechanisms of fatty acid-induced inhibition of glucose uptake. *J.Clin.Invest* 1994, 93:2438-2446.
[200] Santomauro AT, Boden G, Silva ME, Rocha DM, Santos RF, Ursich MJ, Strassmann PG, Wajchenberg BL: Overnight lowering of free fatty acids with Acipimox improves insulin resistance and glucose tolerance in obese diabetic and nondiabetic subjects. *Diabetes* 1999, 48:1836-1841.
[201] Carvalho E, Rondinone C, Smith U: Insulin resistance in fat cells from obese Zucker rats--evidence for an impaired activation and translocation of protein kinase B and glucose transporter 4. *Mol.Cell Biochem.* 2000, 206:7-16.
[202] Wei Y, Sowers JR, Clark SE, Li W, Ferrario CM, Stump CS: Angiotensin II-induced skeletal muscle insulin resistance mediated by NF-kappaB activation via NADPH oxidase. *Am.J.Physiol Endocrinol.Metab* 2008, 294:E345-E351.
[203] Habibi J, Whaley-Connell A, Hayden MR, DeMarco VG, Schneider R, Sowers SD, Karuparthi P, Ferrario CM, Sowers JR: Renin inhibition attenuates insulin resistance, oxidative stress, and pancreatic remodeling in the transgenic Ren2 rat. *Endocrinology* 2008, 149:5643-5653.
[204] Csibi A, Communi D, Muller N, Bottari SP: Angiotensin II inhibits insulin-stimulated GLUT4 translocation and Akt activation through tyrosine nitration-dependent mechanisms. *PLoS.One.* 2010, 5:e10070.
[205] Satoh M, Fujimoto S, Arakawa S, Yada T, Namikoshi T, Haruna Y, Horike H, Sasaki T, Kashihara N: Angiotensin II type 1 receptor blocker ameliorates uncoupled endothelial nitric oxide synthase in rats with experimental diabetic nephropathy. *Nephrol.Dial.Transplant.* 2008, 23:3806-3813.
[206] Conde J, Scotece M, Gomez R, Lopez V, Gomez-Reino JJ, Lago F, Gualillo O: Adipokines: biofactors from white adipose tissue. A complex hub among inflammation, metabolism, and immunity. *Biofactors* 2011, 37:413-420.
[207] Kubota N, Terauchi Y, Yamauchi T, Kubota T, Moroi M, Matsui J, Eto K, Yamashita T, Kamon J, Satoh H, Yano W, Froguel P, Nagai R, Kimura S, Kadowaki T, Noda T: Disruption of adiponectin causes insulin resistance and neointimal formation. *J.Biol.Chem.* 2002, 277:25863-25866.
[208] Fasshauer M, Paschke R, Stumvoll M: Adiponectin, obesity, and cardiovascular disease. *Biochimie* 2004, 86:779-784.
[209] Kern PA, Di Gregorio GB, Lu T, Rassouli N, Ranganathan G: Adiponectin expression from human adipose tissue: relation to obesity, insulin resistance, and tumor necrosis factor-alpha expression. *Diabetes* 2003, 52:1779-1785.
[210] Asayama K, Hayashibe H, Dobashi K, Uchida N, Nakane T, Kodera K, Shirahata A, Taniyama M: Decrease in serum adiponectin level due to obesity and visceral fat accumulation in children. *Obes.Res.* 2003, 11:1072-1079.
[211] Gueugnon C, Mougin F, Simon-Rigaud ML, Regnard J, Negre V, Dumoulin G: Effects of an in-patient treatment program based on regular exercise and a balanced diet on

high molecular weight adiponectin, resistin levels, and insulin resistance in adolescents with severe obesity. *Appl.Physiol Nutr.Metab* 2012, 37:672-679.

[212] Thundyil J, Pavlovski D, Sobey CG, Arumugam TV: Adiponectin receptor signalling in the brain. *Br.J.Pharmacol.* 2012, 165:313-327.

[213] Bjursell M, Ahnmark A, Bohlooly Y, William-Olsson L, Rhedin M, Peng XR, Ploj K, Gerdin AK, Arnerup G, Elmgren A, Berg AL, Oscarsson J, Linden D: Opposing effects of adiponectin receptors 1 and 2 on energy metabolism. *Diabetes* 2007, 56:583-593.

[214] Bullen JW, Jr., Bluher S, Kelesidis T, Mantzoros CS: Regulation of adiponectin and its receptors in response to development of diet-induced obesity in mice. *Am.J.Physiol Endocrinol.Metab* 2007, 292:E1079-E1086.

[215] Inukai K, Nakashima Y, Watanabe M, Takata N, Sawa T, Kurihara S, Awata T, Katayama S: Regulation of adiponectin receptor gene expression in diabetic mice. *Am.J.Physiol Endocrinol.Metab* 2005, 288:E876-E882.

[216] Ran J, Hirano T, Fukui T, Saito K, Kageyama H, Okada K, Adachi M: Angiotensin II infusion decreases plasma adiponectin level via its type 1 receptor in rats: an implication for hypertension-related insulin resistance. *Metabolism* 2006, 55:478-488.

[217] Iwai M, Kanno H, Tomono Y, Inaba S, Senba I, Furuno M, Mogi M, Horiuchi M: Direct renin inhibition improved insulin resistance and adipose tissue dysfunction in type 2 diabetic KK-A(y) mice. *J.Hypertens.* 2010, 28:1471-1481.

[218] Pscherer S, Heemann U, Frank H: Effect of Renin-Angiotensin system blockade on insulin resistance and inflammatory parameters in patients with impaired glucose tolerance. *Diabetes Care* 2010, 33:914-919.

[219] Premaratna SD, Manickam E, Begg DP, Rayment DJ, Hafandi A, Jois M, Cameron-Smith D, Weisinger RS: Angiotensin-converting enzyme inhibition reverses diet-induced obesity, insulin resistance and inflammation in C57BL/6J mice. *Int.J.Obes.(Lond)* 2012, 36:233-243.

[220] Schupp M, Janke J, Clasen R, Unger T, Kintscher U: Angiotensin type 1 receptor blockers induce peroxisome proliferator-activated receptor-gamma activity. *Circulation* 2004, 109:2054-2057.

[221] Prasannarong M, Santos FR, Henriksen EJ: ANG-(1-7) reduces ANG II-induced insulin resistance by enhancing Akt phosphorylation via a Mas receptor-dependent mechanism in rat skeletal muscle. *Biochem.Biophys.Res.Commun.* 2012, 426:369-373.

[222] Munoz MC, Giani JF, Burghi V, Mayer MA, Carranza A, Taira CA, Dominici FP: The Mas receptor mediates modulation of insulin signaling by angiotensin-(1-7). *Regul.Pept.* 2012, 177:1-11.

[223] Leehey DJ, Singh AK, Bast JP, Sethupathi P, Singh R: Glomerular renin angiotensin system in streptozotocin diabetic and Zucker diabetic fatty rats. *Transl.Res.* 2008, 151:208-216.

[224] Gupte M, Boustany-Kari CM, Bharadwaj K, Police S, Thatcher S, Gong MC, English VL, Cassis LA: ACE2 is expressed in mouse adipocytes and regulated by a high-fat diet. *Am.J.Physiol Regul.Integr.Comp Physiol* 2008, 295:R781-R788.

[225] Lambert DW, Yarski M, Warner FJ, Thornhill P, Parkin ET, Smith AI, Hooper NM, Turner AJ: Tumor necrosis factor-alpha convertase (ADAM17) mediates regulated ectodomain shedding of the severe-acute respiratory syndrome-coronavirus (SARS-CoV) receptor, angiotensin-converting enzyme-2 (ACE2). *J.Biol.Chem.* 2005, 280:30113-30119.

In: Renin-Angiotensin System
Editors: Ayako Himura and Takeshi Sato

ISBN: 978-1-62417-788-0

Chapter IV

Cross-Talk between Renin-Angiotensin System and LOX-1: Implications in Cardiovascular Diseases

Zufeng Ding[1], Fenxi Zhang[2], Yao Dai[1], J. L. Mehta[1] and Xianwei Wang*[1]

[1]Division of Cardiology, University of Arkansas for Medical Sciences and the Central Arkansas Veterans Healthcare System, Little Rock, AR, US

[2]Department of Anatomy, Sanquan college, Xinxiang Medical university, Xinxiang, P.R. China

Abstract

The renin-angiotensin system (RAS) is a major hormonal system that plays an essential role in regulating salt-water balance and blood pressure. Angiotensin II (Ang II) is the major active mediator of RAS. Ang II exerts its effects by activating a number of receptors, primarily type 1 (AT1R) and type 2 (AT2R). The role of both of these receptors in cardiovascular physiology and pathology has been widely studied. Besides stimulating salt and water retention via aldosterone, AT1R activation is thought to promote vasoconstriction, inflammation, oxidant stress and smooth muscle cell hypertrophy, whereas AT2R is believed to oppose the actions of AT1R. Lectin-like oxidized low density lipoprotein scavenger receptor-1 (LOX-1) is one of the major receptors responsible for binding, internalizing and degrading oxidized low density lipoprotein (ox-LDL). The activation of LOX-1 is also known to be related to the pathogenesis of several cardiovascular diseases. Recent findings, including those from our laboratory, have indicated that LOX-1 and Ang II receptors, especially AT1R, have a mutually facilitative interaction in the genesis of atherosclerosis, hypertension, myocardial ischemia, and cardiac remodeling. In this review, we summarize the interplay between LOX-1 and AT1R or AT2R in the pathogenesis of several cardiovascular diseases.

---

* Address for correspondence: Xianwei Wang, MD, PhD; Cardiovascular Division, UAMS; Little Rock, AR 72205; XWang2@uams.edu; Phone: 501-257-4849.

Keywords: Angiotensin II receptors, LOX-1, Atherosclerosis, Hypertension, Cardiac remodeling

Abbreviations

ACE2	angiotensin-converting enzyme 2
Ang	angiotensin
AMI	myocardial infarction
AP-1	activator protein 1
ARB	AT1R blocker
AT1R	angiotensin II type I receptor
AT2R	angiotensin II type II receptor
CRP	C-reactive protein
ECs	Endothelial cells
EGFR	epidermal growth factor receptor
ERK 1/2	extracellular-signal-regulated kinase 1/2
HCAECs	human coronary artery endothelial cells
HUVECs	human umbilical vein endothelial cells
ICAM-1	intercellular cell adhesion molecule-1
IL	interleukin
JNK	c-Jun N-terminal kinase
KO	knock-out
LCA	left coronary artery
LPS	lipopolysaccharide
LV	Left ventricular
MAPK	Mitogen-activated protein kinase
MDA	malondialdehyde
MMPs	matrix metalloproteinases
NADPH	nicotinamide adenine dinucleotide phosphate
NF-kB	nuclear factor-kappa B
OLR-1	oxidized low density lipoprotein receptor-1
ox-LDL	oxidized low density lipoprotein
PDGF	platelet-derived growth factor
p38MAPK	p38 mitogen-activated protein kinase
RAS	renin-angiotensin system
ROS	reactive oxygen species
SAPK	stress-activated protein kinase
TBARS	thiobarbituric acid reactive substances
TGF	transforming growth factor
VEGF	vascular endothelial growth factor
VEGF-R	VEGF receptor
VSMCs	Vascular smooth muscle cells

I. Introduction

Renin-angiotensin system (RAS) plays a key role in several physiological and pathophysiological processes involving the cardiovascular system [1]. RAS not only functions as an endocrine system, but it also plays functions in paracrine and autocrine patterns [2]. As the main active mediator of RAS, angiotensin II (Ang II), has been identified to function in nearly all organs, including heart, kidney, vasculature, and brain [2]. In utero, Ang II plays a major role in the cardiovascular development in the fetus [3]. Exogenous administration of Ang II in the adult increases salt/water retention, vascular tone and blood pressure, while long-term exposure to Ang II induces vascular smooth muscle cell (VSMC) and fibroblast growth [2]. Ang II exerts its effects by activating its many receptors. However, it is thought that activation of type I receptor (AT1R) and type II receptor (AT2R) mediates most of the known functions of RAS [4]. Both receptors belong to G protein-coupled receptor superfamily (GPCRs) and play their role via activation of G protein-mediated signaling pathway [5]. AT1R and AT2R only share 30% structural similarity [6], and their functions and signaling pathways are quite different [4].

Generally, AT1R is viewed to mediate most of the molecular and cellular actions of Ang II, and AT2R is thought to oppose these actions [7]. Ang II and its receptors are the major physiological regulators for electrolyte-fluid balance, blood pressure, secretion of aldosterone, cell proliferation, angiogenesis, inflammation and tissue remodeling, and play a central role in the pathophysiology of hypertension, acute myocardial infarction (AMI), cardiac remodeling after AMI, ischemic stroke, congestive heart failure, and atherogenesis [8].

Oxidized low density lipoprotein (ox-LDL) is formed after LDL particles are bombarded with free radical, nascent oxygen or so called 'reactive oxygen species (ROS)'. Several ROS generating systems, including nicotinamide adenine dinucleotide phosphate (NADPH) oxidase, mitochondrial electron transport enzymes, xanthine oxidase, lipoxygenase, cyclo-oxygenase, cytochrome P450 enzymes, are responsible for the formation of ox-LDL [9]. Generally, ox-LDL formation is increased in various pathological states such as dyslipidemia, metabolic syndrome, diabetes, obesity, aging and atherosclerosis [9].

Lectin-like oxidized low-density lipoprotein receptor-1 (LOX-1), a specialized receptor for ox-LDL, also known as oxidized low density lipoprotein receptor-1 (OLR-1), has been identified to be expressed on several cell lines including endothelial cells (ECs), macrophages, VSMCs, fibroblasts, monocytes, and cardiomyocytes [10, 11]. LOX-1, particularly in ECs, is responsible for uptake and internalization of ox-LDL and plays a fundamental role in the genesis and progression of atherosclerosis and its complications [12]. The well-known risk factors for atherosclerosis, such as hypertension, dyslipidemia, diabetes mellitus and smoking, are also associated with increase in plasma levels of ox-LDL, enhanced oxidative stress and increased LOX-1 expression [13].

There is increasing evidence for a cross-talk between RAS (mainly Ang II and AT1R activation) and oxidized lipids (mainly ox-LDL and LOX-1 activation) in atherosclerosis and probably other cardiovascular diseases such as hypertension, myocardial ischemia, and cardiac remodeling following sustained hypertension or AMI. There is increased RAS activation in hyperlipidemia, and RAS activation in turn upregulates and activates LOX-1, and then facilitates cellular uptake of ox-LDL [4].

II. Inter-Regulatory Interaction between LOX-1 and AT1R in Cardiovascular System

A growing body of evidence shows a reciprocal regulation between LOX-1 and AT1R in cardiovascular system. Morawietz et al. showed that Ang II stimulated LOX-1 expression in the cultured human umbilical vein endothelial cells (HUVECs) [14]. Simultaneously, other laboratories independently observed the similar phenomena in other cell lines, including human VSMCs, human coronary artery endothelial cells (HCAECs), monocytes and macrophages [15-17]. Ang II-stimulated LOX-1 expression can be inhibited by AT1R blocker losartan, not by AT2R blocker PD123319, which indicates that LOX-1 upregulation by Ang II is mediated by AT1R activation, not by AT2R [17]. In animal and clinical studies, AT1R blockade has been observed to effectively inhibit LOX-1 expression and activation [18, 19]. Long-term exposure to Ang II enhances ox-LDL uptake and induces endothelial dysfunction and injury [14]. Ang II-stimulated ox-LDL uptake boosts the proatherosclerotic processes.

On the other hand, activation of LOX-1 was shown to stimulate the expression of AT1R. A number of investigators have observed that high levels of serum cholesterol, especially LDL-cholesterol, cause an upregulation of AT1R in the blood vessels [20]. In studies in our laboratory, AT1R expression was found to be markedly up-regulated in the cultured HCAECs and cardiomyocytes exposed to ox-LDL, and the expression of AT1R paralleled LOX-1 expression [21]. Animal studies demonstrated an increased AT1R transcription in rabbits and mice fed a high cholesterol diet.

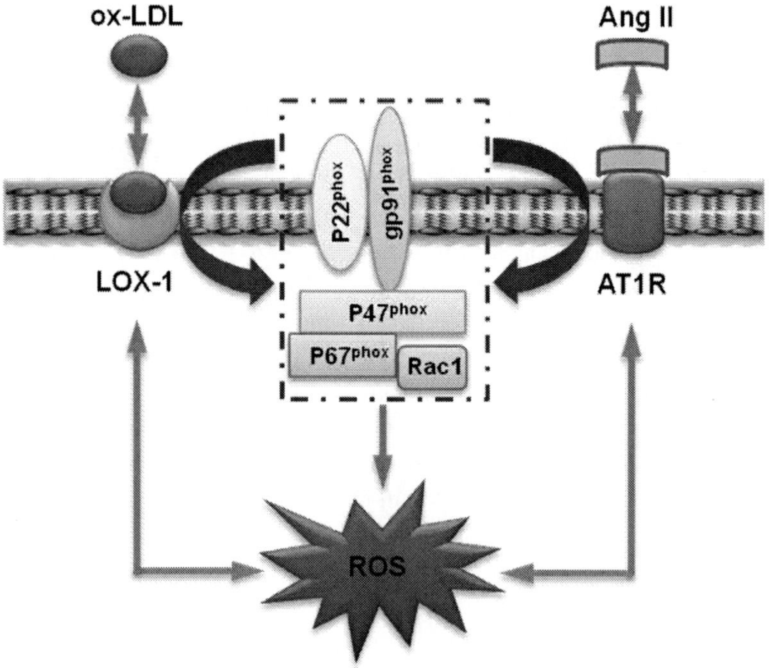

Figure 1. Reciprocal regulation between LOX-1 and AT1R in cardiovascular cells. Ox-LDL (via LOX-1) and Ang II (via AT1R) regulate expression and activation of NADPH subunits, and then promote ROS generation, and the increased cellular ROS further stimulate LOX-1 and AT1R expression, which form a regulatory feedback loop.

Yang et al. reported several-fold increased expression of total Ang II receptors content in the aortic intima, primarily in VSMCs, of hypercholesterolemic rabbits [20]. The increase in Ang II receptors was a result of marked upregulation of AT1R [20].

ROS are oxygen-derived small molecules, some being oxygen radicals and non-radicals. ROS represent common cellular signals that stimulate transduction of a series of down-stream cellular signals, such as p38 mitogen-activated protein kinase (p38MAPK), extracellular-signal-regulated kinase 1/2 (ERK1/2), c-Jun N-terminal kinase (JNK) and nuclear factor-kappa B (NF-kB). Ox-LDL, via activating LOX-1, stimulates ROS generation. There is a positive feedback loop between ROS and LOX-1. ROS enhance LOX-1 expression, and LOX-1 activation in turn enhances ROS generation. Some studies suggest that LOX-1 activation triggers the activation NADPH oxidase-MAPKs-NF-κB pathway [22]. NADPH oxidase system is the most potent oxidant enzyme system for ROS generation in vascular cells as well as in many other cell lines [23]. AT1R functions in the same manner as LOX-1 to stimulate ROS generation in cardiovascular system. Actually, AT1R and LOX-1 share the same NADPH oxidase-ROS-MAPK-NF-kB pathway to induce cardiovascular dysfunction. Studies from our and other laboratories have demonstrated that AT1R blockers and LOX-1 inhibitors attenuate Ang II-mediated ROS and the NADPH oxidase ($p40^{phox}$ and $gp91^{phox}$ subunits) [21, 24]. Zhang et al. [25] reported that angiotensin-converting enzyme 2 (ACE2) regulated both AT1R and LOX-1 expressions in the abdominal aorta of rabbits fed a high cholesterol diet. They also observed that an overexpression ACE2 inhibited the expressions of LOX-1 and AT1R at transcription and translation levels. These authors showed that the effect of ACE2 on AT1R and LOX-1 expression depend on ROS generation.

III. Cross-Talk between LOX-1 and AT1R in Endothelial Activation/Dysfunction

Several lines of evidence suggest that excess activation of LOX-1 or/and AT1R would cause endothelial activation/dysfunction, including angiogenesis, apoptosis and inflammation. The effects of AT1R or/and LOX-1 on endothelial dysfunction and injury depends on the extent of ROS generation [2, 26, 27]. ROS is the "signal bridge" to link LOX-1 and AT1R in endothelial activation/dysfunction. Ox-LDL, especially in low concentrations, has been known to induce endothelial proliferation. An in vitro study showed that 1-10μg/ml ox-LDL promoted proliferation of HUVECs, with the most optimal concentration being 5μg/ml [28]. Further study showed that the effect of ox-LDL on endothelial proliferation was dependent on the expression of $p27^{Kip1}$, as its knockdown significantly inhibited cell proliferation [28]. Besides HUVECs, ox-LDL (and LOX-1 activation) has also been observed to stimulate proliferation of HCAECs, SMCs, cardiomyocytes, macrophages and fibroblasts [29-32]. Recently, we found that deletion of LOX-1 gene inhibited cardiac fibroblast proliferation via regulation of cytoskeleton organization [33]. All these observations suggest that low concentrations of ox-LDL via LOX-1 induce proliferation of endothelial cells and other cardiovascular system cell lineages. Studies from our group and others show that low physiologic concentrations of Ang II also stimulate proliferation of endothelial cells [34-36], as well as other cell lines, such as SMCs [37], cardiomyocytes [32], fibroblasts [38], stem cells [39], hematopoietic progenitor cells [40], and cancer cells [41].

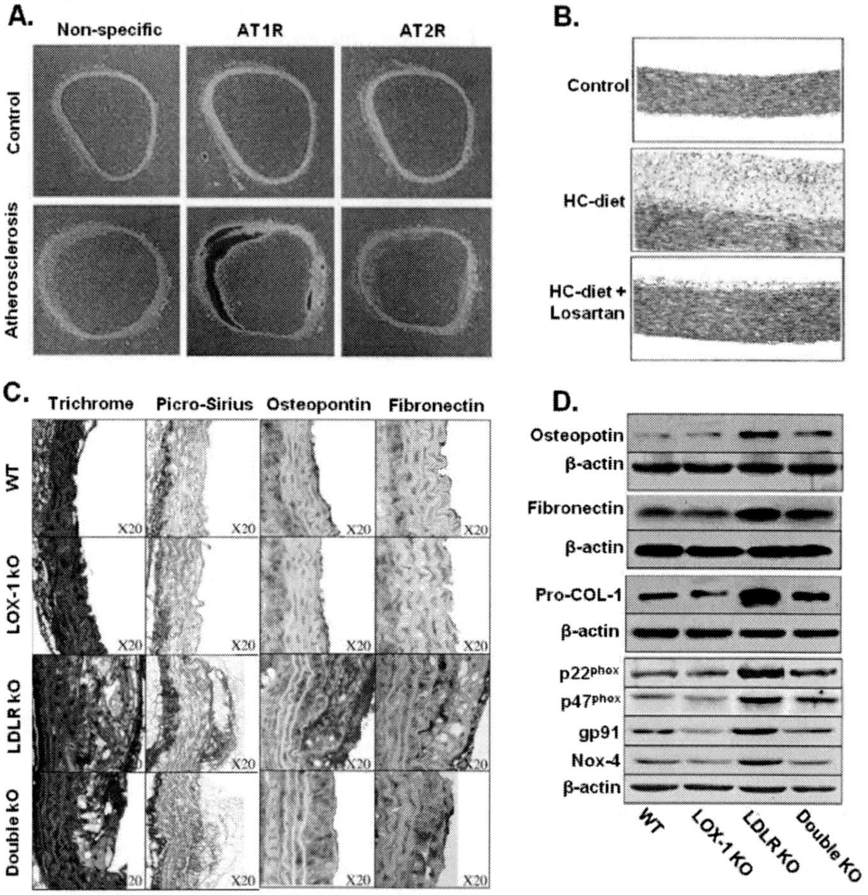

Figure 2. AT1R and LOX-1 function in atherosclerosis. A. AT1R expression in the control aorta (rabbits fed with normal-diet) and atherosclerotic aorta (rabbits fed with high cholesterol-diet). B. AT1R blocker losartan inhibits the formation of atherosclerotic plaques. C. LOX-1 deletion inhibits the progress of atherosclerosis and blood vessel (aorta) fibrosis in LDLR knockout mice fed with high-fat diet. D. Osteoptin, fibronection and pro-collagen-1 exppression and NADPH subunits ($p22^{phox}$, $p47^{phox}$, gp91 and Nox-4) expression in wild-type mice (WT), LOX-1 knockout (LOX-1 KO), low-density lipoprotein receptor knockout (LDLR KO) and LOX-1 and LDLR knockout (double KO) mice fed a high-cholesterol diet.

Some studies also suggest an interplay between Ang II and LOX-1 in the regulation of cell proliferation. Inhibition of LOX-1 is observed to reduce Ang II-induced cardiomyocyte proliferation [32], and LOX-1 overexpression upregulates AT1R expression and promotes cardiomyocyte growth [42], as well as Ang II induces LOX-1 expression and cell proliferation [42].

Ang II and ox-LDL (mainly via their receptors, AT1R and LOX-1) have been shown to promote angiogenesis. Low concentrations of ox-LDL (< 5 ug/ml) and Ang II (< 1 nmol/L) have been shown to induce capillary formation from cultured ECs. Ang II via induction of expression of vascular endothelial growth factor (VEGF) and its receptor (VEGF-R) regulates the development of new blood vessels [43, 44]. The formation of new blood vessels by Ang II seems to depend on AT1R activation, not AT2R [44]. AT2R activation actually attenuates angiogenesis by inhibition of epidermal growth factor receptor (EGFR) phosphorylation [44]. Recent studies from our group showed that Ang II-induced capillary formation from ECs is mediated to some part via LOX-1 sensitive redox-sensitive pathway [22].

Ang II and ox-LDL also trigger cell apoptosis, by activating their specific receptors AT1R (sometime AT2R) and LOX-1, respectively. The pro-apoptotic effect seems to requite high concentrations of Ang II. Dimmeler et al. showed that 1 μM Ang II induced apoptosis of HUVECs via activation of caspase cascade; further, the pro-apoptotic effect of Ang II in these studies was shown to be attenuated by both AT1R and AT2R blockers [45]. Li et al. also observed that exposure of HCAECs to 1 μM Ang II for 24 hour significantly increased apoptotic cell number, but the pro-apoptotic effect of Ang II in HCAECs could be inhibited by AT1R blocker losartan, but not by the AT2R blocker PD-123177, which suggests that Ang II-mediated HCAEC apoptosis is mainly via activation of AT1R [46].

This study and others also showed that the activation of phospholipase C/protein kinase C (PLC/PKC), one of downstream signals of AT1R activation, is mainly responsible for AT1R-mediated EC apoptosis [46, 47]. Besides ECs, Ang II has also been shown to induce apoptosis of SMCs, cardiomyocytes and renal proximal tubular cells [48-50], but to suppress the apoptosis of some cancer cell lines [51, 52]. While there is some variability in the role of AT2R in endothelial cell apoptosis [44, 45]. Ang II-triggered apoptosis in VSMCs is primarily mediated by activation of AT2R, not AT1R, because this effect is only blocked by AT2R inhibition [53, 54].

LOX-1 activation upon binding of ox-LDL is also known to stimulate apoptosis of many cell lines, including vascular ECs. Li et al. from our group firstly showed ox-LDL triggered apoptosis of HCAECs, which could be inhibited by antisense to LOX-1 mRNA and by LOX-1 inhibitors [55].

Further studies from our group demonstrated that ox-LDL/LOX-1-mediated endothelial cell apoptosis involved down-regulation of c-IAP-1 and Bcl-2, release of cytochrome *c* and Smac, activation of caspase-9 and caspase-3 [56]. In general, low concentrations of ox-LDL (<5 μg/ml) do not cause cell apoptosis, however, high concentrations of ox-LDL (>20 μg/ml) significantly enhance apoptosis [9].

Our in vivo studies also showed that LOX-1 was co-localized within the apoptotic cells in the advanced atherosclerotic carotid arteries [57]. LOX-1 activation also plays an important role in Ang II-induced cell apoptosis. Ox-LDL and Ang II synergistically interact to induce endothelial injury and apoptosis [58].

Both these mediators of cell response to oxidant stress can also stimulate the uptake of ox-LDL and then lead to apoptosis [58]. In consonance with these studies, Xu et al. recently demonstrated that LOX-1 plays a critical role in Ang II-induced renal tubular epithelial dysfunction [59].

Activation of AT1R and LOX-1 stimulates endothelial inflammation via generation of ROS, which is one of the early events in the progress of atherosclerosis. Griendling et al [60] showed that Ang II elicited ROS generation that subsequently increased the expression of monocyte chemoattractant protein-1 (MCP-1), a factor that facilitates monocytes migration into subendothelial layer.

Tummala et al [61] found that Ang II increased the expression of vascular cell adhesion molecule-1 (VCAM-1), which is an important promoter for adhesion of monocyte /macrophage to EC lining. Activation of LOX-1 following exposure of ECs to ox-LDL has been shown to stimulate the expression of MCP-1 and VCAM-1 in ECs [62,63]. Actually,

LOX-1 itself is known to be a pro-inflammatory molecule as LOX-1 inhibition seems to reduce inflammatory response in a variety of situations [64-66]. In addition, several investigators have shown that activation of LOX-1 and AT1R is directly involved in the alteration of normal EC phenotype quiescent anti-inflammatory to an inflammatory phenotype, and this involves change in shape and internal structure [67-69].

In conclusion, Ang II and ox-LDL have a synergistic or complementary effect on ECs and SMCs which leads to cell proliferation, apoptosis, inflammation and angiogenesis. The dysfunction and injury of these cells are causally involved in the pathogenesis of atherosclerosis and other vascular diseases. The NADPH oxidase-ROS signaling pathway is the "bridge" in their interplay.

IV. Cross-Talk between LOX-1 and AT1R in Atherosclerosis

It is generally acknowledged that atherosclerosis is a multifactoral pathological process, and there is considerable evidence that dyslipidemia, especially increase in ox-LDL, and activation of RAS play a considerable role in initiation of atherosclerosis [9, 70]. Ox-LDL and Ang II cause oxidative injury to ECs and SMCs in the arterial wall, and initiate an inflammatory state [9, 71-73]. Increasing evidence suggests that both LOX-1 and AT1R are upregulated in atherosclerotic tissues, and their interplay via ROS generation, cell apoptosis, inflammation and fibrosis, is critically important in the pathophysiology of atherosclerosis.

Clinical and experimental studies show that LOX-1 expression and activation are also increased in atherosclerotic intima [74]. Ox-LDL accumulation accelerates atherosclerotic plaque formation. Intracellular ox-LDL causes oxidative damage in endothelial ECs, SMCs and macrophages, and promotes their apoptosis [75]. LOX-1 mediates ox-LDL internalization, which leads to lipid accumulation, oxidative injury, endothelial dysfunction and foam cell formation. Vascular dysfunction and foam cell formation are the early first step of atherogenesis.

RAS plays an important role in atherogenesis, and several of RAS modulators, like ACE inhibitors and AT1R blocker (ARB), are frequently used in clinic to prevent the progress of atherosclerosis. Accumulating evidence suggests that all components of RAS are upregulated in atherosclerotic tissues [76]. Chronic infusion of Ang II has been demonstrated to promote the atherosclerotic lesion formation in arch, thoracic, and abdominal aorta in the LDL receptor (LDLr) null mice [77].

Pharmacologic intervention with ACE inhibitors or ARBs has been shown to interfere with atherogenesis. Our group observed that use of ARBs, such as rosuvastatin and candesartan, decreased atherosclerosis (by 23 and 26%, respectively) in mice fed a high cholesterol-diet. Others have also shown that ACE inhibitors and ARBs prevent the progression of atherosclerosis [78]. Recent studies show that a direct renin inhibitor Aliskiren inhibits atherosclerotic development and improves plaque stability in APOE*3Leiden.CETP mice [79]. Although different ARBs inhibit atherogenesis through somewhat different mechanisms, generally all ARBs inhibit NADPH oxidase expression and ROS generation, thereby attenuate lipoprotein oxidation.

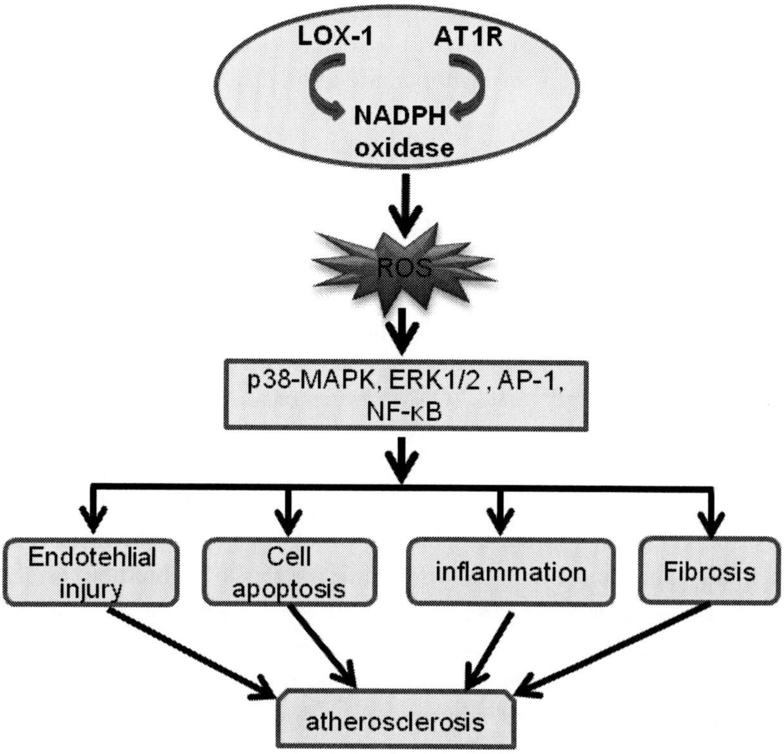

Figure 3. Summary of the signaling and roles of AT1R and LOX-1 in atherosclerosis. AT1R and LOX-1 both stimulate ROS generation by NADPH oxidase, and then trigger the activation of p38MAPK, ERK1/2, AP-1 an NF-κB, which causes endothelial injury, cell apoptosis, inflammation, and fibrosis in aorta, and finally initiates the formation of atherosclerosis.

In addition, ARBs may influence atherogenesis by inhibition of inflammation. Recently, Matsumura et al. reported that telmisartan, but not other ARBs, inhibited inflammatory gene expression and ox-LDL-induced macrophage migration [80].

ROS is involved in the initiation and progression of atherosclerosis. High levels of ROS are present in vascular tissues destined to develop atherosclerosis. Actually, atherosclerosis is thought to result in part from a balance between oxidative stress and antioxidants in the arterial wall. Some investigators have reported that antioxidant drugs prevent the progress of atherosclerosis [23, 71, 81, 82]. For example, Zhao et al. showed that dietary supplementation with vitamin E attenuated atherosclerosis in apoE-/- mice [81]. Chen et al from our laboratory showed that the calcium channel blocker amlodipine and the 3-hydroxy-3-methyl-glutaryl-CoA (HMG-CoA) reductase inhibitor reduced atherogenesis in the New Zealand White (NZW) rabbits fed a high-cholesterol diet, and postulated that the inhibition of LDL oxidation contributed to the anti-atherosclerotic effect of these agents [82]. However, other studies failed to show inhibition of atherogenesis by vitamin E [83-85]. Other recent studies have shown that candesartan modestly reduces ROS generation and LOX-1 expression with a concurrent reduction of atherosclerosis in the ApoE -/- mice; importantly the HMG CoA reducatse inhibitor rosuvastatin also reduced ROS generation, LOX-1 expression and atherosclerosis. Most importantly, simultaneous administration had a dramatic effect on inhibition of ROS generation and LOX-1 expression and on the extent of atherosclerosis [86].

As mentioned previously, ROS is the 'signal bridge' between LOX-1 and AT1R, and also the foundation of the interplay of the two receptors in atherogenesis. Activation of both receptors promotes atherogenesis through increase of oxidative stress and inflammation in the arterial tissues.

Apoptosis is seen in ECs, SMCs and macrophages in the developing atherosclerotic plaque as well as in fully developed plaque, particularly in the unstable region. Recent studies have suggested that *a*poptosis plays different roles in the different stages of atherosclerosis. In the early stage, apoptosis inhibits the progression of atherosclerotic plaques; however, in the advanced stage, apoptosis promotes the development of necrotic-core in the plaque, and makes the plaques unstable and prone to rupture [87]. Ox-LDL causes cell apoptosis in vascular system via increase of oxidative stress and oxidative damages [88]. Studies from our laboratory have demonstrated that LOX-1 is extensively expressed in ECs, SMCs, macrophages and new-formed blood vessels in the core of advanced atherosclerotic lesions, and significantly increased in atherosclerotic grafted vein and carotid artery specimens [57]. In the plaque, LOX-1 expression is mainly localized in apoptotic cells [57]. Ang II also triggers apoptosis in the atherosclerotic plaques, which accelerates the onset and progression of atherosclerosis. The potent anti-atherosclerotic effects of inhibition of RAS by ACE inhibitors and AT1R antagonists are, at least in part, based on their interference with apoptotic and angiogenic processes leading ultimately to plaque stabilization and reduced coronary event rate. On the other hand, some studies suggest that strategies that enhance the regression or inhibit progression of atherosclerosis are associated with increased apoptosis [89]. The precise role of apoptosis in atherosclerosis, therefore, at this time remains unclear.

Basic and clinical research shows that inflammation and atherosclerosis proceed in parallel [90]. Inflammation has been identified at all stages of atherosclerosis [91]. Actually, atherosclerosis is a result of chronic inflammatory reaction of the arterial wall. The early stage of atherogenesis is characterized by activation of ECs resulting in expression of adhesion molecules. Blood leukocytes, mediators of inflammation, are also found localizing in the earliest lesions of atherosclerosis [91]. Leukocyte adhesion to ECs is a key step in the formation of atherosclerotic plaques and acceleration of atherogenesis [92], since deletion of a number of inflammatory steps has been shown to limit atherogenesis [9, 94]. Many cells within the atherosclerotic intima highly express intercellular cell adhesion molecule-1 (ICAM-1) and VCAM-1 [95]. Up-regulation of adhesion molecules, especially VCAM-1 in ECs and VSMCs is believed to be a specific molecular marker of initial of atherogenesis [90].

Activation of LOX-1 initiates inflammation. LOX-1 activation via ox-LDL induces the phosphorylation of p38MAPK and activates NF-κB signaling, which then stimulates the expression of inflammatory molecules such as interleukins and adhesion molecules in ECs, and enhances leukocytes adhesion [96]. A recent study shows that LOX-1 is one of the receptors for C-reactive protein (CRP), a recognized factor for atherosclerosis [97]. Shih et al. observed the direct binding of CRP with LOX-1 in human EC membrane and induction of inflammatory genes including interleukin 8 (IL-8), ICAM-1, and VCAM-1 [90]. In addition, LOX-1 itself is also an adhesive molecule and displays adhesive properties. As such, it has been identified as one of pro-inflammatory genes.

Ang II is also a critical factor in inflammation [98, 99]. It via AT1R stimulates the expression of a number of pro-inflammatory genes such as interleukins, VCAM-1 and MCP-1, and promotes vascular dysfunction and facilitates the development of atherosclerotic plaques [98,100]. Pan et al. reported that Ang II promotes inflammatory gene expression in cultured human ECs and VSMCs, which can be abrogated by pretreatment of cells with an ARB. In vivo studies showed that AT1R activation led to vascular inflammation in animal model [99]. We have recently observed that Ang II can upregulate its own receptors- such as AT1R and AT2R [38]. It should also be mentioned that AT2R activation serves to modulate the inflammation caused by AT1R expression [101]. In cardiovascular disease states, like atherosclerosis and myocardial ischemia, expression of both AT1R and AT2R is activated; AT2R expression may reduce the tissues injurious effect of AT1R upregulation.

In addition, LOX-1 and AT1R expressions have also been observed to be upregulated by inflammatory factors, such as tumor necrosis factor-a (TNF-a), transforming growth factor (TGF), lipopolysaccharide (LPS). Both LOX-1 and AT1R are up-regulated in inflammatory states and/or in atherosclerotic arteries, and their activation accelerates the inflammatory progress in atherogenesis [61].

It is known that the presence of fibrous elements and collagen accumulation in the arterial wall is one of the determinants of atherogenesis and its clinical presentations [102]. Collagens are important components of atherosclerotic plaques and constitute about 60% of the total plaque protein. The formation of collagens contributes to plaque growth and accelerates arterial lumen narrowing [102]. Collagens to some extent stimulate atherosclerotic lesion formation and progression via modulation of EC and macrophage functions and SMC proliferation [102]. A firm fibrotic plaque is a hallmark of a stable lesion. A stable plaque forms with a thick fibrous cap and a small lipid core. The unstable plaque has a higher probability to rupture than fibrotic plaque.

LOX-1 activation also promotes the accumulation of collagen. Hu et al. reported that LOX-1 expression regulated collagen accumulation [103]. These authors found that $TGF\beta_1$-mediated collagen formation in fibroblasts was a critical component of LOX-1's function, especially in the state of NADPH oxidase activation and increased ROS generation.

Further studies by these authors showed that LOX-1 deletion could decrease collagen accumulation in atherosclerotic plaques in LDLr null mice. LOX-1 deletion could normalize the expression and activity of matrix metalloproteinases (MMPs). Of note, direct blockade of LOX-1 using LOX-1 antibodies or deletion of LOX-1 attenuates collagen formation in fibroblasts or in atherosclerotic plaque in LOX-1 KO mice fed a high-cholesterol diet [103, 104].

Accumulating evidence suggests that Ang II promotes myocardial and perivascular fibrosis [105]. Many studies have demonstrated that Ang II induces proliferation in cardiac fibroblasts via activation of AT1R [106, 107]. Crabos et al. reported Ang II induces c-fos expression and increases collagen DNA, RNA and protein expressions in cardiac fibroblasts [107]. Ang II also induces secretion of MMPs in cardiac fibroblasts. Chen et al. found AT1R activation via Ang II induces procallagen-1 expression, which is mediated by the increase of ROS followed by the activation p38MAPK, ERK1/2, activator protein 1 (AP-1) and NF-κB [108]. Use of antioxidants, pravastatin and pioglitazone, significantly reduces procollagen-1 expression [108]. More importantly, Ang II has been also found to promote aortic adventitial fibroblasts proliferation and collagen synthesis [62, 63].

Other recent studies have shown that AT1R activation increases the expression of collagens and MMPs in ECs as well as in VSMCs [109, 110]. Activation of both LOX-1 and AT1R enhances collagen formation, and blockade of both receptors is necessary for inhibition of cardiac and arterial fibrosis.

These observations suggest a cross-talk between LOX-1 and AT1R in relation to development of fibrosis, the process of atherogenesis proceeds.

In conclusion, both ox-LDL and Ang II play a key role in the pathogenesis of atherosclerosis. Ox-LDL and Ang II induce changes that lead to EC dysfunction and apoptosis, ROS generation, oxidative damage, acute or chronic inflammation, cell proliferation and migration and fibrosis through activating their receptors, mainly LOX-1 and AT1R. All these harmful features are important for atherogenesis.

Blocking LOX-1 and AT1R, or deletion of LOX-1 and AT1R has been demonstrated to mitigate atherosclerosis. Drugs acting on RAS and certain antioxidants delay the progress of atherosclerosis. The cross-talk between LOX-1 and AT1R in atherogenesis suggests that a combination therapy designed to block RAS and LOX-1 may be more useful than the one that affects only one pathway.

V. Cross-Talk between LOX-1 and AT1R in Hypertension

Activation of AT1R induces vasoconstriction, sodium and water retention, neurohumoral activation, increases vascular ROS production, and leads to increase of blood pressure [4, 26]. Increased renin production and angiotensinogen expression can activate AT1R, leading to high blood pressure, associated with typical organ complications [4, 26]. In human, there is an ongoing debate whether gene polymorphisms within the ACE, renin, or AT1R genes – which could presumably increase AT1R activation – contributes to the development of hypertension or cardiovascular events.

The correlation between these gene alterations and blood-pressure elevation is usually not overwhelmingly tight, supposedly because hypertension is a disease initiated by multiple exogenous and endogenous factors. In contrast to the predominant essential hypertension, some forms of secondary hypertension are often exclusively driven by an activated RAS.

For example, renal diseases and renovascular stenotic diseases are propagated by increased renin production and subsequently enhanced AT1R stimulation by increased levels of circulating Ang II. In addition, hypertensive patients with signs of an activated RAS, as evidenced by increased circulating renin levels, experience higher cardiovascular event rates. Thus, RAS along with the AT1R activation contributes significantly to the onset and progression of most forms of hypertension, although the precise role of the RAS in the etiology of essential hypertension remains obscure.

Additional evidence for the pivotal relevance of the AT1R in hypertension is derived from multiple clinical trials which show effective blood-pressure reduction by ACE inhibitors and ARBs. Moreover, a recent interventional study revealed superiority of an ARB in comparison with traditional blood-pressure-lowering drugs, suggesting that besides mere blood-pressure reduction, blockade of the AT1R offers additional benefits for vascular and myocardial biology [111]. Although LOX-1 mRNA expression is minimal in normal arterial tissues, it is markedly upregulated in vascular tissues of spontaneously hypertensive animals, suggesting a possible role of LOX-1 in hypertension [26, 112]. Hu et al indeed showed recently that LOX-1 null mice have attenuated hypertensive response to Ang II [113]. These findings suggest that LOX-1 participates in the progression of hypertension. This concept is also supported by in vitro observations that ox-LDL stimulates AT1R expression.

Cardiac remodeling is initially an adaptive response to several forms of cardiac stress states, such as hypertension. RAS and its effector hormone, Ang II, have well-known endocrine properties that contribute to cardiac remodeling and heart failure [112].

Work in our laboratory showed that the Ang II (AT1R)-ROS-LOX-1 loop directly regulates the development of cardiac remodeling in mice with Ang II–induced hypertension. Chen et al had previously shown that the overexpression of LOX-1 in rat cardiac fibroblasts enhances the expression of collagen I and the phosphorylation of p38MAPK [114].

As discussed earlier, studies have also shown that Ang II via AT1R activation stimulates the expression of LOX-1. In turn, activation of LOX-1 increases AT1R expression. Activation of both AT1R and LOX-1 induces a state of oxidative stress. In addition, activation of both AT1R and LOX-1 enhances the growth of cardiac fibroblasts and promotes collagen synthesis [4].

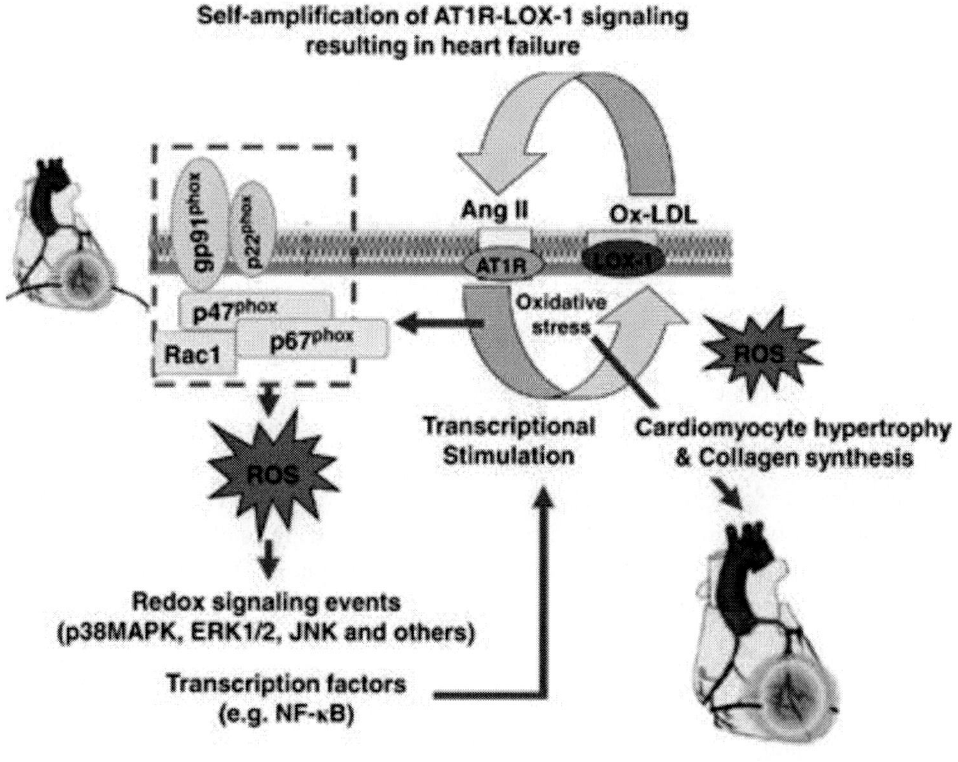

Figure 4. Feedback between AT1R, LOX-1 and NADPH oxidase in heart failure. ROS play an important role in the cross-talk between LOX-1 and AT1R. Angiotensin II induces oxidative stress and ROS generation via AT1R transcription. This process is NADPH oxidase-dependent. Intense oxidant stress, particularly in the infarct-prone region (AAR), induces the upregulation of NF-κB, leading to LOX-1 transcription and activation in the ischemic myocardium. The upregulation of LOX-1 further stimulates ROS generation, which enhances AT1R transcription and activation. The so-called 'ischemia begets ischemia' concept may be the result of a positive feedback between AT1R, LOX-1 and NADPH oxidase. Of note, this positive feedback triggers pathological cardiac remodeling. Our work shows that LOX-1 inhibition provides protection against AT1R-mediated oxidant stress and LV functional deterioration during chronic ischemia and improves animal survival.

VI. Cross-Talk between LOX-1 and AT1R in Myocardial Ischemia and Remodeling

Heart failure is the leading cause of morbidity in the world, and chronic myocardial ischemia is perhaps the most common cause of heart failure [115]. Post-myocardial infarct remodeling has been divided into an early phase (within 72 h) and a late phase (after 72 h). The early phase involves expansion of the infarct zone. The non-infarcted zone undergoes progressive pathological remodeling 1-2-months after the acute ischemic injury, when cardiomyocyte hypertrophy and interstitial fibrosis ensue, resulting in progressive left ventricular (LV) enlargement. The process of cardiac remodeling is initiated and amplified by a host of biochemical alterations with a major role for RAS. Accordingly, RAS modulators are frequently used in the treatment of patients with heart failure.

ROS are released in large amounts in the ischemic myocardium and lead to oxidant stress [116-118]. ROS generation and release, although high in the early phase of myocardial ischemia, can be detected in the circulating blood of animals for a long time after myocardial ischemia. The ischemic myocardium shows intense expression of AT1R and AT2R as well as LOX-1. It is possible that the upregulation of AT1R, AT2R and LOX-1 is a response to ROS release [119]. Regardless of the precise contribution, oxidant load in response to AT1R and LOX-1 activation plays a key role in cardiomyocyte hypertrophy and growth of fibroblasts, which are precursors to the syndrome of heart failure [120]. As mentioned previously, LOX-1 and AT1R activation both are potent stimuli for endothelial and cardiomyocyte apoptosis [121]. Accordingly, LOX-1 deletion (by gene knockout or use of antibody) or AT1R blockers can reduce oxidant stress and inflammation, and modify infarct size and LV hemodynamics in animals subjected to brief period of myocardial ischemia [122].

While the role of LOX-1 activation during acute ischemia was documented many years back [122], the contribution of LOX-1 in chronic ischemia and the development of structural and molecular aspects of heart failure became evident only recently. Lu et al [119] performed total left coronary artery (LCA) occlusion in wild-type and LOX-1 null mice and followed these mice for 4 weeks. There was a marked improvement in the survival rate in LOX-1 null mice (vs the wild-type mice) over the first 6 h period following total LCA occlusion [121]. This probably reflects a marked reduction in ROS release in the LOX-1 null mice during the early phase of myocardial ischemia. The inflammatory response in the ischemic myocardium was also suppressed, in keeping with the results of a previous study that showed that rodents pretreated with LOX-1 antibody had improved survival after lipopolysaccharide administration, and implicated a markedly reduced inflammatory activity as the basis of this phenomenon [64].

During chronic ischemia, mice missing LOX-1 had smaller infarcts after LCA occlusion, despite similar area at risk (AAR) as the wild-type mice, and had improved survival. Importantly, cardiomyocyte hypertrophy and interstitial fibrosis were less marked in the LOX-1 null mice, suggesting a role for LOX-1 in cardiac remodeling process. The reduction in cardiomyocyte hypertrophy and interstitial fibrosis resulted in improved cardiac function, as assessed by echocardiographic and direct LV hemodynamic measurements. Further, these authors found that AT1R upregulated in the chronically ischemic hearts, and LOX-1 deletion reduced AT1R expression. Our in vitro studies showed that AT1R over-expression is the basis of cardiomyocyte hypertrophy and this phenomenon can be blocked by LOX-1 blockade [21].

It is of note that AT2R expression also upregulated in the chronically ischemic wild type mouse hearts studied by Lu et al [119]. The role of AT2R in this setting until now was unclear except that it has been postulated for a long time that AT2R opposes the effect of AT1R activation [7]. It is worth noting that besides reduction in AT1R expression, AT2R expression was also reduced in LOX-1 null mice subjected to ischemia. To define the precise role of AT1R and AT2R in cardiomyocyte hypertrophy, Wang et al transduced the cultured cardiomyocytes with AT1R and AT2R genes. Forced overexpression of AT1R, but not AT2R, resulted in enhanced NADPH activity, cardiomyocyte hypertrophy as well as LOX-1 expression.

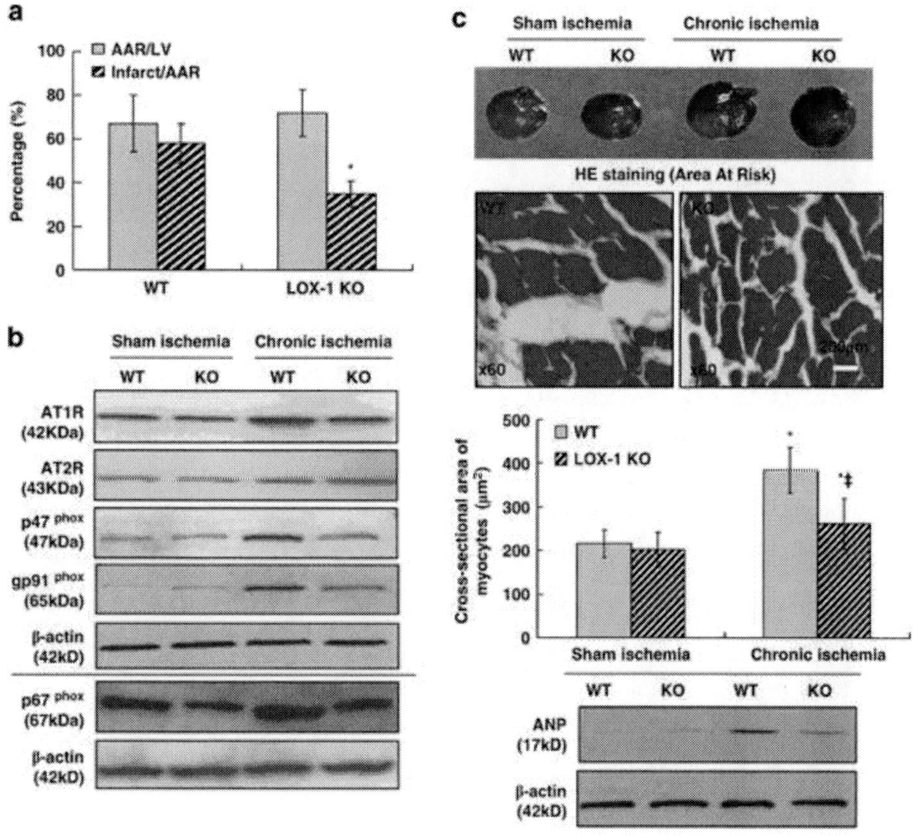

Figure 5. Amelioration of cardiac hypertrophy in LOX-1 KO mice as compared with wild-type (WT) mice. (a) Summary data on myocardial AAR and infarct size in WT chronic ischemia group and LOX-1 KO chronic ischemia group (n=6 in each group). There were no differences in AAR/LV between wild-type and LOX-1 KO mice groups. However, the LOX-1 KO mice had smaller infarcts than WT mice (38.2±6.7% vs 61.7±8.9% of AAR, *P<0.05). (b) Representative western blots of AT1R, AT2R, p47phox and gp91phox subunits of NADPH oxidase, atrial natriuretic peptide and β-actin expression in the four groups of mice (western blot analysis, n=4 in each group). (c) Representative pictures of hearts and histological sections of cardiomyocytes in AAR (magnification, × 600). Summary data on cardiomyocyte size are expressed as mean±s.d., based on 200 cardiomyocytes examined in each slice, and at least four slices examined in each heart. *P<0.05 compared to corresponding sham ischemia group; ‡P<0.05 compared to WT chronic ischemia.

Of note, overexpression of AT2R resulted in the downregulation of p67^{phox} subunits of NADPH oxidase and a small but significant reduction in LOX-1 expression in the cultured cardiomyocytes. These observations from transduction of cardiomyocytes in vitro suggest that AT2R overexpression in chronically ischemic hearts may serve to limit LOX-1 activation in vivo.

Other studies in chronically ischemic mice showed that the wild type mice developed extensive fibrosis in the perivascular region and between cardiac myocytes; this phenomenon was much less marked in the LOX-1 null mice [119]. Simultaneously performed in vitro studies showed that LOX-1 inhibition or abrogation can reduce fibroblast growth and collagen formation by cardiac fibroblasts via inhibition of NADPH oxidase activity [123]. NADPH oxidase activates MAPKs (p38, p44/42 and stress-activated protein kinase (SAPK)/JNK) and, thereafter, induces translocation of the redox-sensitive transcription factor NF-kB [124]. In keeping with this well-defined signaling pathway, Wang et al identified a marked increase in the expression of phos-p38MAPK, phos-JNK and phos-NF-kB p65 in the wild-type mice ischemic hearts, but not in the LOX-1 null mice hearts (vs wild-type mice) [119]. We believe this study is the first one to document persistent activation of this pathway in the LV during sustained ischemia and its attenuation in the LOX-1 null mice resulting in improved cardiac function.

Conclusion

Here, we summarized the latest findings on cross-talk between LOX-1 and RAS in cardiovascular system. LOX-1 and RAS activate each other and play a synergistic effect in the genesis and progress of atherosclerosis, hypertension, myocardial ischemia and remodeling. The cross-talk between LOX-1 and RAS (especially AT1R) in cardiovascular diseases suggests that combination of therapies designed to block RAS and LOX-1 may be more useful than those that affect only one pathway.

References

[1] Abd El-Aziz TA, Hussein YM, Mohamed RH, Shalaby SM. Renin-angiotensin system genes polymorphism in Egyptians with premature coronary artery disease. *Gene.* 2012, 498: 270-275.

[2] Mehta PK, Griendling KK. Angiotensin II cell signaling: physiological and pathological effects in the cardiovascular system. *Am. J. Physiol. Cell Physiol.* 2007, 292: C82-C97.

[3] Lamparter S, Sun Y, Weber KT. Angiotensin II receptor blockade during gestation attenuates collagen formation in the developing rat heart. *Cardiovasc. Res.* 1999, 43: 165-172.

[4] Wang X, Phillips MI, Mehta JL. LOX-1 and angiotensin receptors, and their interplay. *Cardiovasc. Drugs Ther.* 2011, 25: 401-417.

[5] Dimitrijevic I, Rissler P, Luts L, Edvinsson L. Reduced expression of angiotensin II and angiotensin receptor type 1 and type 2 in resistance arteries from nasal lesions in granulomatosis with polyangiitis (Wegener's granulomatosis). *Scand. J. Rheumatol.* 2011, 40: 448-452.

[6] Sander GE, MaKinnie JJ, Greenberg SS, Giles TD. Angiotensin-converting enzyme inhibitors and angiotensin II receptor antagonists in the treatment of heart failure caused by left ventricular systolic dysfunction. *Prog. Cardiovasc. Dis.* 1999, 41: 265-300.

[7] Karpe PA, Gupta J, Marthong RF, Ramarao P, Tikoo K. Insulin resistance induces a segmental difference in thoracic and abdominal aorta: differential expression of AT1 and AT2 receptors. *J. Hypertens.* 2012, 30: 132-146.

[8] Jia L, Li Y, Xiao C, Du J. Angiotensin II induces inflammation leading to cardiac remodeling. *Front Biosci.* 2012, 17: 221-231.

[9] Mitra S, Deshmukh A, Sachdeva R, Lu J, Mehta JL. Oxidized low-density lipoprotein and atherosclerosis implications in antioxidant therapy. *Am. J. Med. Sci.* 2011, 342: 135-142.

[10] Sawamura T, Kume N, Aoyama T, Moriwaki H, Hoshikawa H, Aiba Y, Tanaka T, Miwa S, Katsura Y, Kita T, Masaki T. An endothelial receptor for oxidized low-density lipoprotein. *Nature.* 1997, 386: 73-77.

[11] Murphy JE, Tedbury PR, Homer-Vanniasinkam S, Walker JH, Ponnambalam S. Biochemistry and cell biology of mammalian scavenger receptors. *Atherosclerosis.* 2005, 182: 1-15.

[12] Sawamura T, Kakino A, Fujita Y. LOX-1: a multiligand receptor at the crossroads of response to danger signals. *Curr. Opin. Lipidol.* 2012, 23: 439-445.

[13] Yamagata K, Miyashita A, Chino M, Matsufuji H. Apigenin inhibits tumor necrosis factor alpha plus high glucose-induced LOX-1 expression in human endothelial cells. *Microvasc. Res.* 2011, 81: 60-67.

[14] Morawietz H, Rueckschloss U, Niemann B, Duerrschmidt N, Galle J, Hakim K, Zerkowski HR, Sawamura T, Holtz J. Angiotensin II induces LOX-1, the human endothelial receptor for oxidized low-density lipoprotein. *Circulation.* 1999, 100: 899-902.

[15] Keidar S, Attias J. Angiotensin II injection into mice increases the uptake of oxidized LDL by their mcrophages via a proteoglycan-mediated pathway. *Biochem. Biophys. Res. Commun.* 1997, 239: 63-67.

[16] Keidar S, Kaplan M, Hoffman A, Aviram M. Angiotensin II stimulates macrophages mediated oxidation of low density lipoproteins. *Atherosclerosis.* 1995, 115: 201-215.

[17] Li D, Zhang YC, Philips MI, Sawamura T, Mehta JL. Upregulation of endothelial receptor for oxidized low-density lipoprotein (LOX-1) in cultured human coronary artery endothelial cells by angiotensin II type 1 receptor activation. *Circ. Res.* 1999, 84: 1043-1049.

[18] Ge J, Huang D, Liang C, Luo Y, Jia Q, Wang K. Upregulation of lectinlike oxidized low-density lipoprotein receptor-1 expression contributes to the vein graft atherosclerosis: modulation by losartan. *Atherosclerosis.* 2004, 177: 263-268.

[19] Nickenig G, Wassmann S, Böhm M. Regulation of the angiotensin AT1 receptor by hypercholesterolaemia. *Diabetes Obes. Metab.* 2000, 2: 223-228.

[20] Yang BC, Phillips MI, Mohuczy D, Meng H, Shen L, Mehta P, Mehta JL. Increased angiotensin II type 1 receptor expression in hypercholesterolemic atherosclerosis in rabbits. *Arterioscler. Thromb. Vasc. Biol.* 1998, 18: 1433-1439.

[21] Kang BY, Mehta JL. Rosuvastatin attenuates Ang-II mediated cardiomyocyte hypertrophy via inhibition of LOX-1. *J. Cardiovasc. Pharmacol. Ther.* 2009, 14: 283-291.

[22] Dandapat A, Hu C, Sun L, Mehta JL. Small concentrations of oxLDL induce capillary tube formation from endothelial cells via LOX-1-dependent redox-sensitive pathway. *Arterioscler. Thromb. Vasc. Biol.* 2007, 27: 2435-2442.

[23] Bedard K, Krause KH. The NOX family of ROS-generating NADPH oxidases: physiology and pathophysiology. *Physiol. Rev.* 2007, 87: 245-313.

[24] Han C, Liu J, Liu X, Li M. Angiotensin II induces C-reactive protein expression through ERK1/2 and JNK signaling in human aortic endothelial cells. *Atherosclerosis.* 2010, 212: 206-212.

[25] Zhang C, Zhao YX, Zhang YH, Zhu L, Deng BP, Zhou ZL, Li SY, Lu XT, Song LL, Lei XM, Tang WB, Wang N, Pan CM, Song HD, Liu CX, Dong B, Zhang Y, and Cao Y. Angiotensin-converting enzyme 2 attenuates atherosclerotic lesions by targeting vascular cells. *Proc. Natl. Acad. Sci. U S A.* 2010, 107: 15886–15891.

[26] Lu J, Mitra S, Wang X, Khaidakov M, Mehta JL. Oxidative stress and lectin-like ox-LDL-receptor LOX-1 in atherogenesis and tumorigenesis. *Antioxid. Redox. Signal.* 2011, 15: 2301-2333.

[27] Mehta JL, Chen J, Hermonat PL, Romeo F, Novelli G. Lectin-like, oxidized low-density lipoprotein receptor-1 (LOX-1): a critical player in the development of atherosclerosis and related disorders. *Cardiovasc. Res.* 2006, 69: 36-45.

[28] Seibold S, Schürle D, Heinloth A, Wolf G, Wagner M, Galle J. Oxidized LDL induces proliferation and hypertrophy in human umbilical vein endothelial cells via regulation of p27Kip1 expression: role of RhoA. *J. Am. Soc. Nephrol.* 2004, 15: 3026-3034.

[29] Hamilton JA, Myers D, Jessup W, Cochrane F, Byrne R, Whitty G, Moss S. Oxidized LDL can induce macrophage survival, DNA synthesis, and enhanced proliferative response to CSF-1 and GM-CSF. *Arterioscler. Thromb. Vasc. Biol.* 1999, 19: 98-105.

[30] Zettler ME, Prociuk MA, Austria JA, Masaeli H, Zhong G, Pierce GN. OxLDL stimulates cell proliferation through a general induction of cell cycle proteins. *Am. J. Physiol. Heart Circ. Physiol.* 2003, 284: H644-H653.

[31] Yu S, Wong SL, Lau CW, Huang Y, Yu CM. Oxidized LDL at low concentration promotes in-vitro angiogenesis and activates nitric oxide synthase through PI3K/Akt/eNOS pathway in human coronary artery endothelial cells. *Biochem. Biophys. Res. Commun.* 2011, 407: 44-48.

[32] Kang BY, Khan JA, Ryu S, Shekhar R, Seung KB, Mehta JL. Curcumin reduces angiotensin II-mediated cardiomyocyte growth via LOX-1 inhibition. *J. Cardiovasc. Pharmacol.* 2010, 55:176-183.

[33] Wang X, Khaidakov M, Ding Z, Mitra S, Lu J, Dai Y, Mehta JL. LOX-1 and cardiac fibroblast growth. *Hypertension.* 2012, 60: 1437-1442.

[34] Hu C, Dandapat A, Mehta JL. Angiotensin II induces capillary formation from endothelial cells via LOX-1 dependent redox-sensitive pathway. *Hypertension.* 2007, 50: 952-957.

[35] Yang LL, Li DY, Zhang YB, Zhu MY, Chen D, Xu TD. Salvianolic acid A inhibits angiotension II-induced proliferation of human umbilical vein endothelial cells by attenuating the production of ROS. *Acta Pharmacol. Sin.* 2012, 33: 41-48.
[36] Herr D, Rodewald M, Fraser HM, Hack G, Konrad R, Kreienberg R, Wulff C. Regulation of endothelial proliferation by the rennin-angiotension system in human vein endothelial cells. *Reproduction.* 2008, 136: 125-130.
[37] Daemen MJ, Lombardi DM, Bosman FT, Schwartz SM. Angiotensin II induces smooth muscle cell proliferation arterial wall. *Circ. Res.* 1991, 68: 450-456.
[38] Wang X, Lu J, Khaidakov M, Mitra S, Ding Z, Raina S, Goyal T, Mehta JL. Aspirin suppresses cardiac fibroblast proliferation and collagen formation through downregulation of angiotensin type 1 receptor transcription. *Toxicol. Appl. Pharmacol.* 2012, 259: 346-354.
[39] Kim YH, Han HJ. Synergistic effect of high glucose and ANG II on proliferation of mouse embryonic stem cells: involvement of PKC and MAPKs as well as AT1 receptor. *J. Cell Physiol.* 2008, 215: 374-382.
[40] Rodgers KE, Xiong S, Steer R, diZerega GS. Effect of angiotensin II on hematopoietic progenitor cell proliferation. *Stem Cells.* 2000, 18: 287-294.
[41] Du N, Feng J, Hu LJ, Sun X, Sun HB, Zhao Y, Yang YP, Ren H. Angiotension II receptor type 1 blockers suppress the cell proliferation effects of angiotensin II in breast cancer cells by inhibiting AT1R signaling. *Oncol. Rep.* 27: 1893-1903.
[42] Kang BY, Hu C, Ryu S, Khan JA, Biancolella M, Prayaga S, Seung KB, Novelli G, Mehta P, Mehta JL. Genomics of cardiac remodeling in angiotensin II-treated wild-type and LOX-1-deficient mice. *Physiol. Genomics.* 2010, 42: 42-54.
[43] Fernandez LA, Twickler J, Mad A. Neovascularization produced by angiotension II. *J. Lab. Clin. Med.* 1985, 105: 141-145.
[44] Fujiyama S, Matsubara H, Nozawa Y, Maruyama K, Mori Y, Tsuysumi Y, Masaki H, Uchiyama Y, Koyama Y, Nose A, Iba O, Tateishi E, Ogata N, Jyo N, Higashiyama S, Iwasaka T. Angiotensin AT(1) and AT(2) receptors differentially regulate angiopoietin-2 and vascular endothelial growth factor expression and angiogenesis by modulating heparin binding-epidermal growth factor (EGF)-mediated EGF receptor transactivation. *Circ. Res.* 2001, 88: 22-29.
[45] Dimmeler S, Rippmann V, Weiland U, Haedeler J, Zeiher AM. Angiotensin induces apoptosis of human endothelial cells. Protective effect of nitric oxide. *Cir. Res.* 1997, 81: 970-976.
[46] Li D, Yang B, Philips MI, Mehta JL. Proapoptotic effects of ANG II in human artery endothelial cells: role of AT1 receptor and PKC activation. *Am. J. Physiol.* 1999, 276: H786-H792.
[47] Vivar R, Soto C, Copaja M, Mateluna F, Aranguiz P, Muñoz JP, Chiong M, Garcia L, Letelier A, Thomas WG, Lavandero S, Díaz-Araya G. Phospholipase C/protein kinase C pathway mediates angiotensin II-dependent apoptosis in neonatal rat cardiac fibroblasts expressing AT1 receptor. *J. Cardiovasc. Pharmacol.* 2008, 52: 184-190.
[48] Bascands JL, Girolami JP, Troly M, Escargueil-Blanc I, Nazzal D, Salvayre R, Blaes N. Angiotensin II induces phenotype-dependent apoptosis in vascular smooth muscle cells. *Hypertension.* 2001, 38: 1294-1299.

[49] Grishko V, Pastukh V, Solodushko V, Gillespie M, Azuma J, Schaffer S. Apoptotic cascade initiated by angiotensin II in neonatal cardiomyocytes: role of DNA damage. *Am. J. Physiol. Heart Circ. Physiol.* 2003, 285: H2364-2372.

[50] Bhaskaran M, Reddy K, Radhakrishanan N, Franki N, Ding G, Singhal PC. Angiotensin II induces apoptosis in renal proximal tubular cells. *Am. J. Physiol. Renal. Physiol.* 2003, 284: F955-F965.

[51] Zhao Y, Chen X, Cai L, Yang Y, Sui G, Wu J. Angiotensin II suppresses adriamycin-induced apoptosis through activation of phosphatidylinositol 3-kinase/Akt signaling in human breast cancer cells. *Acta Biochim. Biophys. Sin.* 2008, 40: 304-310.

[52] Amaya K, Ohta T, Kitagawa H, Kayahara M, Takamura H, Fujimura T, Nishimura G, Shimizu K, Miwa K. Angiotensin II activates MAP kinase and NF-kappaB through angiotensin II type I receptor in human pancreatic cancer cells. *Int. J. Oncol.* 2004, 25: 849-856.

[53] Nagashima H, Sakomura Y, Aoka Y, Uto K, Kameyama Ki, Ogawa M, Aomi S, Koyanagi H, Ishizuka N, Naruse M, Kawana M, Kasanuki H. Angiotensin II type 2 receptor mediates vascular smooth muscle cell apoptosis in cystic medial degeneration associated with Marfan's syndrome. *Circulation.* 2001, 104: 1282-1287

[54] Tan NY, Li JM, Stocker R, Khachiqian LM. Angiotensin II-inducible smooth muscle cell apoptosis involves the angiotensin II type 2 receptor, GATA-6 activation, and FasL-Fas engagement. *Circ. Res.* 2009, 105: 422-430.

[55] Li D, Mehta JL. Upregulation of endothelial receptor for oxidized LDL (LOX-1) by oxidized LDL and implications in apoptosis of human coronary artery endothelial cells: evidence from use of antisense LOX-1 mRNA and chemical inhibitors. *Arterioscler. Thromb. Vasc. Biol.* 2000, 20: 1116-1122.

[56] Chen J, Mehta JL, Haider N, Zhang X, Narula J, Li D. Role of caspases in ox-LDL-induced apoptotic cascade in human coronary artery endotelial cells. *Circ. Res.* 2004, 94: 370-376.

[57] Li DY, Chen HJ, Staples ED, Ozaki K, Annex B, Singh BK, Vermani R, Mehta JL. Oxidized low-density lipoprotein receptor LOX-1 and apoptosis in human atherosclerotic lesions. *J. Cardiovasc. Pharmacol. Ther.* 2002, 2: 147-153.

[58] Li D, Mehta JL. Intracellular signaling of LOX-1 in endothelial cell apoptosis. *Circ. Res.* 2009, 104: 566-568.

[59] Xu Y, Ruan S, Xie H, Lin J. Role of LOX-1 in Ang II-induced oxidative functional damage in renal tubular epithelial cells. *Int. J. Mol. Med.* 2010, 25: 679-690.

[60] Griendling KK, Ushio-Fukai M, Lassègue B, Alexander RW. Angiotensin II signaling in vascular smooth muscle cells: new concepts. *Hypertension.*1997, 29: 366-373.

[61] Tummala PE, Chen XL, Sundell CL, Laursen JB, Hammes CP, Alexander RW, Harrison DG, Medford RM. Angiotensin II induces vascular cell adhesion molecule-1 expression in rat vasculature: potential link between the renin-angiotensin system and atherosclerosis. *Circulation.*1999, 100: 1223-1229.

[62] Mackness B, Hine D, Liu Y, Mastorikou M, Mackness M. Paraoxonase-1 inhibits oxidised LDL-induced MCP-1 production by endothelial cells. *Biochem. Biophys. Res. Commun.* 2004, 318: 680-683.

[63] Aikawa M, Sugiyama S, Hill CC, Voglic SJ, Rabkin E, Fukumoto Y, Schoen FJ, Witztum JL, Libby P. Lipid lowering reduces oxidative stress and endothelial cell activation in rabbit atheroma. *Circulation.* 2002, 106: 1390-1396.

[64] Honjo M, Nakamura K, Yamashiro K, Kiryu J, Tanihara H, McEvoy LM, Honda Y, Butcher EC, Masaki T, Sawamura T. Lectin-like oxidized LDL receptor-1 is a cell-adhesion molecule involved in endotoxin-induced inflammation. *Proc. Narl. Acad. Sci. U S* A. 2003, 100: 1274-1279.

[65] Li D. Williams V, Liu L, Chen H, Sawamura T, Antakli T, Mehta JL. LOX-1 inhibition in myocardial ischemia-reperfusion injury: modulation of MMP-1 and inflammation. *Am. J. Physiol. Heart Circ. Physiol.* 2002, 283: H1795-H1801.

[66] Wu Z, Sawamura T, Kurdowska AK, Ji HL, Idell S, Fu J. LOX-1 deletion improves neutrophil responses, enhances bacterial clearance, and reduces lung injury in a murine polymicrobial sepsis model. *Infect. Immun.* 2011, 79: 2865-2870.

[67] Dworakowski R, Anilkumar N, Zhang M, Shah AM. Redox signalling involving NADPH oxidase-derived reactive oxygen species. *Biochem. Soc. Trans.* 2006, 34: 960-964.

[68] Irani K. Oxidant signaling in vascular cell growth, death, and survival: a review of the roles of reactive oxygen species in smooth muscle and endothelial cell mitogenic and apoptotic signaling. *Circ. Res.* 2000, 87: 179-183.

[69] Li JM, Shah AM. Endothelial cell superoxide generation: regulation and relevance for cardiovascular pathophysiology. *Am. J. Physiol. Regul. Integr. Comp. Physiol.* 2004, 287: R1014–R1030.

[70] Grote K, Drexler H, Schieffer B. Renin-angiotensin system and atherosclerosis. *Nephrol. Dial Transplant.* 2004, 19: 770-773.

[71] Ricciarelli R, Zingg JM, Azzi A. Vitamin E reduces the uptake of ooxidized LDL by inhibiting CD36 scavenger receptor expression in the cultured aortic smooth muscle cells. *Circulation.* 2000, 102: 82-87.

[72] Thatcher SE, Zhang X, Howatt DA, Lu H, Gurley SB, Daugherty A, Cassis LA. Angiotensin II-converting enzyme 2 deficiency in whole body or bone marrow-derived cells increases atherosclerosis in low-density lipoprotein receptor-/- mice. *Arterioscer. Thromb. Vasc. Biol.* 2011, 31: 758-765.

[73] Cha J, Ivanov V, Ivanova S, Kalinovsky T, Rath M, Niedzwiecki A. Evolution of angiotensin II-mediated atherosclerosis in ApoE KO mice. *Mol. Med. Report.* 2010, 3: 565-570.

[74] Kataoka H, Kume N, Miyamoto S, Minami M, Moriwaki H, Murase T, Sawamura T, Masaki T, Hashimoto N, Kita T. Expression of lectinlike oxidized low-density lipoprotein receptor-1 in human atherosclerotic lesions. *Circulation.* 1999, 99: 3110-3117.

[75] Boullier A, Bird DA, Chang MK, Dennis EA, Friedman P, Gillotre-taylor K, Hörkkö S, Palinski W, Quehenberger O, Shaw P, Steinberg D, Terpstra V, Witztum JL. Scavenger receptors, oxidized LDL, and atherosclerosis. *Ann. N. Y. Acad. Sci.* 2001, 947: 214-223.

[76] Weiss D, Sorescu D, Taylor WR. Angiotensin II and atherosclerosis. *Am. J. Cardiol.* 2001, 87: 25C-32C.

[77] Daugherty A, Cassis L. Chronic angiotensin II infusion promotes atherogenesis in low density lipoprotein receptor -/- mice. *Ann. N. Y. Acad. Sci.* 1999, 892: 108-118.

[78] Schiffrin EL, Canadian Institutes of Health Research Multidisciplinary Research Group on Hypertension. Beyond blood pressure: the endothelium and atherosclerosis progression. *Am. J. Hypertens.* 2002, 15: 115S-122S.

[79] Kühnast S, van der Hoorn JW, van den Hoek AM, Havekes LM, Liau G, Jukema JW, Princen HM. Aliskiren inhibits atherosclerosis development and improves plaque stability in APOE*Leiden.CETP transgenic mice with or without treatment with atorvastatin. *J. Hypertens*. 2012, 30: 107-116.

[80] Matsumura T, Kinoshita H, Ishii N, Fukuda K, Motoshima H, Senokuchi T, Taketa K, Kawasaki S, Nishimaki-Mogami T, Kawada T, Nishikawa T, Araki E. Telmisartan exerts antiatherosclerotic effects by activationg peroxisome proliferation-activated receptor-γ in macrophages. *Arterioscler. Thromb. Vasc. Biol.* 2011, 31: 1268-1275.

[81] Zhao L, Praticó D, Rader DJ, Funk CD. 12/15 -Lipoxygenase gene disruption and vitamin E administration diminish atherosclerosis and oxidative stress in apolipoprotein E deficient mice through a final common pathway. *Prostaglandins Other. Lipid Mediat.* 2005, 78: 185-193.

[82] Chen L, Haught WH, Yang B, Saldeen TG, Parathasarathy S, Mehta JL. Preservation of endogenous antioxidant activity and inhibition of lipid peroxidation as common mechanisms of antiatherosclerotic effects of vitamin E, lovastatin and amlodipine. *J. Am. Coll. Cardiol.* 1997, 30: 569-575.

[83] Chan AC. Vitamins and atherosclerosis. *J. Nutr*. 1998, 128: 1593-1596.

[84] Hasty AH, Gruen ML, Terry ES, Surmi BK, Atkinson RD, Gao L, Morrow JD. Effects of vitamin E on oxidative stress and atherosclerosis in an obese hyperlipidemic mouse model. *J. Nutr. Biochem*. 2007, 18: 217-133.

[85] Hatziqueorqiou C, Taylor AJ, Feuerstein IM, Bautista L, O'Malley PG. Antioxidant vitamin intake and subclinical coronary atherosclerosis. *Prev. Cardiol.* 2006, 9: 75-81.

[86] Chen J, Li D, Schaefer R, Mehta JL. Cross-talk between dyslipidemia and rennin-angiotensin system and the role of LOX-1 and MAPK in atherogenesis studies with the combined use of rosuvastatin and candesartan. *Atherosclerosis*. 2006, 184: 295-301.

[87] Stoneman VE, Bennett MR. Role of apoptosis in atherosclerosis and its therapeutic implications. *Clin. Sci.* (Lond). 2004, 107: 343-354.

[88] Novelli G, Mango R, Vecchione L, Mariotti E, Borgiani P, Mehta JL. Romeo F. New insights in atherosclerosis research: LOX-1, leading actor of cardiovascular disease. *Clin. Ter.* 2007, 158: 239-248.

[89] Purushothaman KR, Purushothaman M, Levy AP, Lento PA, Evrard S, Kovacic JC, Briley-Saebo KC, Tsimikas S, Witztum JL, Krishnan P, Kini A, Fayad ZA, Fuster V, Sharma SK, Moreno PR. Increased expression of oxidation-specific epitopes and apoptosis are associated with haptoglobin genotype: possible implications for plaque progression in human atherosclerosis. *J. Am. Coll. Cardiol*. 2012, 60: 112-129.

[90] Libby P. Inflammation in atherosclerosis. *Nature*. 2002, 420: 868-874.

[91] Libby P, Ridker PM, Maseri A. Inflammation and atherosclerosis. *Circulation*. 2001, 105: 1135-1143.

[92] Wright AP, Öhman MK, Hayasaki T, Luo W, Russo HM, Guo C, Eitzman DT. Atherosclerosis and leukocyte-endothelial adhesive interactions are increased following acute myocardial infarction in apolipoprotein E deficient mice. *Atherosclerosis*. 2010, 212: 414-417.

[93] Han X, Kitamoto S, Wang H, Biosvert WA. Interleukin-10 overexpression in macrophages suppresses atherosclerosis in hyperlipidemic mice. *FASEB J.* 2010, 24: 2869-2880.

[94] Charo IF, Taub R. Anti-inflammatory therapeutics for the treatment of atherosclerosis. *Nat. Rev. Drug Discov.* 2011, 10: 365-376.

[95] Libby P, Li H. Vascular cell adhesion molecule-1 and smooth muscle cell activation during atherogenesis. *J. Clin. Invest.* 1993, 92: 538-539.

[96] Lee WJ, Ou HC, Hsu WC, Chou MM, Tseng JJ, Hsu SL, Tsai KL, Sheu WH. Ellagic acid inhibits oxidized LDL-mediated LOX-1 expression, ROS generation, and inflammation in human endothelial cells. *J. Vasc. Surg.* 2010, 52: 1290-1300.

[97] Shih HH, Zhang S, Cao W, Hahn A, Wang J, Paulsen JE, Harnish DC. CRP is a novel ligand for the oxidized LDL receptor LOX-1. *Am. J. Physiol. Heart Circ. Physiol.* 2009, 296: H1643-H1650.

[98] Phillips MI, Kagiyama S. Angiotensin II as a pro-inflammatory mediator. *Curr. Opin. Investig. Drugs.* 2002, 3: 569-577.

[99] Pan P, Fu H, Zhang L, Huang H, Luo F, Wu W, Guo Y, Liu X. Angiotensin II upregulates the expression of placental growth factor in human vascular endothelial cells and smooth muscle cells. *BMC Cell Biol.* 2010, 11: 36.

[100] Nyby MD, Abedi K, Smutko V, Eslami P, Tuck ML. Vascular angiotensin type 1 receptor expression is associated with vascular dysfunction, oxidative stress and inflammation in fructose-fed rats. *Hypertens. Res.* 2007, 30: 451-457.

[101] Wang X, Lu J, Khaidakov M, Ding Z, Mitra S, Lu J, Liu S, Mehta JL. Cross-talk between inflammation and angiotensin II: Studies based on direct transfection of cardiomyocytes with AT1R and AT2R cDNA. *Exp. Biol. Med.* [Epub ahead of print].

[102] Rekhter MD. Collagen synthesis in atherosclerosis: too much and not enough. *Cardiovasc. Res.* 1999, 41: 376-384.

[103] Hu C, Dandapat A, Sun L, Khan JA, Liu T, Hermonat PL, Mehta JL. Regulation of TGFbeta1-mediated collagen formation by LOX-1: studies based on forced overexpression of TGFbeta1 in wild-type and lox-1 knock-out mouse cardiac fibroblasts. *J. Biol. Chem.* 2008, 283: 10226-10231.

[104] Hu C, Dandapat A, Sun L, Chen J, Marwali MR, Romeo F, Sawamura T, Mehta JL. LOX-1 deletion decreases collagen accumulation in atherosclerotic plaque in low-density lipoprotein receptor knockout mice fed a high-cholesterol diet. *Cardiovasc. Res.* 2008, 79: 287-293.

[105] Gelband CH, Katovich MJ, Raizada MK. Current perspectives on the use of gene therapy for hypertension. *Circ. Res.* 2000, 87: 1118-1122.

[106] Liou JY, Hong HJ, Sung LC, Chao HH, Chen PY, Cheng TH, Chan P, Liu JC. Nicorandil inhibits angiotensin-II-induced proliferation of cultured rat cardiac fibroblasts. *Pharmacology.* 2011, 87: 144-151.

[107] Crabos M, Roth M, Hahn AW, Erne P. Characterization of angiotensin II receptors in cultured adult rat cardiac fibroblasts. Coupling to signaling systems and gene expression. *J. Clin. Invest.* 1994, 93: 2372-2378.

[108] Chen J, Mehta JL. Angiotensin II-mediated oxidative stress and procollagen-1 expression in cardiac fibroblasts: blockade by pravastatin and pioglitazone. *Am. J. Physiol. Heart Cir. Physiol.* 2006, 291: H1738-H1745.

[109] Dab H, Kacem K, Hachani R, Dhaouadi N, Hodroj W, Sakly M, Randon J, Bricca G. Physiological regulation of extracellular matrix collagen and elastin in the arterial wall of rats by noradrenergic tone and angiotensin II. *J. Renin. Angiotensin Aldosterone Syst.* 2012, 13: 19-28.

[110] Arenas IA, Xu Y, Lopez-Jaramillo P, Davidge ST. Angiotensin II-induced MMP-2 release from endothelial cells is mediated by TNF-alpha. *Am. J. Physiol. Cell Physiol.* 2004, 286: C779-C784.
[111] Whaley-Connell A, Habibi J, Cooper SA, Demarco VG, Hayden MR, Stump CS, Link D, Ferrario CM, Sowers JR. Effect of renin inhibition and AT1R blockade on myocardial remodeling in the transgenic Ren2 rat. *Am. J. Physiol. Endocrinol. Metab.* 2008, 295: E103-E109.
[112] Paul M, Poyan Mehr A, Kreutz R. Physiology of local renin-angiotensin systems. *Physiol. Rev.* 2006, 86: 747-803.
[113] Hu C, Kang BY, Megyesi J, Kaushal GP, Safirstein RL, Mehta JL. Deletion of LOX-1 attenuates renal injury following angiotensin II infusion. *Kidney Int.* 2009, 76: 521-527.
[114] Chen K, Chen J, Liu Y, Xie J, Li D, Sawamura T, Hermonat PL, Mehta JL. Adhesion molecule expression in fibroblasts: alteration in fibroblast biology after transfection with LOX-1 plasmids. *Hypertension.* 2005, 46: 622-627.
[115] Ferdinandy P, Schulz R, Baxter GF. Interaction of cardiovascular risk factors with myocardial ischemia/reperfusion injury, preconditioning, and postconditioning. *Pharmacol. Rev.* 2007, 59: 418-58.
[116] Sorescu D, Griendling KK. Reactive oxygen species, mitochondria, and NAD(P)H oxidases in the development and progression of heart failure. *Congest Heart Fail.* 2002, 8: 132-140.
[117] Liu X, Gai Y, Liu F, Gao W, Zhang Y, Xu M, Li Z. Trimetazidine inhibits pressure overloadinduced cardiac fibrosis through NADPH oxidase-ROS-CTGF pathway. *Cardiovasc. Res.* 2010, 88: 150–158.
[118] Doerries C, Grote K, Hilfiker-Kleiner D, Luchtefeld M, Schaefer A, Holland SM, Sorrentino S, Manes C, Schieffer B, Drexler H, Landmesser Ul. Critical role of the NAD(P)H oxidase subunit p47phox for left ventricular remodeling/dysfunction and survival after myocardial infarction. *Circ. Res.* 2007, 100: 894–903.
[119] Lu J, Wang X, Wang W, Muniyappa H, Hu C, Mitra S, Long B, Das K, Mehta JL. LOX-1 abrogation reduces cardiac hypertrophy and collagen accumulation following chronic ischemia in the mouse. *Gene. Ther.* 2012, 19: 522-531.
[120] Gao L, Mann GE. Vascular NAD(P)H oxidase activation in diabetes: a double-edged sword in redox signalling.Cardiovasc Res. 2009, 82: 9-20.
[121] Hu C, Dandapat A, Chen J, Fujita Y, Inoue N, Kawase Y, Jishage K, Suzuki H, Sawamura T, Mehta JL. LOX-1 deletion alters signals of myocardial remodeling immediately after ischemia–reperfusion. *Cardiovasc. Res.* 2007, 76: 292-302.
[122] Li D, Williams V, Liu L, Chen H, Sawamura T, Romeo F, Mehta JL.. Expression of lectin-like oxidized low-density lipoprotein receptors during ischemia–reperfusion and its role in determination of apoptosis and left ventricular dysfunction. *J. Am. Coll. Cardiol.* 2003, 41: 1048-55.
[123] Hu CP, Dandapat A, Liu Y, Hermonat PL, Mehta JL. Blockade of hypoxia-reoxygenation-mediated collagen type I expression and MMP activity by overexpression of TGF-beta1 delivered by AAV in mouse cardiomyocytes. *Am. J. Physiol. Heart Circ. Physiol.* 2007, 293: H1833-H1838.
[124] Levitan I, Volkov S, Subbaiah PV. Oxidized LDL: diversity, patterns of recognition, and pathophysiology. *Antioxid. Redox. Signal.* 2010, 13: 39-75.

In: Renin-Angiotensin System
Editors: Ayako Himura and Takeshi Sato
ISBN: 978-1-62417-788-0

Chapter V

Intensive Blockade of Renin-Angiotensin System

Nicolás Roberto Robles*
University of Salamanca School of Medicine, Salamanca, Spain

Abstract

The intensive blockade of renin-angiotensin system has been tested in the treatment of renal disease associated to micro or macroalbuminuria, in congestive heart failure and also after myocardial infarction. Several authors have reported a superior effect of the combination of ACE inhibition and ARBs on microalbuminuria and on clinical proteinuria in patients with primary nephropathies as well as in type 1 and type 2 diabetic patients. A systematic review and meta-analysis has addressed this issue suggesting that concomitant therapy with an ARBs and an ACE inhibitor leads to greater reductions in proteinuria than monotherapy.

Nevertheless, there is no evidence that this kind of therapy can reduce renal disease progression to end stage renal failure. The ONTARGET trial cast some shadows on the use of dual blockade of renin-angiotensin system in ischemic cardiopathy. The combination of the ACE inhibitor and ARBs was associated with more adverse events without an increase in benefit in terms of cardiovascular mortality and morbidity reduction. On December, 20th 2011 Novartis announced that following the interim review of data from the ALTITUDE study a decision to terminate the trial has been taken on the recommendation of the independent Data Monitoring Committee overseeing the trial. Is this the end for dual blockade as therapeutic resource? Some could reasonably think that this is the safer position. But, are there alternative treatments for proteinuria? Unfortunately, the answer is no. In most patients there is not an ethiological treatment for proteinuric renal disease, at least at this moment. It could be argued that ARBs megadosage could be the alternative to dual blockade. There are some reports on the use of a very high dosage of ARBs for the treatment of proteinuria; nevertheless there has been no adequate, head to head comparison which has shown whether this option is more or less effective than dual blockade and, most importantly, whether it is safer.

* Cardiovascular Risk Chair, University of Salamanca School of Medicine, Salamanca, Spain, e-mail: *nrrobles@yahoo.es*.

Why Try Intenstive Blockade of Renin-Angiotensin System?

The renin–angiotensin system (RAS) preserves fluid volume during periods of restricted dietary salt, and also prevents ischaemia during acute volume loss. The main effector peptide of the RAS is angiotensin II. It induces vasoconstriction and sympathetic activation, raises aldosterone levels, and promotes renal salt and water retention via the angiotensin II type 1 (AT1) receptor [1]. 1 Over the last few decades, the RAS has been a drug target of particular interest because of its involvement in cardiovascular and renovascular disease. Cardiovascular and renovascular disease can be understood as a continuum of risk factors, target organ damage, events, and mortality. Risk factors (such as hypertension, dyslipidaemia, diabetes, and smoking) lead to the development of target organ damage including atherosclerosis, left ventricular hypertrophy, and renal impairment. Target organ damage progressively worsens, leading ultimately to myocardial infarction, heart failure, end-stage renal disease, stroke, or death [2]. Angiotensin II, the main effector peptide of the RAS, plays an active role during all stages of this continuum. The first step in the RAS cascade is the formation of angiotensin I from the precursor angiotensinogen under the action of renin; indeed, early evidence for the importance for the RAS in cardiovascular disease came from the consistent finding that renin activity is predictive of the risk for cardiovascular events. Angiotensin I is then converted to angiotensin II, the principal effector peptide of the RAS, by ACE. In addition, angiotensin II can be produced in tissues by enzymes such as chymase. This locally produced angiotensin II which is believed to mediate paracrine and autocrine functions. Angiotensin II acts via 2 receptor subtypes: angiotensin type 1 (AT1) and AT2. Activation of AT1 receptors results in vasoconstriction, aldosterone and vasopressin secretion, sodium retention, and decreased renal perfusion. Hence, these receptors mediate the deleterious effects of angiotensin II, including elevated blood pressure and cardiac and vascular remodeling [3]. The effects of the AT2 receptors have been less clearly defined because of the limited expression of these receptors in adults, because of their unconventional signaling pathways, and because many AT2-mediated actions are masked by opposing AT1-mediated effects. However, it is now recognized that AT2 receptors generally oppose the actions of AT1 receptors, mediating various antiproliferative and anti-inflammatory effects and promoting tissue differentiation and regeneration and apoptosis [4].

Additional components of the RAS have been identified in the last decade, including bioactive angiotensin peptides, such as angiotensin III, angiotensin IV, and angiotensin-(1-7), the effects of which have not yet been fully elucidated for the cardiovascular and renal system [5]. The discovery of the renin receptor has shed further light on the biology of the RAS. Renin, simply considered until recently as the rate-limiting enzyme of RAS activation, has also turned out to be the ligand for a protein known as the renin/prorenin receptor, which binds renin and prorenin about equally, regardless of their biologic activities. Prorenin, which represents 70%–90% of total circulating renin, when bound to the receptor, induces an increase in the catalytic efficiency of angiotensinogen conversion to angiotensin I, which contributes to local production of angiotensin II and it's systemic levels, as well as binding of renin/prorenin to the renin/prorenin receptor, exerting physiologic effects that are independent of angiorensin II, including activation of intracellular signal pathways, enhanced synthesis of

DNA, and stimulation of the release of plasminogen activator inhibitor (PAI-1), collagen-1, fibronectin, and transforming growth factor beta-1 [6].

The two major classes of drugs that target the RAS are the angiotensin-converting enzyme (ACE) inhibitors and the selective AT1 receptor blockers (ARBs). Although both of these drug classes target angiotensin II, the differences in their mechanisms of action have implications for their effects on other pathways and receptors that may have therapeutic implications [7]. Both ACE inhibitors and ARBs are effective antihypertensive agents that have been shown to reduce the risk of cardiovascular and renal events. Direct inhibition of renin—the most proximal aspect of the renin-angiotensin system—became clinically feasible from 2007 with the introduction of aliskiren (Rasilez; Novartis Pharmaceuticals, Switzerland). Aliskiren has been shown to be efficacious for the management of hypertension, congestive heart failure, and proteinuria either as monotherapy or in combination with ACE inhibitors or angiotensin receptor blockers [8].

Angiotensin Converting Enzyme Inhibitors

The ACE inhibitors reduce RAS activation by blocking the conversion of angiotensin I to angiotensin II, leading to decreased activation of both AT1 and AT2 receptors. Angiotensin II type 1 receptors predominantly mediate the pathological effects of angiotensin II, including vasoconstriction and other mechanisms that raise blood pressure as well as vascular hypertrophy, endothelial dysfunction, atherosclerosis, inflammation, and apoptosis.5 Angiotensin II type 2 receptors, in contrast, mediate mostly opposing and beneficial effects, promoting anti-proliferation, differentiation, regeneration, antiinflammation, and apoptosis. In addition to blocking the conversion of angiotensin I to angiotensin II, ACE inhibitors block the enzymatic degradation of bradykinin. Increased levels of bradykinin contributes to the positive effects of ACE inhibitors since activation of ϕ2 receptor leads to release of nitric oxide, with vasodilatory and tissue protective results. In addition, evidence is accumulating that ACE itself can act as a cell-surface receptor and that binding of an ACE inhibitor to the enzyme triggers a signaling cascade that leads ultimately to PGI2 generation and additional vasodilatory effects [9].

Although acute treatment with an ACE inhibitor reduces circulating angiotensin II to negligible levels, chronic treatment has been associated with reemergence of angiotensin II, a phenomenon referred to as 'reactivation'. In a study of patients with congestive heart failure on long-term ACE inhibitor therapy, reactivation of angiotensin II occurred in approximately one in every six patients and reactivation of aldosterone in about one in every three patients [10]. These late changes in patients that were receiving ACE inhibitors have been linked to poorer outcomes [11].

Angiotensin-converting enzyme inhibition has been associated with angio-oedema (very uncommon, 0.1%) and cough [12, 13]. A theoretical disadvantage of ACE inhibition is that it reduces activity of the AT2 receptor along with the AT1 receptor. Despite their drawbacks, ACE inhibitors are an important drug class because of their proven effectiveness for reducing cardiovascular events and mortality in patients with advanced cardiovascular disease evidenced by CHF or a history of myocardial infarction (MI). However, ACE inhibitors may also reduce cardiovascular risk in patients with less advanced coronary heart disease. This was demonstrated in the Heart Outcomes Prevention Evaluation (HOPE) study, which compared ramipril with placebo [14].

Angiotensin Receptor Blockers

The ARBs block the RAS by antagonizing the binding of angiotensin II to the AT1 receptor. Because the ARBs are selective for the AT1 receptor, these agents have a greater potential for providing a complete inhibition of the RAS than ACE inhibitors. In addition, ARBs have minimal affinity for the AT2 and thus permit activation of the AT2 receptor by angiotensin II, possibly providing beneficial (but unproven) anti-proliferative and anti-inflammatory effects.

Unlike ACE inhibitors, ARBs have no effects on bradykinin accumulation and do not induce NO and PGI_2 via the B2 receptor. The clinical implications of this difference between the ARBs and the ACE inhibitors, aside from the absence of kinin-related cough with ARBs, are not known. The ARBs have been associated with a highly favourable tolerability profile, better than that of any of the other classes of antihypertensives [15]. The clinical evidence for the efficacy of ARBs in reducing cardiovascular events has become quite strong as a result of recent major outcome trials [16].

Direct Renin Inhibitors

Renin is not only the rate-limiting step in angiotensin II formation, but also shows remarkable substrate specificity for angiotensinogen making it an attractive target for therapeutic inhibition. Furthermore, the recent identification of a renin receptor in the glomerular mesangium and in arterial subendothelium suggests the possibility of additional advantages of renin inhibition beyond those of ACE inhibitors and ARBs [17]. For instance, binding of renin to this receptor not only increases its catalytic efficiency in angiotensin I formation but also converts otherwise inert pro-renin into an active moiety. Moreover, the interaction of either renin or pro-renin with its receptor, in the absence of angiotensin peptide formation, leads to activation of the potentially pathogenetic mitogen-activated protein kinase (MAPK) pathway, [18].

Aliskiren is an orally active renin inhibitor, which became the first drug in its class to receive regulatory approval for the treatment of hypertension in 2007. Aliskiren inhibits the first rate-limiting step in the RAS cascade, the conversion of angiotensinogen to angiotensin I and thereby reducing synthesis of all subsequent components of the cascade. In contrast, use of an ACE inhibitor or ARB leads to a compensatory rise in the upstream components of the RAS cascade, including plasma renin activity [19].

Clinical studies in hypertension patients with aliskiren have demonstrated impressive reductions in BP, with similar safety and tolerability to ARBs. This study also demonstrated that side effects in the aliskiren-treated group were comparable to those seen in placebo-treated patients. In clinical trials thus far, the most common adverse events reported have been headache, diarrhea, dizziness, fatigue and back pain; the frequencies of these are similar to both ARBs and placebo [20].

Strategies to Get Maximal Blockade of R.A.S.

So that, although these three classes of drugs act blocking the RAS the mechanism is different in each case and, so that, using a *combination of treatment* could improve the effectiveness of RAS blockade with, at least in theory, positive clinical consequences. The results of these combined treatments will be discussed below.

On the other hand, the extremely good tolerance of the ARBs which have seldom untoward effects has led to develop a second strategy of treatment using *maximal dosage of ARB* above the recommended dosage (i.e. irbesartan, 900 mg daily).

Dual Blockade of R.A.S. Using Ace Inhibitors Associated with Arbs

Dual blockade of renin-angiotensin system has been tested for cardiovascular morbidity prevention, after myocardial infarction, in the treatment of renal disease associated to micro or macroalbuminuria, and in congestive heart failure.

Cardiovascular Prevention

Dual blockade of RAS do not seem to reduce blood pressure intensively [21]. The Ongoing Telmisartan Alone and in Combination with Ramipril Global Endpoint Trial (ONTARGET) evaluated whether the ARB telmisartan was not inferior to the ACE inhibitor ramipril and whether a combination of the two drugs was superior to ramipril alone as a treatment to prevent vascular events in high-risk patients who had cardiovascular disease or diabetes mellitus but did not have heart failure. The conclusions were that telmisartan was equivalent to ramipril in patients with vascular disease or high risk diabetes and was associated with less angioedema. The combination of the two drugs was associated with more adverse events without an increase in benefit [22]. The superiority of dual blockade of RAS for the treatment of hypertension in patients with high cardiovascular risk could not be proved. Moreover, these results prompted an urgent reappraisal of the European Guidelines on Hypertension Management due to the finding of a clear J curve effect on cardiovascular morbidity and mortality [23].

Ischemic Cardiopathy

The ONTARGET trial cast some shadows on the use of dual blockade RAS in ischemic cardiopathy, since nearly one half of the sample has previously suffered a myocardial infarction, and one quarter more have other manifestations of coronary artery disease. These results resemble closely those of the VALIANT study, in which the combination of a full dose of captopril plus valsartan (the latter at a lower dose than that used in the valsartan- only group) did not significantly reduce the occurrence of the primary outcome but did increase hypotension [24]. In a double-blind design this trial compared the effect of the ARB valsartan, the ACE inhibitor captopril, and the combination of the two on mortality in this population of patients. Patients receiving conventional therapy were randomly assigned, 0.5 to 10 days after acute myocardial infarction, to additional therapy with valsartan (4909 patients), valsartan plus captopril (4885 patients), or captopril (4909 patients). The primary end point was death from any cause. During a median follow-up of 24.7 months, 979 patients in the valsartan group died, as did 941 patients in the valsartan-and-captopril group and 958 patients in the captopril group (hazard ratio in the valsartan group as compared with the captopril group, 1.00; 97.5 percent confidence interval, 0.90 to 1.11; P=0.98; hazard ratio in the valsartanand- captopril group as compared with the captopril group, 0.98; 97.5 percent confidence interval, 0.89 to 1.09; P=0.73). The upper limit of the one-sided 97.5 percent confidence interval for the comparison of the valsartan group with the captopril group was within the prespecified margin for noninferiority with regard to mortality (P=0.004) and with regard to the composite end point of fatal and nonfatal cardiovascular events (P<0.001). The valsartan-and-captopril group had the most drug-related adverse events. With monotherapy, hypotension and renal dysfunction were more common in the valsartan group, and cough, rash, and taste disturbance were more common in the captopril group. Valsartan was as effective as captopril in patients who are at high risk for cardiovascular events after myocardial infarction, but combining valsartan with captopril increased the rate of adverse events without improving survival. Taken together, the final results of these two studies showed no additive effect of ARBs in conjunction with a full dose of a proven ACE inhibitor to improve the prognosis of coronary artery disease. Contrariwise, a substantial increase of undesirable secondary effects was detected.

Renal Disease

Several authors have reported a superior effect of the combination of ACE inhibition and ARB on microalbuminuria and on clinical proteinuria in patients with primary nephropathies [25, 26, 27, 28, 29] and in type 1 and type 2 diabetic patients [30, 31] (figure 1). A systematic review and meta-analysis has addressed this issue suggesting that concomitant therapy with an ARB and an ACE inhibitor leads to greater reductions in proteinuria than monotherapy [32]. A false report suggested that dual RAS blockade may safely retard progression of non diabetic renal disease compared with either ACE inhibitor or ARB monotherapy [33], but the authors lately recognized that the data were modified to get the desired results.

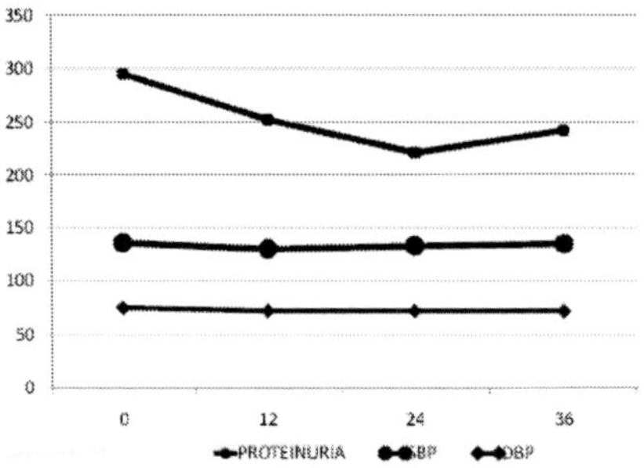

Figure 1. Comparative long term effect of dual blockade with candesartan in proteinuria (100*g/day), SBP and DBP (mmHg). From reference 31.

The renal results of ONTARGET trial were separately reported. The primary renal outcome was a composite of dialysis, doubling of serum creatinine, and death. Analysis was by intention to treat. 784 patients permanently discontinued randomised therapy during the trial because of hypotensive symptoms (406 on combination therapy, 149 on ramipril, and 229 on telmisartan). The number of events for the composite primary outcome was similar for telmisartan (13.4%) and ramipril (13.5%), but was slightly increased with combination therapy (14.5%; p=0·037). The secondary renal outcome, dialysis or doubling of serum creatinine, was similar with telmisartan (2.21%) and ramipril (2.03%) and more frequent with combination therapy (2.49%, p=0.038). Estimated glomerular filtration rate declined less with ramipril compared with telmisartan (−2·82 mL/min/1·73 m^2 vs −4·12, p<0·0001) or combination therapy (−6·11, p<0·0001). Conversely, the increase in urinary albumin excretion was smaller with telmisartan (p=0·004) or with combination therapy (p=0·001) than with ramipril [34].

So that, in people at high vascular risk, telmisartan's effects on major renal outcomes were similar to ramipril and, although combination therapy reduces proteinuria to a greater extent than monotherapy, overall it worsens major renal outcomes. Nevertheless, the results of the ONTARGET were difficult to translate to true renal disease. Most of renal patients have high blood pressure and proteinuric, non-vascular, renal disease. On the other hand the patients recruited in ONTARGET were not hypertensive at recruitment, were older and, as it's antecedents suggest, they have renal microvascular disease highly sensitive to changes in blood pressure levels.

Other reports suggested that, in proteinuric renal disease, dual blockade of the renin-angiotensin system could be useful and secure in most patients even in the stage III or KDOQI Guidelines, although it should be closely monitored [35].

Most recently, Luño et al. [36] reported the results of a multicenter open-label randomized controlled trial to compare the efficacy of combining the angiotensin-converting enzyme inhibitor lisinopril and the angiotensin II receptor blocker irbesartan with that of each drug in monotherapy (at both high and equipotent doses) in slowing the progression of type 2 diabetic nephropathy.

One hundred and thirty three patients with type 2 diabetic nephropathy (age, 66 ± 8 years; 76% men) from 17 centers in Spain. Patients were randomly assigned (1:1:2) to lisinopril (n =35), irbesartan (n = 28), or the combination of both (n = 70). The primary composite outcome was a >50% increase in baseline serum creatinine level, end-stage renal disease, or death.

After a median follow-up of 32 months, 21 (30%) patients in the combination group, 10 (29%) in the lisinopril group, and 8 (29%) in the irbesartan group reached the primary outcome. HRs were 0.96 (95% CI, 0.44-2.05; P = 0.9) and 0.90 (95% CI, 0.39-2.02; P = 0.8) for the combination versus the lisinopril and irbesartan groups, respectively.

There were no significant differences in proteinuria reduction or blood pressure control between groups. The number of adverse events, including hyperkalemia, was similar in all 3 groups. They were unable to show a benefit of the combination of lisinopril and irbesartan compared to either agent alone at optimal high doses on the risk of progression of type 2 diabetic nephropathy.

Therefore, in this moment we can only assure that dual blockade of RAS using an ACE inhibitor and an ARB may get a further decrease in proteinuria but there is no evidence in the long run that this combination could retard CKD progression.

Congestive Heart Failure

Dual blockade of RAS has also been tested in the treatment of chronic heart failure. The prevalence of symptomatic heart failure in the general population ranges from 0.4 to 2% [37] and the prognosis of heart failure is poor and half of the patients will die within 4 years, and in patients with severe heart failure >50% will die within one year [38]. Angiotensin converting enzyme inhibitors remain the first choice for inhibition of the RAS in chronic heart failure, but ARBs can now be considered a reasonable alternative [39].

The combination of an ACE inhibitors and ARBs may produce more reduction of left ventricle size than either agent alone. In the RESOLVD study, the combination of candesartan and enalapril was compared with the respective monotherapies [40]. Left ventricular end-diastolic and end systolic volumes increased to a significantly lesser extent in patients receiving combination therapy than in either of the monotherapy groups. The blood pressure reductions achieved with combination therapy, although modest, were significantly greater than those achieved with either agent alone. Despite the modest reduction in blood pressure found with combination therapy, there was no increase in the heart rate. The addition of enalapril significantly attenuated the increase in plasma angiotensin II concentrations seen in candesartan-treated patients, and plasma concentrations of brain natriuretic peptide were significantly lower with combination therapy than with either candesartan or enalapril monotherapy. Triple neurohormonal blockade with candesartan, enalapril, and metoprolol controlled release resulted in a significant increase in the left ventricular ejection fraction and reductions in the end systolic and end diastolic volumes, compared with dual neurohormonal blockade [41]. As would be expected, the heart rate was decreased significantly in patients treated with metoprolol controlled release, but there was no significant difference in the incidence of hyperkalemia or any increases in serum creatinine between the groups.

In the CHARM-Added trial [42], the use of candesartan over a median follow-up of 41 months resulted in a 15% relative risk reduction of cardiovascular death or heart failure hospitalization, with each of the components contributing. Risk reductions in deaths attributed to worsening heart failure and sudden deaths both contributed to the effect on cardiovascular death. This favourable effect in reducing cardiovascular mortality or CHF hospitalization was evident consistently in patients receiving ACE inhibitors at doses recommended for heart failure as well as in patients on lower doses. A beneficial effect on cardiovascular mortality or hospitalization due to chronic heart failure was also evident with concomitant use of an ACE inhibitor, a beta-blocker, and candesartan. The use of candesartan resulted in a 17% relative risk reduction for chronic heart failure hospitalizations as a first event, and a reduction in the total number of investigator reported chronic heart failure hospitalizations. Symptoms of heart failure as assessed by the NYHA functional class improved in patients treated with candesartan [43]. In spite of these results dual blockade is not recommended in clinical guidelines due to the possible risk associated to simultaneous use of antialdosteronics.

Dual Blockade of R.A.S. Using Direct Renin Inhibitors

In humans, the target organ-protective effects of aliskiren are being investigated in ASPIRE HIGHER, the largest clinical trials program underway in the cardiorenal disease area, involving 14 randomized, double-blind studies including more than 35,000 patients with hypertension, diabetes, heart failure, renal dysfunction, and previous myocardial infarction [44]. Due to ethical issues most of the clinical trials included in this program were developed using dual blockade of the RAS instead of using aliskiren alone.

The most important study that assessed the efficacy of aliskiren in patients with heart failure was the ALOFT (Aliskiren Observation of Heart Failure Treatment) trial [45]. A total of 302 hypertensives who had stable heart failure (New York Heart Association Class II–III) were randomized to 12 weeks of treatment with aliskiren 150 mg or placebo in addition to prior treatment with an ACEI (or ARB) and beta- blocker. Compared with placebo, aliskiren reduced plasma BNP by 25% (P = 0.016), plasma N-terminal proBNP by 25% (P = 0.0106) and urinary aldosterone by 21% (P = 0.015). An improvement in Doppler echocardiographic measurement of left ventricular filling pressure was also observed. Aliskiren was well tolerated and there was no significant difference between aliskiren and placebo for the safety assessment of renal dysfunction, symptomatic hypotension, and hyperkalemia. Because reductions in BNP and plasma N-terminal proBNP with other RAS inhibitors have been associated with improved cardiovascular outcomes in patients with heart failure [46], the neurohormonal results of ALOFT suggest that add-on treatment with aliskiren 150 mg has the potential to reduce morbidity and mortality in these patients.

Left ventricular hypertrophy is a marker of cardiac end organ damage and is associated with increased cardiovascular morbidity and mortality. ALLAY (Aliskiren in Left Ventricular Hypertrophy) was a 36-week study that compared the effects of aliskiren 300 mg and losartan 100 mg alone and in combination on left ventricular hypertrophy (assessed by magnetic resonance imaging) in 465 overweight, hypertensive patients. Aliskiren monotherapy was statistically non inferior to losartan in reducing left ventricular mass index (4.9 g/m2 for aliskiren versus 4.8 g/m2 for losartan). The aliskiren-losartan combination resulted in a greater reduction in left ventricular mass index (5.8 g/m2) compared with losartan monotherapy, although the difference was not statistically significant. These results were independent of BP decrease. Safety and tolerability were similar across all the treatment groups [47].

ASPIRE evaluated the effects of adding aliskiren to standard therapy, including an ACEI or an ARB, on left ventricular volume and function after myocardial infarction. A total of 820 post-myocardial infarction patients were randomly treated with aliskiren or placebo in addition to the best available medical therapy. At 36 weeks of follow-up, echocardiographically assessed left ventricular end-systolic volume (the primary outcome) was reduced by an average of 4.4 mL in the aliskiren group and by 3.5 mL in the placebo group (not statistically significant). No between-group differences were observed in left ventricular end-diastolic volume, infarct segment, or the percentage of patients whose ejection fraction decreased by more than six points. In addition, the combined rates for cardiovascular deaths, hospitalization for heart failure, recurrent heart attack, resuscitated sudden death, and stroke were similar between the aliskiren-treated patients and those given standard therapy. In contrast, patients receiving aliskiren in addition to another RAS blocker had a higher rate of adverse events, particularly hyperkalemia and hypotension. The authors concluded that the use of this combination could not be recommended following myocardial infarction [48]. The results of ASPIRE are consistent with those of ONTARGET and VALIANT trials, dual RAS blockade did not produce any significant clinical advantage in this high-risk population, but significantly increased the risk of hypotension, syncope, renal dysfunction, and hyperkalemia. The first large study to assess the renoprotective effects of aliskiren was AVOID (Aliskiren in the Evaluation of Proteinuria in Diabetes), in which 599 patients with diabetes, nephropathy, and proteinuria were treated with losartan 100 mg followed by the addition of placebo or aliskiren 300 mg. Adding aliskiren to losartan provided a further significant 20% reduction in urinary albumin:creatinine ratio compared with the addition of placebo. Almost twice as many patients in the aliskiren group achieved a reduction in urinary albumin:creatinine ratio of at least 50% from baseline. The additive antiproteinuric effect of combining aliskiren with losartan appeared to be independent of BP reduction, which was similar in the two treatment groups [49]. In a more recent study, Persson et al evaluated the renal effects of aliskiren 300 mg or irbesartan 300 mg alone and in combination in 26 hypertensive patients with Type 2 diabetes and albuminuria. Both monotherapies significantly reduced proteinuria, but the reduction was more pronounced with the aliskiren-irbesartan combination [50].

The rationale and design of the ALTITUDE (Aliskiren Trial in Type 2 Diabetes Using Cardio-Renal Endpoints) study mace it the most important trial on diabetes nephropathy treatment since the Irbesartan Diabetic Nephropathy Trial (IDNT). The primary objective of the ALTITUDE trial was to determine whether aliskiren 300 mg once daily, reduces cardiovascular and renal morbidity and mortality compared with placebo when added to conventional treatment (including ACE inhibitor or ARBs). ALTITUDE was an international, randomized, double-blind, placebo-controlled, parallel-group study, which will include three categories of high-risk patients with type 2 diabetes (aged ≥35 years): those with either urinary albumin/creatinine ratio ≥200 mg/g (i.e. proteinuric patients); microalbuminuria urinary albumin/creatinine ratio ≥20 <200 mg/g and eGFR ≥30 <60 mL/min/1.73 m2; and thirdly, those with a history of cardiovascular disease and eGFR ≥30 <60 mL/min/1.73 m2 with or without microalbuminuria. ALTITUDE randomized 8606 patients with a planned follow-up time of 48 months. The primary outcome measure was time to first event for the composite endpoint of cardiovascular death, resuscitated death, myocardial infarction, stroke, unplanned hospitalization for heart failure, onset of end-stage renal disease or doubling of baseline serum creatinine concentration. Secondary endpoints include a composite cardiovascular endpoint and a composite renal endpoint [51]. As it can be seen, the most striking difference with ONTARGET trial was that ALTITUDE one specifically recruited renal disease patients. Unfortunately, on December 20th, 2011 Novartis announced that following the interim review of data from the ALTITUDE study a decision to terminate the trial has been taken on the recommendation of the independent Data Monitoring Committee overseeing the trial. The committee concluded that patients were unlikely to benefit from treatment added on top of standard anti-hypertensives, and identified higher adverse events in patients receiving rasilez in addition to standard of care in the trial. Specifically, in the trial arm in which rasilez was added to the standard of care there was an increased incidence after 18-24 months of non-fatal stroke, renal complications, hyperkalemia and hypotension in this high-risk study population [52]. One more time the conclusions of ONTARGET on the clinical security of dual RAS blockade were confirmed. The AVANT-GARDE (aliskiren and valsartan to reduce NT-proBNP via renin-angiotensin-aldosterone system blockade) study investigated whether aliskiren, alone or in combination with valsartan, could improve ventricular hemodynamics, as assessed by reductions in NT-proBNP levels. It was a multinational, double-blind trial, that randomized 1101 patients stabilized after ACS without clinical evidence of heart failure or left ventricular function ≤40% but with an increased level of NP 3–10 days after admission to aliskiren, valsartan, their combination, and placebo. The primary endpoint was the change in NT-proBNP from baseline to Week 8. NT-proBNP declined significantly in each treatment arm, including placebo, by week 8, though there were no differences in the reduction between treatment strategies (42% in placebo, 44% in aliskiren, 39% in valsartan, and 36% in combination arm). Although several subgroups had higher baseline levels of NP and greater reductions over the study period, there were no differences among treatment groups in any subgroup. There were no differences in clinical outcomes but there were more adverse events, including serious events and adverse events leading to early study drug discontinuation, in patients treated with active therapy. Thus, there was no evidence for a benefit of early initiation of inhibition of RAAS with valsartan, aliskiren, or their combination compared with placebo with respect to a reduction in NP over 8 weeks of therapy. Moreover, adverse events were reported more frequently in patients assigned to active therapy [53].

We have studied the use of triple blockade with aliskiren (300 mg) in a group of 19 patients. The results were compared with another group of 36 patients where receiving dual blockade where the ACE inhibitor was switched to aliskiren (300 mg). After nine months of treatment proteinuria was decreased in the triple blockade group but remains unchanged in the other one (figure 2). There were no changes in BP, potassium or plasmatic creatinine. Treatment was halted in two patients of the second group due to renal impairment [54].

Harel et al. have performed a meta-analysis of 10 randomised controlled studies with 4814 participants. Combination therapy with aliskiren and angiotensin converting enzyme inhibitors or angiotensin receptor blockers significantly increased the risk of hyperkalaemia compared with monotherapy using angiotensin converting enzymes or angiotensin receptor blockers (relative risk 1.58, 95% confidence interval 1.24 to 2.02) or aliskiren alone (1.67, 1.01 to 2.79). The risk of acute kidney injury did not differ significantly between the combined therapy and monotherapy groups (1.14, 0.68 to 1.89) [55].

After the interruption of ALTITUDE the European Medicines Agency (EMEA) banned the use of dual blockade with aliskiren in diabetics subjects and patients with moderate to severe renal failure [56]. Afterwards, the Food and Drugs Administration (FDA) contraindicated this use in diabetic patients and warning to avoid use of aliskiren with ARBs or ACE inhibitors in patients with moderate to severe renal impairment (i.e., where glomerular filtration rate [GFR] < 60 mL/min) [57].

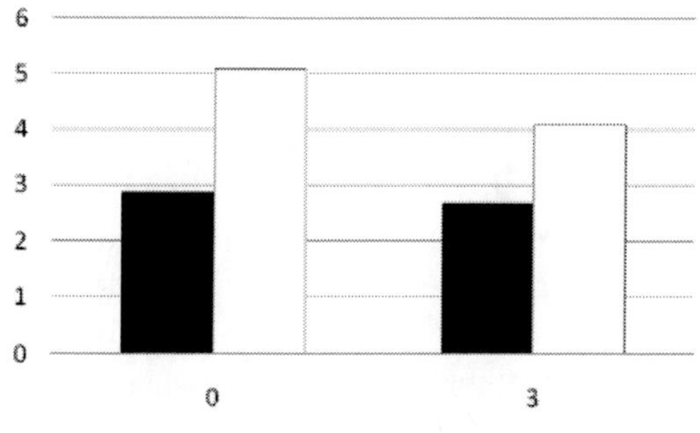

Figure 2. Changes on proteinuria after adding aliskiren to dual blockade (Add on) or switching ACE inhibitor for aliskiren. P = 0.031, ANOVA test.

High Dosage of ARBs

Caution about side effects is probably the most important factor limiting the use of higher doses of antihypertensive drugs in the initial treatment of hypertension. Treatment for hypertension has traditionally been commenced with low doses, with subsequent up-titration as needed. This pattern was primarily due to fear of side effects associated with older therapies, especially adrenergic blockers, which were associated with dose-related side effects such as postural hypotension, drowsiness and dry mouth.

In comparison with these other classes of drugs, side effects associated with ARBs can hardly be differentiated from placebo. Thus, the presumption that high doses automatically mean more side effects, which has limited starting doses with the older classes of antihypertensives, does not appear to be a clinically relevant factor with ARBs [58]. So that, increase the doses of ARBs above the maximal dosage for its antihypertensive effect could be a way to get intensive blockade of RAS. Weinberg et al. observed 48 patients receiving treatment with high doses (1.5-5 times greater than the maximum approved dose) of ARBs, for 40 + 24 months (range 6-98 months).Results: The average ARB dose tended to increase over time and was 3.2 +/- 1.2 times greater at the end of the study than that at the start. SBP was similar at the beginning and end of the study period but diastolic blood pressure showed a decrease throughout the study and was significantly reduced in association with 1.5x and 2x the maximum ARB dose. Serum creatinine concentration was greater ($P < 0.05$) at the periods of 3x and 4x the maximum dose, but this represented increases of only 12 and 20% from baseline, respectively. Potassium did not significantly change. Most important, no significant changes in albumin excretion were detected [59, 60].

Rossing et al evaluated the renoprotective effect of ultrahigh doses of irbesartan in type 2 diabetic patients with microalbuminuria. This double-masked randomized crossover trial included 52 hypertensive type 2 diabetic patients with microalbuminuria on ongoing antihypertensive medication. At inclusion, previous antihypertensive treatment was discontinued and replaced with bendroflumethiazide, 5 mg once daily, for the entire study. Following 2 months wash-out (baseline), patients were treated randomly with irbesartan 300, 600, and 900 mg once daily, each dose for 2 months. All doses of irbesartan significantly reduced albuminuria, ambulatory blood pressure, and GFR from baseline. Reductions in albuminuria from baseline were 52%, 49%, and 59% with increasing doses of irbesartan ($P < 0.01$). No differences in blood pressure reduction were found [61].

Weir et al. studied 392 hypertensive patients with type 2 diabetes and albuminuria (110 African-Americans). All patients received valsartan 160 mg once daily in the morning for 4 weeks, following which patients were randomized to receive one of three valsartan doses: 160, 320 or 640 mg/day. If at week 6, target BP (<130/80 mmHg) was not achieved, then other add-on antihypertensives were allowed. The predominant blood pressure reduction was observed within 4 weeks. Greater reduction in urinary albumin excretion was observed with higher doses of valsartan (320 or 640 mg). At week 30, greater reductions were observed with 320 mg (−50 and −41%, for African–Americans and non-African–Americans, respectively) and 640 mg (−35 and −47% for African–American and non-African–Americans, respectively) as compared with 160 mg (−24 and −22% for African–Americans and non-African–Americans, respectively). The proportion of patients who normalized their albuminuria was similar between African–Americans and non-African–Americans at 160 mg

(19 vs. 12%, respectively) and 320 mg (19 vs. 18%, respectively) but was higher for non-African–American (29%) as compared with African–American patients (16%) at 640 mg [62]. Schmieder et al. [63] designed a randomized, double-blind trial with parallel group design to analyze the antiproteinuric effect of candesartan at high doses. Patients with normal or mildly impaired renal function, protein excretion rate of 1 to 10 g/day, and treatment with an angiotensin-converting enzyme inhibitor or angiotensin receptor blocker for 3 months were eligible. After a 4-wk treatment with 16 mg/d candesartan, patients (n = 32) were allocated to double-blind therapy with either 32 or 64 mg/day candesartan for 12 weeks, followed again by 4 weeks of candesartan 16 mg/day. Proteinuria at study entry was similar in both groups (32 mg/d candesartan 2.14 g/day; 64 mg/day candesartan 2.54 g/day). After the double-blind treatment phase, proteinuria was reduced to 1.42 g/day in the 64-mg/day group (P = 0.017), without any change in the 32-mg/day group (2.02 g/day. After downtitration to 16 mg/day candesartan, proteinuria increased again to 2.38 g/d in the 64-mg/day group (P = 0.001) but remained unchanged in the 32-mg/day group (2.04 g/day). No change in BP was noticed in response to the different doses of candesartan.

A multicenter Canadian trial evaluated whether supramaximal dosages of candesartan would reduce proteinuria to a greater extent than the maximum approved antihypertensive dosage. The authors randomly assigned 269 patients who had persistent proteinuria (≥1 g/day) despite 7 weeks of treatment with the highest approved dosage of candesartan (16 mg/d) to 16, 64, or 128 mg/d candesartan for 30 weeks. The median serum creatinine level was 1.47 mg/dl and the median urinary protein excretion was 2.66 g/d; most (53.9%) patients had diabetic nephropathy. The mean difference of the percentage change in proteinuria for patients receiving 128 mg/d candesartan compared with those receiving 16 mg/d candesartan was −33.05% (95% confidence interval −45.70 to −17.44; $P < 0.0001$). Reductions in BP were not different across the three treatment groups. Elevated serum potassium levels ($K+ > 5.5$ mEq/L) led to the early withdrawal of 11 patients, but there were no dosage-related increases in adverse events [64].

Aranda et al. conducted an open randomized study intended to evaluate the long-term renoprotective effects of "standard" (80 mg once daily) versus "high" (80 mg twice daily) doses of telmisartan in 78 hypertensive patients without diabetes with biopsy-proven chronic proteinuric nephropathies. Blood pressure control did not differ between groups during follow-up. In the group administered telmisartan, 80 mg once daily, serum creatinine level increased from 1.6 to 2.7 mg/dl whereas in those administered 80 mg twice daily, serum creatinine did not change during the study. The decrease in proteinuria was more pronounced ($P < 0.01$) in patients administered the high dose of telmisartan compared with those treated with the standard dose. Serum potassium levels and lipid profiles did not change significantly in either group [65].

Rabbani et al. tried to assess the effect of the angiotensin II receptor blocker Irbesartan on protein damage by glycation, oxidation and nitration in patients with type 2 diabetes and microalbuminuria. In a double-masked randomized crossover trial of 52 hypertensive type 2 diabetic patients, antihypertensive treatment was replaced with bendroflumethiazide. After 2-months wash-out, patients were treated randomly with Irbesartan 300, 600, and 900 mg o.d., each dose for 2 months in a three-way crossover study. Treatment with Irbesartan decreased urinary excretion of advanced glycation endproducts (AGEs)--methylglyoxal- and glyoxal-derived hydroimidazolones, MG-H1 and G-H1. Urinary AGEs were decreased by 30-32%.

In plasma protein, treatment with Irbesartan increased content of glycation adducts Nε-fructosyl-lysine, AGEs Nε-carboxymethyl-lysine, Nε-carboxyethyl-lysine and pentosidine, and also increased content of oxidation markers N-formylkynurenine and dityrosine. This was attributed to decreased clearance of plasma protein modified by Nε-fructosyl-lysine and oxidative markers through the glomerular filter tightened by Irbesartan treatment [66].

Lethen et al. examined 36 hypertensive patients without coronary artery or systemic disease. Coronary flow velocity reserve (CFR) was measured using transthoracic Doppler echocardiography in 18 men (54±9 years) before and after 3 months of treatment with 600 mg/d of irbesartan and in 18 controls (55±11 years). Carotid intima-media thickness (IMT) was evaluated with high-resolution echocardiography. Baseline CFR did not differ between groups. CFR significantly improved in the irbesartan group (from 2.87±.42 to 3.78±.32; P<.001), but remained unchanged in controls (from 2.94±.61 to 3.06±.72; P=not significant). CFR improved with treatment independent of associated risk factors. BP decreased from 150±18 mm Hg to 129±25 mm Hg (P<.001) during treatment, whereas IMT and left ventricular mass index showed no significant differences at the end of the follow-up period in both groups. The three-month irbesartan treatment significantly increased CFR in patients with hypertension. Patients with lower baseline CFR tended to show a more pronounced CFR response [67].

Table 1 resumes the experience with ultrahigh dosage of ARBs. Taken all together it seems to reduce urinary albumin excretion but any other benefits have been not demonstrated. On the other hand have yet to make any head to head comparisons to evaluate whether ultrahigh dosage of ARBs is more effective or safer than the dual blockade of R.A.S.

Resume

Indications

Hypertension.	Blood pressure decrease is small. Combining other kinds of drugs gets better results.
Renal disease.	Dual blockade combining R.A.S. blocking drugs reduce proteinuria but there is no evidence that can retard renal disease progression.
Coronary disease.	There is no benefit for dual blockade.
Congestive heart failure.	Dual blockade may improve clinical status but antialdosteronic diuretic are preferred as treatment.

Contraindications

1. Combining direct renin inhibitors and any other RAS blocking drug is banned in diabetic patients.
2. Combining direct renin inhibitors and any other RAS blocking drug is not recommended in non diabetic patients when GFR is <60 ml/min.
3. Never use dual blockade whenever hiperkaliemia is present.
4. Avoid the dual therapy when blood pressure is low.
5. Close monitoring of renal function is needed in patients with GFR < 60 ml/min when ACE inhibitors and ARBs are combined to treat proteinuria.

Table 1. Comparative Of Ultrahigh Dosage Of ARBs

Author	N	ARBs (daily dosage)	Objective	Results
Weinberg et al.	48	Several.	Microalbuminuria.	No benefit
Rossing et al.	52	Irbesartan (900 mg).	Microalbuminuria.	Decrease
Weir et al.	392	Valsartan (640 mg).	Microalbuminuria.	Decrease
Schmieder et al.	32	Candesartan (64 mg).	Proteinuria > 1 g/day.	Decrease
Burgess et al.	269	Candesartan (128 mg).	Proteinuria > 1 g/day.	Decrease
Aranda et al.	78	Telmisartan(160 mg).	Proteinuria.	Decrease
Rabbani et al.	52	Irbesartan (900 mg).	Biomarkers.	Decrease
Lethen et al.	18	Irbesartan (600 mg).	Coronary reserve.	Improve

References in text [60-67].

References

[1] Werner C., Baumhakel M., Teo K. K., Schmieder R., Mann J., Unger T., Yusuf S., Bo¨hm M., R. A. S. blockade with A. R. B. and A. C. E. inhibitors: current perspective on rationale and patient selection. *Clin. Res. Cardiol.* 2008;97:418–431.

[2] Unger T. Targeting cardiovascular protection: the concept of dual renin–angiotensin system control. *Medscape J. Med.* 2008; 10(Suppl.):S4.

[3] Steckelings U. M., Kaschina E., Unger T. The AT2receptor – a matter of love and hate. *Peptides*. 2005;26:1401–1409.

[4] Cesari M., Rossi G. P., Pessina A. C. Biological properties of the angiotensin peptides other than angiotensin II: Implications for hypertension and cardiovascular diseases. *J. Hypertens*. 2002;20:793–799.

[5] Dan Janser A. H., Batenburg W., van Esch J. H. Prorenin and the (pro)renin receptor – an update. *Nephrol Dial Transplant*. 2007;22: 1288–1292.

[6] Kaschina E., Grzesiak A., Li J., Foryst-Ludwig A., Timm M., Rompe F., et al. Angiotensin II type 2 receptor stimulation: a novel option of therapeutic interference with the renin–angiotensin system in myocardial infarction? *Circulation* 2008;118: 2523–2532.

[7] Jadhav M., Yeola C., Zope G., Nabar A. Aliskiren, the first direct renin inhibitor for treatment of hypertension: the path of its development. *J. Postgrad. Med.* 2012;58:32-8.

[8] Fleming I., Kohlstedt K., Busse R. New fACEs to the renin–angiotensin system. *Physiology* (Bethesda) 2005;20:91–95.

[9] MacFadyen R. J., Lee A. F., Morton J. J., Pringle S. D., Struthers A. D. How often are angiotensin II and aldosterone concentrations raised during chronic A. C. E. inhibitor treatment in cardiac failure? *Heart* 1999;82: 57–61.

[10] Swedberg K., Eneroth P., Kjekshus J., Wilhelmsen L. Hormones regulating cardiovascular function in patients with severe congestive heart failure and their relation to mortality. Consensus Trial Study Group. *Circulation* 1990;82:1730–1736.

[11] Dicpinigaitis P. V. Angiotensin-converting enzyme inhibitor-induced cough: A. C. C. P. evidence-based clinical practice guidelines. *Chest* 2006;129:169S–173S.

[12] Sondhi D., Lippmann M., Murali G. Airway compromise due to angiotensin-converting enzyme inhibitor-induced angioedema: clinical experience at a large community teaching hospital. *Chest* 2004; 126: 400–404.

[13] Yusuf S., Sleight P., Pogue J., Bosch J., Davies R., Dagenais G. Effects of an angiotensin-converting-enzyme inhibitor, ramipril, on cardiovascular events in high-risk patients. The Heart Outcomes Prevention Evaluation Study Investigators. *N. Engl. J. Med.* 2000;342: 145–153.

[14] Greathouse M. K., Weir M. R. The role of ARBs alone or with H. C. T. Z. in the treatment of hypertension and prevention of cardiovascular and renal complications. *Postgrad. Med.* 2012; 124: 40-52.

[15] Turnbull F. Effects of different blood-pressure-lowering regimens on major cardiovascular events: results of prospectively-designed overviews of randomised trials. *Lancet* 2003;362:1527–1535.

[16] Oliver J. A. Receptor-mediated actions of renin and prorenin. *Kidney Int.* 2006; 69: 13–5.

[17] Nguyen G., Burckle C., Sraer J. D. The renin receptor: the facts, the promise and the hope. *Curr. Opin. Nephrol. Hypertens* 2003;12: 51–5.

[18] Staessen J. A., Li Y., Richart T. Oral renin inhibitors. *Lancet* 2006;368: 1449-1456.

[19] Ferro A., Gilbert R., Krum H. Importance of renin in blood pressure regulation and therapeutic potential of renin inhibition. *Int. J. Clin. Pract.*, 2006, 60; 577–581,

[20] MacKinnon M., Shurraw S., Akbari A., Knoll G. A., Jaffey J., Clark H. D. Combination therapy with an angiotensin receptor blocker and an A. C. E. inhibitor in proteinuric renal disease: a systematic review of the efficacy and safety data. *Am. J. Kidney Dis.* 2006; 48: 8-20.

[21] The ONTARGET Investigators. Telmisartan, Ramipril, or Both in Patients at High Riskfor Vascular Events. *N. Engl. J. Med.* 2008;358: 1547-1559.

[22] Mancia G., Laurent S., Agabiti-Rosei E., Ambrosioni E., Burnier M., Caulfield M. J., et al. Reappraisal of European guidelines on hypertension management: a European Society of Hypertension Task Force document. *Blood Press.* 2009;18(6): 308-47.

[23] Pfeffer M. A., McMurray J. J. V., Velazquez E. J., et al. Valsartan, captopril, or both in myocardial infarction complicated by heart failure, left ventricular dysfunction, or both. *N. Engl. J. Med.* 2003;349:1893-1906.

[24] Russo D., Minutolo R., Pisani A., Esposito R., Signorello G., Andreucci M. et al. Coadministration of losartan and enalapril exerts additive antiproteinuric effect in IgA nefropathy. *Am. J. Kidney Dis.* 2001; 38: 18-25.

[25] Ruilope L. M., Aldigier J. C., Ponticelli C., Oddou-Stock P., Botteri F., Mann J. F. Safety of the combination of valsartan and benazepril in patients with chronic renal disease. European Group for the Investigation of Valsartan in Chronic Renal Disease. *J. Hypertens* 2000;18: 89-95.

[26] Luño J., Barrio V., Goicoechea M. A., Gonzalez C., Garcia de Vinuesa S., Gomez F., et al. Effects of dual blockade of the renin-angiotensin system in primary proteinuric nephropathies. *Kidney Int.* 2002; 62 (Suppl. 82): S47–S52.

[27] Robles N. R., Ruiz Jiménez B., Hernandez Gallego R., Ruiz Calero R., Sanchez Casado E., Cubero J. J. Dual renin-angiotensin system blockade in patients with single functioning kidey and proteinuria. *Eur. J. Intern. Med.* 2009; 20: 186-189.

[28] Robles N. R., Fernandez-Carbonero E., Romero B., Sanchez Casado E., Cubero J. J., Long-term antiproteinuric effect of dual renin-angiotensin system blockade. *Cardiovasc. Ther.* 2009; 27: 101-107.
[29] Jacobsen P., Andersen S., Rossing K., Hansen B. V., Parving H. H. Dual blockade of the renin-angiotensin system in type 1 patients with diabetic nephropathy. *Nephrol Dial Transplant.* 2002; 17:1019-1024.
[30] Mogensen C. E., Neldam S., Tikkanen I., Oren S., Viskoper R., Watts R. W., Cooper M. E. for the C. A. L. M. study group. Randomised controlled trial of dual blockade of renin-angiotensin system in patients with hypertension, microalbuminuria, and non-insulin dependent diabetes: the candesartan and lisinopril microalbuminuria (C. A. L. M.) study. *B. M. J.* 2000; 321:1440–1444.
[31] Kunz R., Friedrich C., Wolbers M., Mann J. F. E. Meta-analysis: Effect of Monotherapy and Combination Therapy with Inhibitors of the Renin–Angiotensin System on Proteinuria in Renal Disease. *Ann. Intern. Med.* 2008;148:30-48.
[32] Nakao N., Yoshimura A., Morita M., Kayano T., Ideura T. Combination treatment of angiotensin-II receptor blocker and angiotensin-converting-enzyme inhibitor in non-diabetic renal disease (COOPERATE): A randomised controlled trial. *Lancet.* 2003; 361: 117-124.
[33] Mann J. F. E., Schmieder R. E., McQueen M., Dyal L., Shumacher H., Pogue J., et al. Renal outcomes with telmisartan, ramipril, or both, in people at high vascular risk (the ONTARGET study): a multicentre, randomised, double-blind, controlled trial. *Lancet.* 2008; 372: 547-553.
[34] Robles N. R., Cancho B., Barroso S., Martin M. V., Sanchez Casado E. Untoward effects of dual rennin-angiotensis system blockade: Influence of previous chonic renal failure. *Int. J. Clin. Pract.* 2006; 60: 1035-1039.
[35] Fernandez Juarez G., Luño J., Barrio V., de Vinuesa S. G., Praga M., Goicoechea M., et al.; P. R. O. N. E. D. I. Study Group. Effect of Dual Blockade of the Renin-Angiotensin System on the Progression of Type 2 Diabetic Nephropathy: A Randomized Trial. *Am. J. Kidney Dis.* 2012 Aug. 28. [Epub ahead of print].
[36] Mosterd A., Hoes A. W., de Bruyne M. C., Deckers J. W., Linker D. T., Hofman A., Grobbee D. E. Prevalence of heart failure and left ventricular dysfunction in the general population; The Rotterdam Study. *Eur. Heart J.* 1999; 20: 447-455.
[37] Cleland J. G., Gemmell I., Khand A., Boddy A. Is the prognosis of heart failure improving?. *Eur. J. Heart Fail.* 1999; 1:229-241.
[38] Hunt S. A., Abraham W. T., Chin M. H., Feldman A. M., Francis G. S., Ganiats T. G. et al. ACC/AHA 2005 Guideline Update for the Diagnosis and Management of Chronic Heart Failure in the Adult A Report of the American College Cardiology/American Heart Association Task Force on Practice Guidelines (Writing Committee to Update the 2001 Guidelines for the Evaluation and Management of Heart Failure): Developed in Collaboration With the American Society College of Chest Physicians and the International Society for Heart and Lung of Transplantation: Endorsed by the Heart Rhythm Cardiology/American Heart Association. *Circulation* 2005;112: e154-e235.
[39] McKelvie R. S., Yusuf S., Pericak D., Avezum A., Burns R. J., Probstfield J., et al. Comparison of candesartan, enalapril and their combination in congestive heart failure: Randomized Evaluation of Strategies for Left Ventricular Dysfunciton

(R. S. O. L. V. D.) pilot study. The R. E. S. O. L. V. D. Pilot Study Investigators. *Circulation* 1999; 100:1056–1064.

[40] McKelvie R. S., Rouleau J. L., White M., Afzal R., Young J. B., Maggioni A. P., et al. Comparative impact of enalapril, candesartan or metoprolol alone or in combination on ventricular remodeling in patients with congestive heart failure. *Eur. Heart J.* 2003; 24:1727–1734.

[41] McMurray J. J. V., O. ¨ stergren J., Swedberg K., Granger C. B., Held P., Michelson E. L., et al. Effects of candesartan in patients with chronic heart failure and reduced left-ventricular systolic function taking angiotensin-convertingenzyme inhibitors: the CHARM-Added trial. *Lancet* 2003; 362:767–771.

[42] O'Meara E., Solomon S., McMurray J., Pfeffer M., Yusuf S., Michelson E., et al. Effect of candesartan on New York Heart Association functional class. Results of the Candesartan in Heart failure: Assessment of Reduction in Mortality and morbidity (C. H. A. R. M.) programme. *Eur. Heart J.* 2004; 25:1920–1926.

[43] ASPIRE HIGHER clinical program expands to 35,000 patients in 14 trials, the largest cardio-renal outcomes program ever. [Accessed on Jun. 25, 2010]. Available from: *http://www.novartis.be/downloads/nl/pers-media/berichten/reports/2008-0717 financial-report_s1-2008_en.pdf.*

[44] McMurray J., Pitt B., Latini R., et al. Effects of the oral direct renin inhibitor aliskiren in patients with symptomatic heart failure. *Circ. Heart Fail.* 2008;1:17–24.

[45] Latini R., Masson S., Anand I., et al. Effects of valsartan on circulating brain natriuretic peptide and norepinephrine in symptomatic chronic heart failure: The Valsartan Heart Failure Trial (Val-HeFT) *Circulation.* 2002;106:2454–2458.

[46] Solomon S. D., Appelbaum E., Manning W. J., et al. Aliskiren in Left Ventricular Hypertrophy (A. L. L. A. Y.) Trial Investigators. Effect of the direct renin inhibitor aliskiren, the angiotensin receptor blocker losartan, or both on left ventricular mass in patients with hypertension and left ventricular hypertrophy. *Circulation.* 2009;119: 530–537.

[47] Solomon S. D. Effect of the direct renin inhibitor aliskiren on left ventricular remodelling following myocardial infarction with left ventricular dysfunction: ASPIRE. Presented at: American College of Cardiology 59th Annual Scientific Sessions; Atlanta, G. A. Mar. 13–16, 2010.

[48] Parving H. H., Persson F., Lewis J. B., Lewis E. J., Hollengerg N. H. Aliskiren combined with losartan in Type 2 diabetes and nephropathy. *N. Engl. J. Med.* 2008;358:2433-2446.

[49] Persson F., Rossing P., Reinhard H., et al. Renal effects of aliskiren compared with and in combination with irbesartan in patients with Type 2 diabetes, hypertension and albuminuria. *Diabetes Care.* 2009;32:1873-1879.

[50] Parving H. H., Brenner B. M., McMurray J. J., de Zeeuw D., Haffner S. M., Solomon S. D., et al. Aliskiren Trial in Type 2 Diabetes Using Cardio-Renal Endpoints (ALTITUDE): rationale and study design. *Nephrol. Dial Transplant.* 2009; 24: 1663-1671.

[51] *http://www.novartis.com/newsroom/media-releases/en/2011/1572562.shtml* Acceded December, 24th, 2011.

[52] Scirica B. M., Morrow D. A., Bode C., Ruzyllo W., Ruda M., Oude Ophuis A. J., et al. Patients with acute coronary syndromes and elevated levels of natriuretic peptides: the results of the AVANT GARDE-TIMI 43 Trial. *Eur. Heart J.* 2010;31: 1993-2005.

[53] Martinez del Viejo C., Villa J., Robles N. R., Sanchez Casado E., Cubero J. J. Efecto antiproteinúrico de los inhibidores directos de la renina. XL Reunión de la Sociedad Española de Nefrologia. Abstract. *Nefrologia.* 2010; 30 (Suppl.1): 13.

[54] Harel Z., Gilbert C., Wald R., Bell C., Perl J., Juurlink D., Beyene J., Shah P. S. The effect of combination treatment with aliskiren and blockers of the renin-angiotensin system on hyperkalaemia and acute kidney injury: systematic review and meta-analysis. *B. M. J.* 2012 Jan. 9;344:e42. doi: 10.1136/bmj.e42 (Published 9 January 2012).

[55] *http://www.ema.europa.eu/docs/en_GB/document_library/Press_release/2011/12/WC500119982.pdf.*

[56] *http://www.fda.gov/drugs/drugsafety/ucm300889.htm.*

[57] Düssing R. Angiotensin II receptor blockers dosage: How high should we go? *Int. J. Clin. Pract.*, February 2006, 60, 2, 179–183.

[58] Weinberg A. J., Zappe D. H., Ashton M., Weinberg M. S. Safety and tolerability of high-dose angiotensin receptor blocker therapy in patients with chronic kidney disease: a pilot study. *Am. J. Nephrol.* 2004; 24: 340–5.

[59] Weinberg A. J., Zappe D. H., Ashton M., Weinberg M. S. Safety and tolerability of high-dose angiotensin receptor blocker therapy in patients with chronic kidney disease: a pilot study. *Am. J. Nephrol.* 2004; 24: 340-345.

[60] Rossing K., Schjoedt K. J., Jensen B. R., Boomsma F., Parving H. H. Enhanced Renoprotective effects of ultrahigh doses of irbesartan in patients with type 2 diabetes and microalbuminuria. *Kidney Int.* 2005;68: 1190–1198.

[61] Weir M. R., Hollenberg N. K., Zappe D. H., Meng X., Parving H. H., Viberti G., et al. Antihypertensive effects of double the maximum dose of valsartan in African-American patients with type 2 diabetes mellitus and albuminuria. *J. Hypertens.* 2010;28:186–193.

[62] Schmieder R. E., Klingbeil A. U., Fleischmann E. H., Veelken R., Delles C. Additional antiproteinuric effect of ultrahigh dose candesartan: a double-blind, randomized, prospective study. *J. Am. Soc. Nephrol.* 2005; 16: 3038-3045.

[63] Burgess E., Muirhead N., Rene de Cotret P., Chiu A., Pichette V., Tobe S. Supramaximal dose of candesartan in proteinuric renal disease. *J. Am. Soc. Nephrol.* 2009;20:893–900.

[64] Aranda P., Segura J., Ruilope L. M., Aranda F. J., Frutos M. A., López V., López de Novales E. Long-term renoprotective effects of standard versus high doses of telmisartan in hypertensive nondiabetic nephropathies. *Am. J. Kidney Dis.* 2005; 46: 1074-1079.

[65] Rabbani N., Adaikalakoteswari A., Rossing K., Rossing P., Tarnow L., Parving H. H., Thornalley P. J. Effect of Irbesartan treatment on plasma and urinary markers of protein damage in patients with type 2 diabetes and microalbuminuria. *Amino Acids.* 2012; 42: 1627-39.

[66] Lethen H., Tries H. P., Kersting S., Bramlage P., Lambertz H. Improvement of coronary microvascular function after Angiotensin receptor blocker treatment with irbesartan in patients with systemic hypertension. *J. Clin. Hypertens* (Greenwich). 2011; 13: 155-61.

In: Renin-Angiotensin System
Editors: Ayako Himura and Takeshi Sato
ISBN: 978-1-62417-788-0

Chapter VI

Glomerular Renin-Angiotensin System Activation: Implications in Pathological Glomerular Remodeling

Shoji Kagami*
Department of Pediatrics, The Institute of Health Bioscience,
The University of Tokushima Graduate School, Tokushima, Japan

Abstract

Sustained pathological glomerular remodeling accompanied by prominent cell proliferation and aberrant extracellular matrix (ECM) formation is the central biological feature of progressive glomerulonephritis (GN) leading to glomerular dysfunction and sclerosis. Accumulating evidence from clinical and basic research indicates that multiple mediators participate in the structural alterations of nephritic glomeruli. In particular, angiotensin II (Ang II), the principal bioactive peptide of the renin-angiotensin system (RAS), mediates glomerular hypertension, cell proliferation and pathological ECM remodeling in various types of progressive glomerular diseases. Recently, apart from the systemic Ang II-generating system (systemic RAS), the local (tissue) Ang II-generating system (local RAS) has been recognized and emphasized to be critically involved in Ang II-mediated pathological tissue remodeling (fibrosis). It is now evident that the kidney expresses all elements (renin, angiotensinogen, angiotensins, and angiotensin converting enzymes as well as their receptors) of the RAS, and locally produced Ang II contributes to not only kidney ontogeny but also to regulation of blood pressure (BP) and progression of chronic kidney disease (CKD). The purpose of this chapter is to review the role of kidney RAS, with particular focus on the role of glomerular RAS in the pathological glomerular remodeling observed in progressive GN.

Keywords: Glomerular renin-angiotensin system, angiotensin II, TGF-β, integrin, glomerulosclerosis

---

* Corresponding author: Shoji Kagami, MD., Ph.D Department of Pediatrics, The Institute of Health Bioscience, The University of Tokushima Graduate School, Tokushima, 3-18-15 Kuramoto-cho, Tokushima 770-8503, Japan. Phone: +81-88-633-7135, Fax: +81-886-31-8697 E-mail: kagami@clin.med.tokushima-u.ac.jp.

Introduction

The accumulation of extracellular matrix (ECM), cell proliferation and extracapillary lesions such as synechiae and/or crescent formation in nephritic glomeruli are prominent pathological features responsible for progressive human and rat experimental glomerulonephritis (GN) [1-3]. It has been demonstrated that a variety of mediators including cytokines, physical factors, adhesion molecules, vasoactive peptides and reactive oxygen species (ROS) play important roles in progressive GN [1-5]. Among these mediators involved in such pathological glomerular remodeling, angiotensin II (Ang II) is especially important. Ang II induces not only vasoconstriction and sodium retention but also acts as a multifunctional molecule that mediates cell growth, oxidative cell damage and tissue fibrosis [6, 7].

Historically, the renin- angiotensin system (RAS) that produces Ang II has been established as an endocrine (circulating) system modulating physiological functions that play a fundamental role in the maintenance of sodium and extracellular fluid, and therefore, regulates the arterial blood pressure (BP) [11]. Ang II is the main effector molecule of this system through the transmission of its action by two main G-protein-coupled receptors with seven-transmembrane domains Ang II type 1 receptor and type 2 receptor (AT1R and AT2R). Recently, the overview of this system became more complex because of the discovery of new biologically active Ang peptides, and their receptors, new functions, and new enzymatic pathways of RAS and the local Ang II -generating system for regulation of local tissue functions [8-10]. A body of evidence demonstrates that there are enough amounts of all the elements of RAS in the kidney, and locally produced Ang II contributes to not only kidney development, but also to regulation of BP and the progression of chronic kidney disease (CKD) [11-13]. The objective of this chapter outlines the role of renal tissue RAS, particularly highlighting on the role of glomerular RAS in the pathological glomerular remodeling observed in progressive GN. The clinical issues regarding the involvement of renal RAS in human GN are not fully covered in this chapter.

RAS Biology- An Update

RAS has been traditionally perceived as a circulating hormonal system (circulating RAS) that regulates the BP, sodium balance and fluid homeostasis. Briefly, renin (a protease) secreted from the granular cells of the juxtaglomerular apparatus (JGA) cleaves the liver-borne angiotensinogen (AGT) to form the inactive precursor Ang I [1-10], which is further cleaved by a carboxyl dipeptidase, namely angiotensin- converting enzyme (ACE) released from capillary endothelial cells to convert Ang I to the Ang II [1-8]. Pulmonary endothelial cells are a particularly rich source of ACE. Ang II is considered the major biologically active component of RAS. The actions of Ang II are transmitted by two main G-protein coupled receptors with seven- transmembrane domains, AT1R and AT2R. Most of the biological effects of Ang II are conveyed by the AT1R. Activation of AT1R induces the most classical actions such as increases in blood volume and BP by stimulating vasoconstriction, and adrenal aldosterone secretion, renal sodium reabsorption and sympathetic neurotransmission. Recent advances in cellular and molecular biology, as well as sophisticated physiological and pharmacological techniques, have generated a new landscape through the discovery of new peptides, and their receptors, enzymatic pathways and biological actions of RAS (Figure 1) [8-15]. Additionally the concept of tissue RAS has been emerged based on a large amount of clinical and experimental research. The functional concept of tissue RAS is based on the synthesis of Ang II from AGT within tissue, which is independent of circulating RAS, and the local actions of produced Ang II in a paracrine and autocrine manners. Cathepsin D is known to cleave AGT to Ang I as an alternative angiotensin formation pathway for RAS activation [16-18]. Interestingly, the kidney-tissue RAS is profoundly involved even in the process of renal growth and development [12, 19].

In fact, the use of ACE inhibitors or AT1R antagonists during fetal life, as well as mutations in the genes encoding AGT, renin, ACE, or AT1R in humans, are associated with renal tubular dysgenesis [20]. Genetic inactivation of AGT, renin, ACE, or AT1R in mice causes abnormal glomerular and renal vascular development, pelvic dilation (hydronephrosis), and hypoplastic papilla [19]. The developing kidney expresses all the components of RAS and has the capacity to both generate Ang II and to transmit its actions within the fetal kidney. Many convincing data supports that locally produced Ang II in the mesenchyme, acts as a morphogenic peptide in a paracrine manner on the adjacent AT_1R/AT_2R-expressing ureteric bud to regulate branching formation in vivo [12, 19].

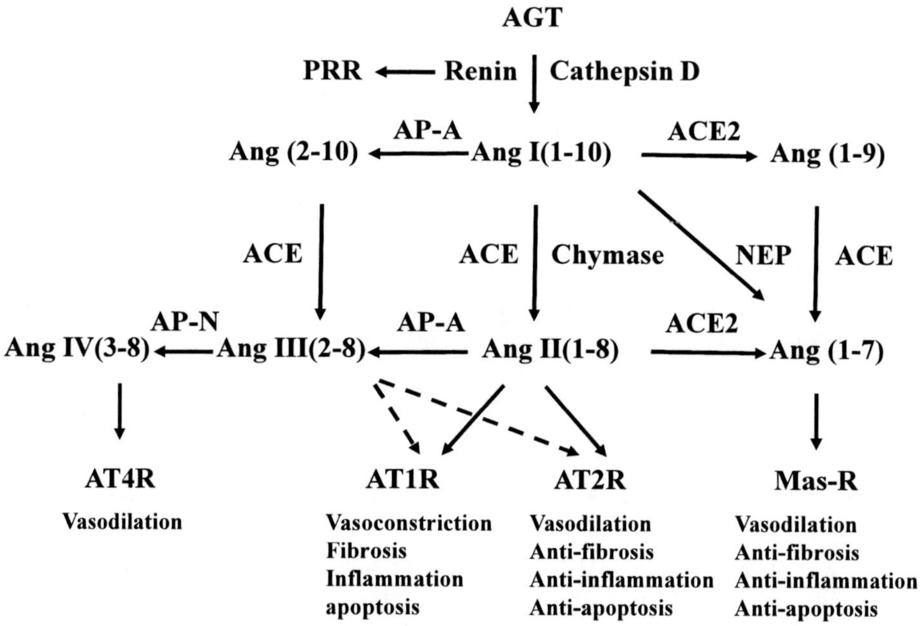

Figure 1. Schema indicating the expanded view of the renin–angiotensin system (RAS). AGT: angiotensinogen, PRR: prorenin/renin receptor, ACE: angiotensin-converting enzyme, ACE2: angiotensin-converting enzyme 2, AP-A: aminopeptidase A, AP-N: aminopeptidase N, NEP: neprilysin, Ang I: angiotensin I, Ang II: angiotensin II, AT1R: angiotensin II type I receptor, AT2R: angiotensin II type 2 receptor, AT4R: angiotensin II type 4 receptor, Mas-R: Mas receptor.

Ang II is now considered to be a multifunctional peptide that induces cell proliferation, hypertrophy, differentiation, apoptosis, superoxide productions, inflammation and ECM production via AT1R signaling [21-25].

These Ang II-AT1R signaling-induced several cell phenotypes are largely mediated through the induction of several cytokines such as transforming growth factor-β (TGF-β), platelet-derived growth factor (PDGF), tumor necrosis factor-α (TNF-α) and monocyte chemoattractant protein-1 (MCP-1) [21, 26-29]. Interestingly, AT2R signaling negatively modulate the actions of AT1R signaling and generally possess beneficial effects such as anti-inflammation, anti- fibrosis and anti-apoptosis on kidney. It has been recently demonstrated that biologically active peptides (Ang (1-7), Ang (2-8)(Ang III) and Ang (3-8)(Ang IV)) in addition to Ang II are generated depending on the activity of ACE, ACE2, a 40% homolog of ACE, and other peptidases such as neprilysin (NEP), aminopeptidase A (AP-A) and AP-N. ACE2 is a monocarboxyl peptidase that metabolizes Ang I to the Ang (1-9) or Ang II to the Ang (1-7) and therefore modulates the amount of Ang II synthesis. Irrespective of a homology with ACE, ACE inhibitors do not inhibit ACE2 activity in clinical practice. Ang (1-9) is further metabolized by ACE to Ang (1-7). Ang (1-9) has been shown to enhance the release of arachidonic acid and nitric oxide (NO) in heart tissues and probably contributes to cardiac functions [30]. The action of Ang (2-10), metabolized from Ang I with AP-A, is also not well characterized but it is implicated in the modulation of vasopressor responses in hypertensive rats [31]. Ang (1-7) is present in the circulation and in many tissues [32, 33], and binds to its G protein-coupled receptor Mas [34]. Recent characterization of ACE2- Ang (1-7) - Mas receptor axis has provided a new pathway that induces vasodilation as well as anti- proliferative and anti-fibrotic actions that are in contrast to the classical ACE-Ang II-AT1R axis of RAS [35]. Similar to Ang II, Ang III interacts with AT1R and AT2R , albeit with lower affinity, and has actions similar to those of Ang II [36]. Furthermore, Ang IV has high affinity for AT4R, an insulin-regulated aminopeptidase (IRAP), and has critical physiological effects in several organ systems such as the heart, kidney and vasculature [37-40]. For an example, Ang IV effects are contradictory to those of the classical ACE-Ang II-AT1R system in the heart [38]. Finally, binding of prorenin to renin/prorenin receptor (PRR) leads to activation of prorenin to active renin by displacement of the prosegment [41]. Stimulation of PRR activates intracellular signaling to upregulate the expression of profibrotic proteins [42]. Overall, the expanded view of RAS is quite complex and multilayered.

Glomerulus-Based Ang II-Generating System

All the components of the RAS have been demonstrated to be expressed within the glomerulus and the resultant product, Ang II, regulates glomerular hemodynamics, capillary wall permeability and participates in glomerular damage leading to the pathological remodeling under the diseased condition [43-45]. Using micropuncture methods, pioneering studies by Seikaly et al reported that the concentrations of total immunoreactive Ang (reflecting Ang II and lesser amounts of the three fragments) in rat glomerular filtrate averaged 32 nM compared with 32 pM in systemic plasma, indicating that the Ang II concentration in the Bowman's space is 1000-fold higher than that in the systemic circulation [46]. Therefore, they suggested the existence of a glomerulus-based Ang II-generating system within the kidney. Subsequently, using isolated glomeruli, they demonstrated that rat glomeruli can produce Ang II independent of neural innervation, vascular attachment, or exogenous influences. These findings firmly support evidence for an Ang II-generating system operating in the glomerulus [47]. Many studies using histochemical techniques, including in situ hybridization and biochemical methods, have been reported that RAS components such as AGT, ACE, ACE2, Ang II, AT1R and AT2R are detected in normal glomeruli of both rats and humans. New analytical methods, such as the matrix-assisted laser desorption ionization time of flight (MALDI-TOF)- mass spectrometry (MS), provides us with the dissection of Ang metabolism in the glomerulus with more specificity and ease than that of previous methods [15]. Recently, Velez et al examined the metabolism of Ang I in freshly isolated intact rat glomeruli using MALDI-TOF-MS (48-50). They showed that there is prominent glomerular conversion of Ang I to Ang (2-10) and Ang (1-7), mediated by AP-A and NEP, respectively, and suspected that the formation of these alternative Ang peptides may be critical to counterbalance the local actions of Ang II within glomeruli. Furthermore, they examined the each contribution of the three glomerular cell types (endothelial cells (GECs), mesangial cells (MCs), podocytes (PODs)) to Ang metabolism using MALDI-TOF-MS in combination with cell culture methods [48-50]. They demonstrated that PODs express a functional intrinsic RAS characterized by AGT, NEP, AP-A, ACE2 and renin activities, which favors formation of Ang (1-7) and Ang (2-10) from Ang I and promotes rapid degradation of Ang II [49]. In contrast, human GECs possess prominent ACE activity leading to Ang II formation and less production of Ang (1-7) through the prolyendopeptidase (PEP) and ACE2 activities [50]. Many additional studies have indicated that MCs also express a functional intrinsic RAS characterized by AGT, prorenin, cathepsin B (an enzyme possibly involved in renin activation), chymase, ACE, and ACE2, which primarily generates Ang II and very small amounts of Ang (1-7) and Ang (1-9) [50-53], Collectively, it appears likely that GECs and MCs (glomerular endocapillary cells) possess prominent Ang II-forming capabilities, while PODs (glomerular extracapillary cells) possess a major Ang II- degrading activity. Therefore, the damage to specific cell types in the glomeruli may lead to distinct effects on the balance of glomerular Ang II synthesis and degradation. In addition, we should consider that the relative abundance of other Ang I matabolites, such as Ang (1-7) and Ang (2-10), within glomeruli also influence the net effects of these Ang peptides on glomerular cells. Detailed analysis of the paramount enzymatic pathway of RAS, which is responsible for the conversion to these Ang peptides should provide new insights into regulation of Ang II actions in glomerular functions and preventing the progression of glomerular disease.

The Ang II-Transforming Growth Factor β (TGF-β) Axis in CKD Progression

In addition to demonstration of the involvement of glomerular RAS activation in local Ang II synthesis, the crucial role of the Ang II- TGF-β axis in CKD progression has been established [26, 54, 55]. Most CKD progression into renal failure, irrespective of primary etiology, begins at the glomerulus. Relentless glomerular injury usually induces glomerulosclerosis (pathological glomerular remodeling) accompanied by massive accumulation of ECM, loss of capillary lumen patency and local tuft adhesion to the Bowman's capsule as observed in synechiae and/or crescent formation (Figure 2). Increased expression of ECM components, such as fibronectin, laminin and collagen type IV (collagen

IV) as well as the neoexpression of collagen I, and III, are characteristically observed in the disfiguring glomeruli [3, 56]. Many studies suggest that several matrix metalloproteinases (MMPs) decreasing ECM degradation and adhesion molecules such as integrins are also involved in this disfiguring morphology of nephritic glomeruli [57-59]. TGF-β serves as a representative cytokine for inducing glomerulosclerosis in CKD as follows. TGF-β1 directly stimulates the expression of many ECM genes in glomerular cells (1). Additionally, TGF-β1 enhances the β 1-integrin- mediated ECM remodeling by MCs [56, 57, 60]. On the other hand, TGF-β1 reduces collagenase production and simultaneously stimulates expression of tissue inhibitors of MMPs, resulting in an overall inhibition of ECM degradation [59].

Collectively, the increased expression of mesangial TGF-β1 induces ECM accumulation via the above mechanisms that are largely mediated by the intracellular Smad and ERK 1/2, ERK5 signaling pathways in damaged glomeruli [61, 62, 63]. It is well established that the loss of PODs is significantly involved in the development of progressive glomerulosclerosis. A loss of PODs leads to 'bare areas' of glomerular basement membrane, leading to the formation of synechiae to Bowman's capsule and then to segmental and finally global glomerular sclerosis [64].

TGF-β1 also plays a major part in POD loss in glomerular diseases. TGF-β1 induces POD apoptosis by the activation of p38 and classic effector caspase-3 [65]. In TGF-β1–overexpressing transgenic mice, PODs undergo apoptosis in situ shortly after the sclerotic lesion appears in the glomerulus [65]. In fact, TGF-β1 expression is enhanced in the PODs of patients with progressive GN such as focal segmental glomerulosclerosis and membranous nephropathy [66].

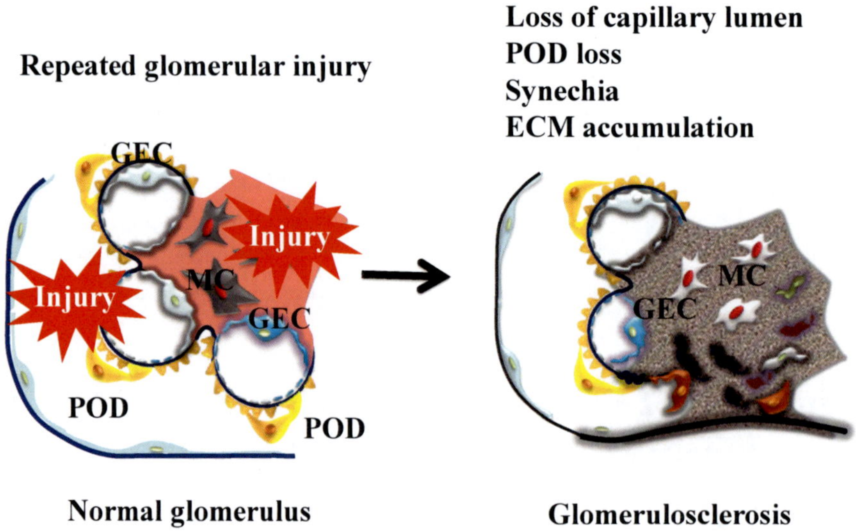

Figure 2. Schema of pathological processes leading to glomerulosclerosis. GEC: glomerular endothelial cell (GEC), MC: glomerular mesangial cell, POD: glomerular podocyte, ECM: extracellular matrix. Repeated glomerular injury causes pathological glomerular remodeling that leads to the development of glomerulosclerosis.

Extensive studies of various human diseases and in animal models have shown that ACE inhibitors (ACEIs) and /or AT1R blockers (ARBs) are superior to other anti-hypertensive agents for protection of the kidney against progressive glomerular deterioration, suggesting that Ang II also plays a pivotal role in CKD progression [67, 68]. There is now accumulating evidence that Ang II is a key molecule that induces glomerulosclerosis in CKD progression (Figure 3) [66–68]. A close expressional link exists between the Ang II and the TGF-β within the diseased kidney [54, 55, 69]. In fact, many profibrotic effects of Ang II on the kidney are mediated by TGF-β stimulation. We initially demonstrated that Ang II stimulates TGF-β1 expression in glomerular cells, including MCs [26]. Moreover, in cultured MCs, Ang II not only stimulates transcription of TGF-β1, but also promotes its conversion to the biologically active form. We further demonstrated by application of a neutralizing anti-TGF-β1 antibody that Ang II markedly increases the expression of ECM component genes as well as the PAI-1 gene that regulates ECM degradation by MCs through the induction of TGF-β1, indicating that the Ang II- TGF-β1 axis is critically involved in pathological glomerular ECM remodeling in CKD [26, 70]. Furthermore, this Ang II -TGF-β1 axis mediates the induction of POD apoptosis in diseased glomeruli (Figure 3) [66].

Indeed, some experimental studies provided evidence that the inhibition of Ang II activity by ARB slows the process of glomerulosclerosis and decreases the expression of TGF-β1 as well as Ang II level in diseased glomeruli [71, 72].

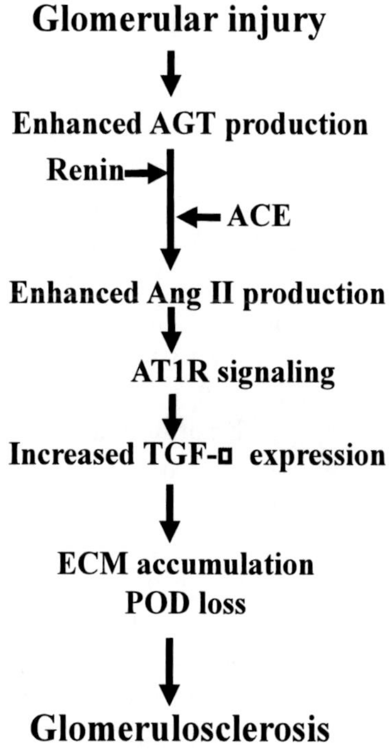

Figure 3. Overview of the Ang II -TGF-β1 axis in the development of glomerulosclerosis. Repeated glomerular injury induces enhanced production of angiotensinogen (AGT) that leads to increased production of angiotensin II (Ang II) (RAS activation) within nephritic glomeruli. Then, Ang II induces TGF-β1 expression, and followed by extracellular matrix (ECM) accumulation and podocyte (POD) apoptosis, finally resulting in the development of glomerulosclerosis.

Contribution of Glomerular RAS Activation to Pathological Glomerular Remodeling in Disease Progression

Recent studies using immunohistochemical and in situ hybridization techniques have shown that the parallel increases of AGT and Ang II are found in the damaged glomeruli of several types of rat and human glomerulopathies, whereas there are inconsistent findings in the remaining RAS components, suggesting that the activity of the glomerular Ang II - generating system is mainly dependent on AGT expression in diseased glomeruli [72-78]. Biochemical analyses of isolated glomeruli from diabetic rats revealed that the level of glomerular Ang II synthesis is increased due to an increase of AGT protein, and an increase in the formation of Ang II is mediated by an unidentified enzymatic pathway other than ACE within diabetic glomeruli [79]. On the other hand, studies of several genetically manipulated animals suggest the involvement of increased glomerular Ang II synthesis in glomerular injury. Rat glomeruli expressing with human renin and AGT genes developed glomerular sclerosis and showed MC activation (α-smooth muscle actin positive) [80]. Upstream stimulatory factor 2 (USF2) transgenic mice show increased renin expression and enhanced renin activity in the kidney, which stimulates glomerular Ang II generation, leading to glomerular hypertrophy and ECM accumulation accompanied by enhanced TGF-βexpression and albuminemia [81]. The transgenic TG (mRen2)27 rat (Ren2 rats), which harbors both the native Ren1 and the murine renin transgene, is indicated as a model of excessive tissue RAS activity (the increased tissue levels of AngII) and develops hypertension, focal segmental glomerulosclerosis, and proteinuria [82-84]. Moreover, increased immunostaining of Ang II and AT1R has been demonstrated in the damaged glomeruli of Ren2 rats [84].

AGT is the only substrate for renin, a rate-limiting enzyme of the RAS. Therefore, the amount of AGT determines the amount of tissue-based Ang II synthesis and tissue RAS activity [11]. The cellular origins of AGT and the activation mode of RAS leading to the Ang II formation within the glomerulus are still not fully understood. Using a rat remnant model, Lee et al reported the triggering of a cascade from glomerular Ang II generation to TGF-β and ECM protein gene expression as a result of hemodynamic changes and injured or activated GEC synthesizes of AGT, leading to development of a segmental glomerular sclerotic lesion [85]. This pathological progression can be prevented by ARB, indicating the central role of the Ang II-AT1R- TGF-β pathway in the disease progression of this rat model. Recently, we performed a histochemical study of renal biopsy samples from patients with IgA nephropathy (IgAN) or minor glomerular abnormalities (MGA) [78]. Glomerular AGT is weakly expressed by GECs in patients with MGA, but strongly induced at endocapillary sites including GECs and MCs in IgAN patients although they had normal GFR and BP. The level of glomerular AGT parallels with the levels of glomerular Ang II and TGF-β expression in the diseased glomeruli, respectively. The levels of glomerular injury including cell proliferation, ECM accumulation and proteinuria are also closely correlated with the levels of AGT and Ang II. Additionally, the AGT level appears to determine the Ang II level in nephritic glomeruli. Furthermore, several cell culture studies, including our own, show that Ang II can stimulate the AGT mRNA and AGT protein biosynthesis by renal cells, suggesting that its action might constitute an auto-amplifying loop of the activity of the intrarenal RAS [11, 78]. Therefore, we postulate that, even in the early stage of IgA nephropathy, glomerular RAS activation occurs because of increased GEC-and MC-AGT expression and results in enhanced local Ang II generation leading to the clinical and pathological abnormalities. A glomerular Ang II-AGT positive feed back loop might drive RAS activation for further glomerular injury. Similarly, Nakamura et al reported that salt – sensitive glomerular injury in eNOS-/- mice is mediated by enhancement of glomerular GEC-AGT-derived Ang II, through the augmentation of glomerular oxidative stress [86]. Thus, GEC-AGT expression may play a key role in glomerular RAS activation followed by glomerular pathological alterations in CKD.

Emerging evidence indicates that glomerular Ang II production is also regulated by the expression ratio of ACE to ACE2 within the glomerulus [75]. ACE2 degrades Ang II to Ang (1-7) that antagonizes Ang II-mediated vasoconstriction, as well as proliferative, and fibrotic actions via the Mas receptor, and therefore has the potential to counterbalance the effects of ACE [35]. ACE2 also degrades Ang I to Ang-(1–9) that is subsequently converted to Ang-(1–7) by ACE. Because of these properties, ACE2 has been postulated to be an endogenous ACE inhibitor [87]. There are many data indicating the role of ACE2 expression and/or activity in glomerular disease progression [75, 88, 89]. In the diabetic mouse and human kidney diseases such as diabetic nephropathy and IgA nephropathy, an increase of the ACE /ACE2 ratio, due largely due to decreased ACE2 expression, is observed in damaged glomeruli, suggesting a potential mechanism that leads to increased glomerular Ang II synthesis [27, 42, 43]. Systemic administration of recombinant human ACE2 or an increase in systemic ACE2 by adenoviral expression induces an improvement of DM nephropathy in rats [90, 91]. In contrast, the male ACE2 mutant (ACE2-/ y) mice show increased levels of renal tissue Ang II, leading to glomerulosclerosis [87]. Both the sensitive indicator of ROS production, lipid peroxidation product and the glomerulosclerosis score are markedly enhanced in these mice, whereas ARB prevents such an enhancement, which strongly supports the potential role of ACE2 in Ang II-induced glomerular injury. More recently, Nadarajah R et al investigated the role of POD-ACE2 expression in DM nephropathy using transgenic mice with the overexpressing human ACE2 in PODs [92]. They reported that after STZ-induced DM, these transgenic mice are protected against the development of proteinuria and show the preservation of PODs, and a reduction of glomerular injury compared with that of control mice. Thus, regulation of the ACE2 activity may represent a potentially exciting target for therapeutic intervention.

An Integrating Viewpoint of Ang II, TGF-β and ROS Actions in Glomerular Disease Progression

Finally, we should address the potential role of ROS in the Ang II–induced pathological glomerular remodeling in GN. ROS has been acknowledged as an important pathogenic factor in the progression of CKD, including DM nephropathy [4, 93]. There are several potential pathways for enhanced generation of ROS in CKD. NADPH oxidases are a family of multi-subunit enzyme complexes with the primary function of generating superoxide and/or hydrogen peroxide [94]. The prototype NADPH oxidase (Nox2 [gp91phox]-containing NADPH oxidase), found in phagocytic cells, possesses cytosolic subunits (p47phox, p67phox, or homologues) and membrane-bound subunits (gp91phox and p22phox), which form a functional enzyme complex upon activation. Seven Nox isoforms (Nox1-7) are expressed in a tissue-specific manner [95]. Currently, several types of NADPH oxidases have been identified as the main generators of ROS in renal cells such as tubular epithelial cells and glomerular cells [4]. ROS induces not only cell and tissue damages directly but also works as signaling molecules to regulate the cellular behaviors such as proliferation, differentiation and apoptosis, thereby contributing to the pathogenesis of many kidney diseases [4, 96]. Additionally, there are several interactions between ROS and nitric oxide (NO), which lead to a decrease of NO bioavailability [93]. The superoxide O2- rapidly reacts with NO, yielding peroxinitrite (ONOO-) that oxidizes the zinc-thiolate center of NO synthase (NOS), resulting in a decrease of NO formation. Glomerular endothelial NOS (eNOS) might be good target for superoxides, and therefore leads to glomerular capillary wall damage in nephritic glomeruli [97]. Of note, it has been reported that the activity of NADPH oxidase is enhanced by several agonists such as Ang II and TGF- β 1 [7, 98]. In turn, ROS mediates TGF-β1 and Ang II signaling involved in in the process of CKD progression [98]. Furthermore, TGF-β and ROS are recognized as potential stimulatory factors for intrarenal AGT expression leading to Ang II synthesis in CKD [99, 100]. Indeed, the significant associations of RAS activity (Ang II generation) with TGF-β1 expression, ROS generation and pathological alterations have been reported in several experimental models of rat GN [71, 72, 101-103].

Recently, we investigated the relationship among RAS activity, TGF-β1 and ROS in the nephritic glomeruli using two rat models of progressive GN in combination with ARB (candesartan) treatment [71, 72, 101]. In the ROS- generating system, we focused on the expression of Nox 2, a major component of the NADPH oxidase in the diseased kidney [72, 101].

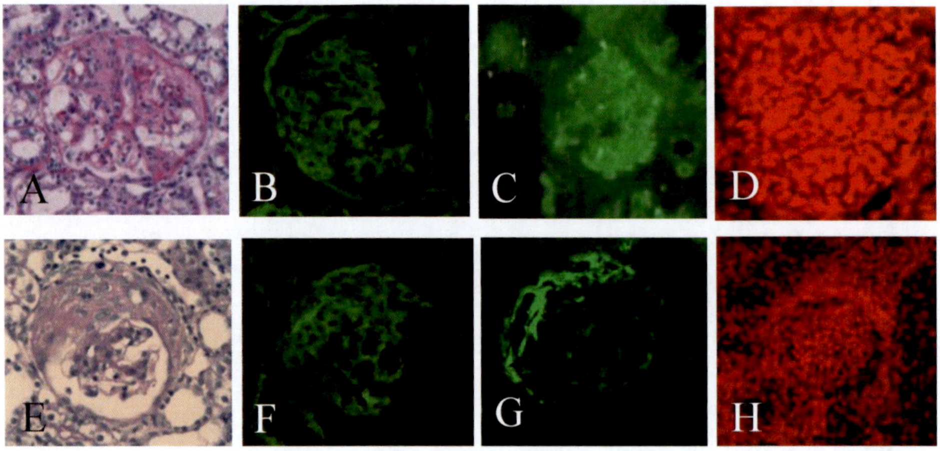

Figure 4. Glomerular alterations, and Ang II, TGF-β1 and ROS expression in two rat models of progressive GN. Immunohistochemical examinations of anti-Thy-1 serum (A-D)- or anti-GBM antibody (E-H)- induced GN in rats. Anti-Thy-1 serum induces severe mesangial proliferative GN with segmental sclerosis and synechiae (A), whereas the anti-GBM antibody. induces severe crescentic GN (E). Enhanced glomerular Ang II synthesis (B, F), TGF-β1 (C, G), production (D, H) are detected in each rat model. Superoxide production was detected by DHE dye. Modified from Ref.71, 72, and 101.

Vehicle-treated nephritic rats shows significant proteinuria and severe GN characterized by severe mesangial proliferation or crescent formation, respectively, while ARB treatment significantly attenuates proteinuria, glomerular Ang II accumulation, superoxide production and such pathological alterations (Figure. 4).

Consistent with histological findings, biochemical analysis of isolated glomeruli revealed that glomerular production of AGT, Ang II, and TGF-β1 and Nox2 is enhanced in a rat model of crescentic GN, whereas ARB treatment significantly reduces each production level in diseased glomeruli to that near the control level.

Therefore, we speculate that the glomerular Ang II-generating system works in vivo for production of Ang II that induces TGF-β1 expression and superoxides, and finally contributes to the development of their respective glomerular lesions observed in the two rat models of GN.

Considering the many data of a mutual stimulatory action among Ang II, TGF-β1 and ROS under the disease condition, combination therapy using drugs that target each mediator may be a potential method to prevent or treat sustained pathological remodeling in GN. Of course, future research should focus on discovery of the integrating point of each mediator-induced complex intracellular signaling pathway in progressive GN.

Conclusion

It is now clear evidence that the glomerulus-based RAS is deeply involved in glomerular physiology and pathophysiology. Enhanced glomerular Ang II actions in diseased glomeruli via ACE-Ang II-AT1R signaling leads to cell proliferation, ECM production and decreased ECM degradation, resulting in pathological glomerular remodeling such as glomerulosclerosis. The glomerular Ang II- AT1R-TGF-β axis is a key molecular cascade for the development of Ang II-induced glomerulosclerosis. A large amount of data concerning animal and human CKD has shown that the use of RAS blockers, such as ACEIs and ARBs, is effective and a promising therapy for attenuating the progression of CKD, beyond the BP lowering effect, which strongly supports the above view of Ang II-mediated progression process of GN. Our recent understanding of glomerular RAS and the molecular interactions among Ang II, TGF-β and NADPH oxidase provides us with new insights regarding the therapeutic strategies for the prevention and treatment of pathological glomerular remodeling in progressive GN. Moreover, the identification of integrating molecules for Ang II, TGF-β and ROS actions that participate in the process of glomerular remodeling would open a new avenue for promising methods to prevent or attenuate the progression of GN.

Acknowledgments

The work of the author was completed with support from a Grant-in-Aid from the Ministry of Education, Culture, Sports, Science and Technology in Japan.

Conflict of interest: The author of this manuscript has no conflict of interest to disclose.

References

[1] BorderWA, Noble NA. Transforming growth factor beta in tissue fibrosis. *N. Engl. J. Med.* 1994 331(19):1286–92.

[2] Atkins RC, Nikolic-Paterson DJ, Song Q, Lan HY. Modulators of crescentic glomerulonephritis. *J. Am. Soc. Nephrol.* 1996 7(11):2271–8.

[3] Kriz W, LeHir M. Pathways to nephron loss starting from glomerular diseases—insights from animal models. *Kidney Int.* 2005 67(2):404–419.

[4] Shah SV, Baliga R, Rajapurkar M, Fonseca VA. Oxidants in chronic kidney disease. *J. Am. Soc. Nephrol.* 2007 18(1):16–28.

[5] Tipping PG, Holdsworth SR. Cytokines in glomerulonephritis. *Semin Nephrol* 2007 27(3):275–85.

[6] Rüster C, Wolf G. Angiotensin II as a morphogenic cytokine stimulating renal fibrogenesis. *J. Am. Soc. Nephrol.* 2011 22(7):1189-99. 2011

[7] Sachse A, Wolf G. Angiotensin II-induced reactive oxygen species and the kidney. *J. Am. Soc. Nephrol.* 2007 18(9):2439-46.

[8] Bader M. Tissue renin-angiotensin-aldosterone systems: targets for pharmacological therapy. *Annu. Rev. Pharmacol. Toxicol.* 2010 50:439–465.

[9] Dzau VJ. Tissue angiotensin and pathobiology of vascular disease: a unifying hypothesis. *Hypertension.* 2001 37(4):1047–1052.

[10] Bader M, Ganten D. Update on tissue renin-angiotensin systems. *J. Mol. Med. (Berl)* 2008 86(6):615–621.

[11] Kobori H, Nangaku M, Navar LG, Nishiyama A. The intrarenal renin-angiotensin system: from physiology to the pathobiology of hypertension and kidney disease. *Pharmacol. Rev.* 2007 59:251–287.

[12] Yosypiv IV. Renin-angiotensin system in ureteric bud branching morphogenesis: insights into the mechanisms. *Pediatr Nephrol.* 2011 26(9):1499–1512.

[13] Lai KN, Leung JC, Tang SC. The renin-angiotensin system (diabetes and the kidney). In: Lai KN, Tang SC, editors. Contributions to nephrology. Basel: Karger; 2011. vol. 170, p. 135–44.

[14] Warner FJ, Lubel JS, McCaughan GW, Angus PW. Liver fibrosis: a balance of ACEs? *Clin. Sci.* (Lond) 2007 113(3):109–118.

[15] Velez JC. The importance of the intrarenal renin-angiotensin system. *Nat. Clin. Pract. Nephrol.* 2009 5(2):89–100.

[16] Morris BJ, Reid IA. A "renin-like" enzymatic action of cathepsin D and the similarity in subcellular distributions of "renin-like" activity and cathepsin D in the midbrain of dogs. *Endocrinology.* 1978 103(4):1289-96.

[17] Fukuda N, Hu WY, Satoh C, Nakayama M, Kishioka H, Kubo A, Kanmatsuse K. Contribution of synthetic phenotype on the enhanced angiotensin II-generating system in vascular smooth muscle cells from spontaneously hypertensive rats. *J. Hypertens.* 1999 17(8):1099-107.

[18] Graciano ML, Cavaglieri Rde C, Dellê H, Dominguez WV, Casarini DE, Malheiros DM, Noronha IL. Intrarenal Renin-Angiotensin system is upregulated in experimental model of progressive renal disease induced by chronic inhibition of nitric oxide synthesis. *J. Am. Soc. Nephrol.* 2004 15(7):1805-15.

[19] Yosypiv IV. Renin-angiotensin system-growth factor cross-talk: a novel mechanism for ureteric bud morphogenesis. *Pediatr. Nephrol.* 2009 24(6): 1113–20.

[20] Lacoste M, Cai Y, Guicharnaud L, Mounier F, Dumez Y, Bouvier R, Dijoud F, Gonzales M, Chatten J, Delezoide AL, Daniel L, Joubert M, Laurent N, Aziza J, Sellami T, Amar HB, Jarnet C, Frances AM, Daïkha-Dahmane F, Coulomb A, Neuhaus TJ, Foliguet B, Chenal P, Marcorelles P, Gasc JM, Corvol P, Gubler MC. Renal tubular dysgenesis, a not uncommon autosomal recessive disorder leading to oligohydramnios: Role of the Renin-Angiotensin system. *J. Am. Soc. Nephrol.* 2006 17(8):2253-63.

[21] Rüster C, Wolf G. Angiotensin II as a morphogenic cytokine stimulating renal fibrogenesis. *J. Am. Soc. Nephrol.* 2011 22(7):1189–99.

[22] Anja Sachse and Gunter Wolf. Angiotensin II–Induced Reactive Oxygen Species and the Kidney *J. Am. Soc. Nephrol.* 2007 18(9): 2439–46.

[23] Lijnen P, Petrov V. Renin-angiotensin system, hypertrophy and gene expression in cardiac myocytes. *J. Mol. Cell Cardiol.* 1999 31(5):949-70.

[24] Müller DN, Fiebeler A, Park JK, Dechend R, Luft FC. Angiotensin II and endothelin induce inflammation and thereby promote hypertension-induced end-organ damage. *Clin. Nephrol.* 2003 60 Suppl 1:S2-12.

[25] Burns WC, Velkoska E, Dean R, Burrell LM, Thomas MC. Angiotensin II mediates epithelial-to-mesenchymal transformation in tubular cells by ANG 1-7/MAS-1-dependent pathways. *Am. J. Physiol. Renal. Physiol.* 2010 299(3):F585-93.

[26] Kagami S, Border WA, Miller DE, Noble NA. Angiotensin II stimulates extracellular matrix protein synthesis through induction of transforming growth factor-beta expression in rat glomerular mesangial cells. *J. Clin. Invest.* 1994 93(6):2431–37.

[27] Urushihara M, Ohashi N, Miyata K, Satou R, Acres OW, Kobori H. Addition of angiotensin II type 1 receptor blocker to CCR2 antagonist markedly attenuates crescentic glomerulonephritis. *Hypertension*. 2011 57(3):586-93.

[28] Tsuchiya K, Yoshimoto T, Hirono Y, Tateno T, Sugiyama T, Hirata Y. Angiotensin II induces monocyte chemoattractant protein-1 expression via a nuclear factor-kappaB-dependent pathway in rat preadipocytes. *Am. J. Physiol. Endocrinol. Metab.* 2006 291(4):E771-8.

[29] Yokoyama T, Sekiguchi K, Tanaka T, Tomaru K, Arai M, Suzuki T, Nagai R. Angiotensin II and mechanical stretch induce production of tumor necrosis factor in cardiac fibroblasts. *Am. J. Physiol.* 1999 Jun;276(6 Pt 2):H1968-76.

[30] Jackman HL, Massad MG, Sekosan M, Tan F, Brovkovych V, Marcic BM, Erdös EG. Angiotensin 1-9 and 1-7 release in human heart: role of cathepsin A. *Hypertension.* 2002 39(5):976-81.

[31] Mustafa MR, Dharmani M, Kunheen NK, Sim MK. Effects of des-aspartate-angiotensin I on the actions of angiotensin III in the renal and mesenteric vasculature of normo- and hypertensive rats. *Regul. Pept.* 2004 120(1-3):15–22.

[32] Gava E, Samad-Zadeh A, Zimpelmann J, Bahramifarid N, Kitten GT, Santos RA, et al. Angiotensin-(1-7) activates a tyrosine phosphatase and inhibits glucose-induced signalling in proximal tubular cells. *Nephrol. Dial Transplant* 2009;24(6):1766–73.

[33] Santos RA, Ferreira AJ, Simões E, Silva AC. Recent advances in the angiotensin-converting enzyme 2-angiotensin(1-7)-Mas axis. *Exp. Physiol.* 2008;93(5):519–27.

[34] Santos RA, Simoes e Silva AC, Maric C, Silva DM, Machado RP, de Buhr I, et al. Angiotensin-(1-7) is an endogenous ligand for the G protein-coupled receptor Mas. *Proc. Natl. Acad. Sci. USA* 2003; 100(14):8258–63.

[35] Ferrario CM, Varagic J. The ANG-(1–7)/ACE2/mas axis in the regulation of nephron function. *Am. J. Physiol. Ren. Physiol.* 2010; 298:F1297–F1305.

[36] Axelband F, Dias J, Miranda F, Ferrão FM, Barros NM, Carmona AK, et al. A scrutiny of the biochemical pathways from Ang II to Ang-(3-4) in renal basolateral membranes. *Regul. Pept.* 2009;158(1–3):47–56.

[37] van Rodijnen WF, van Lambalgen TA, van Wijhe MH, Tangelder GJ, Ter Wee PM. Renal microvascular actions of angiotensin II fragments. *Am. J. Physiol. Renal. Physiol.* 2002 283(1):F86-92.

[38] Yang H, Zeng XJ, Wang HX, Zhang LK, Dong XL, Guo S, Du J, Li HH, Tang CS. Angiotensin IV protects against angiotensin II-induced cardiac injury via AT4 receptor. *Peptides.* 2011 32(10):2108-15.

[39] Esteban V, Ruperez M, Sánchez-López E, Rodríguez-Vita J, Lorenzo O, Demaegdt H, Vanderheyden P, Egido J, Ruiz-Ortega M. Angiotensin IV activates the nuclear transcription factor-kappaB and related proinflammatory genes in vascular smooth muscle cells. *Circ. Res.* 2005 96(9):965-73.

[40] Chai SY, Fernando R, Peck G, Ye SY, Mendelsohn FA, Jenkins TA, et al. The angiotensin IV/AT4 receptor. *Cell Mol. Life Sci.* 2004;61:2728–2737.

[41] Nguyen G, Delarue F, Burcklé C, Bouzhir L, Giller T, Sraer JD. Pivotal role of the renin/prorenin receptor in angiotensin II production and cellular responses to renin. *J. Clin. Invest.* 2002;109:1417–1427.

[42] Nguyen G, Muller DN. The biology of the (pro)renin receptor. *J. Am. Soc. Nephrol.* 2010;21:18–23.

[43] Leehey DJ, Singh AK, Bast JP, Sethupathi P, Singh R. Glomerular renin - angiotensin system in streptozotocin diabetic and Zucker diabetic fatty rats. *Transl. Res.* 2008 Apr;151(4):208-16.

[44] Kagami S. Involvement of glomerular renin-angiotensin system (RAS) activation in the development and progression of glomerular injury. *Clin. Exp. Nephrol.* 2012 16(2):214-20.

[45] Harrison-Bernard LM, Chappell MC. Unraveling the glomerular RAS: one peptidase at a time. *Am. J. Physiol. Renal. Physiol.* 2012 303(3):F373-4.

[46] Seikaly MG, Arant BS, Jr, Seney FD., Jr Endogenous angiotensin concentrations in specific intrarenal fluid compartments of the rat. *J. Clin. Invest.* 1990;86:1352–1357.

[47] Atiyeh BA, Arant BS, Jr, Henrich WL, Seikaly MG. In vitro production of angiotensin II by isolated glomeruli. *Am. J. Physiol.* 1995;268(2 Pt 2):F266–F272.

[48] Velez JC, Ryan KJ, Harbeson CE, Bland AM, Budisavljevic MN, Arthur JM, et al. Angiotensin I is largely converted to angiotensin (1–7) and angiotensin (2–10) by isolated rat glomeruli. *Hypertension.* 2009;53:790–797.

[49] Velez JC, Bland AM, Arthur JM, Raymond JR, Janech MG. Characterization of renin-angiotensin system enzyme activities in cultured mouse podocytes. *Am. J. Physiol. Ren. Physiol.* 2007;293:F398–F407.

[50] Velez JC, Ierardi JL, Bland AM, Morinelli TA, Arthur JM, Raymond JR, Janech MG. Enzymatic processing of angiotensin peptides by human glomerular endothelial cells. *Am. J. Physiol. Renal. Physiol.* 2012 302(12):F1583-94.

[51] Singh R, Singh AK, Alavi N, Leehey DJ. Mechanism of increased angiotensin II levels in glomerular mesangial cells cultured in high glucose. *J. Am. Soc. Nephrol.* 2003;14:873–880.

[52] Cristovam PC, Arnoni CP, Andrade MC, Casarini DE, Pereira LG, Schor N, et al. ACE-dependent and chymase-dependent angiotensin II generation in normal and glucose-stimulated human mesangial cells. *Exp. Biol. Med.* 2008;233:1035–1043.

[53] Aragão DS, Cunha TS, Arita DY, Andrade MC, Fernandes AB, Watanabe IK, et al. Purification and characterization of angiotensin converting enzyme 2 (ACE2) from murine model of mesangial cell in culture. *Int J Biol Macromol.* 2011;49:79–84.

[54] Border WA, Noble NA. Interactions of transforming growth factor- and angiotensin II in renal fibrosis. *Hypertension.* 1998 31(1 Pt 2):181-8.

[55] Wolf G. Renal injury due to renin-angiotensin-aldosterone system activation of the transforming growth factor- b pathway. *Kidney Int.* 2006 70(11):1914-9.

[56] Kagami S, Urushihara M, Kondo S, Hayashi T, Yamano H, Löster K, Vossmeyer D, Reutter W, Kuroda Y. Effects of anti-alpha1 integrin subunit antibody on anti-Thy-1 glomerulonephritis. *Lab. Invest.* 2002 82(9):1219-27.

[57] Kagami S, Kondo S. β 1-integrins and glomerular injury. *J. Med. Invest.* 2004 51(1-2):1-13.

[58] Borza CM, Pozzi A. The role of cell-extracellular matrix interactions in glomerular injury. *Exp. Cell Res.* 2012 318(9):1001-10.

[59] Lenz O, Elliot SJ, Stetler-Stevenson WG. Matrix metalloproteinases in renal development and disease. *J. Am. Soc. Nephrol.* 2000 11(3):574-81.

[60] Kagami S, Kondo S, Löster K, Reutter W, Kuhara T, Yasutomo K, Kuroda Y. Alpha1beta1 integrin-mediated collagen matrix remodeling by rat mesangial cells is differentially regulated by transforming growth factor-beta and platelet-derived growth factor-BB. *J. Am. Soc. Nephrol.* 1999 10(4):779-89.

[61] Poncelet AC, de Caestecker MP, Schnaper HW. The transforming growth factor- b /SMAD signaling pathway is present and functional in human mesangial cells. *Kidney Int.* 1999 56(4):1354-65.

[62] Hayashida T, Poncelet AC, Hubchak SC, Schnaper HW. TGF-b1 activates MAP kinase in human mesangial cells: a possible role in collagen expression. *Kidney Int.* 1999 56(5):1710-20.

[63] Dorado F, Velasco S, Esparís-Ogando A, Pericacho M, Pandiella A, Silva J, López-Novoa JM, Rodríguez-Barbero A. The mitogen-activated protein kinase Erk5 mediates human mesangial cell activation. *Nephrol. Dial Transplant.* 2008 23(11):3403-11

[64] Lemley KV. Protecting podocytes: how good do we need to be? *Kidney Int.* 2012 81(1):9-11.

[65] Schiffer M, Bitzer M, Roberts IS, Kopp JB, ten Dijke P, Mundel P, Böttinger EP. Apoptosis in podocytes induced by TGF-beta and Smad7. *J. Clin. Invest.* 2001 108(6):807-16.

[66] Lee HS. Mechanisms and consequences of TGF-ß overexpression by podocytes in progressive podocyte disease. *Cell Tissue Res.* 2012 347(1):129-40.

[67] Taal MW, Brenner BM. Renoprotective benefits of RAS inhibition: from ACEI to angiotensin II antagonists. *Kidney Int.* 2000;57(5):1803–1817.

[68] Wühl E, Schaefer F. Therapeutic strategies to slow chronic kidney disease progression. *Pediatr Nephrol.* 2008;23(5):705–716.

[69] Mezzano SA, Ruiz-Ortega M, Egido J. Angiotensin II and renal fibrosis. *Hypertension.* 2001 38(3 Pt 2):635-8.

[70] Kagami S, Kuhara T, Okada K, Kuroda Y, Border WA, Noble NA. Dual effects of angiotensin II on the plasminogen/plasmin system in rat mesangial cells. *Kidney Int.* 1997 51(3):664-671.

[71] Urushihara M, Takamatsu M, Shimizu M, Kondo S, Kinoshita Y, Suga K, Kitamura A, Matsuura S, Yoshizumi M, Tamaki T, Kawachi H, Kagami S. ERK5 activation enhances mesangial cell viability and collagen matrix accumulation in rat progressive glomerulonephritis. *Am. J. Physiol. Renal. Physiol.* 2010 298(1):F167-176.

[72] Kinoshita Y, Kondo S, Urushihara M, Suga K, Matsuura S, Takamatsu M, Shimizu M, Nishiyama A, Kawachi H, Kagami S. Angiotensin II type I receptor blockade suppresses glomerular renin-angiotensin system activation, oxidative stress, and progressive glomerular injury in rat anti-glomerular basement membrane glomerulonephritis. *Transl. Res.* 2011 158(4):235-248.

[73] Lai KN, Leung JC, Lai KB, To WY, Yeung VT, Lai FM. Gene expression of the renin-angiotensin system in human kidney. *J. Hypertens.* 1998;16(1):91–102.

[74] Prete D, Gambaro G, Lupo A, Anglani F, Brezzi B, Magistroni R, Graziotto R, Furci L, Modena F, Bernich P, Albertazzi A, D'Angelo A, Maschio G. Precocious activation of genes of the renin-angiotensin system and the fibrogenic cascade in IgA glomerulonephritis. *Kidney Int.* 2003;64(1):149–159.

[75] Ye M, Wysocki J, WilliAm. J., Soler MJ, Cokic I, Batlle D. Glomerular localization and expression of angiotensin-converting enzyme 2 and angiotensin-converting enzyme: implications for albuminuria in diabetes. *J. Am. Soc. Nephrol.* 2006;17(11):3067–75.

[76] Wagner J, Gehlen F, Ciechanowicz A, Ritz E. Angiotensin II receptor type 1 gene expression in human glomerulonephritis and diabetes mellitus. *J. Am. Soc. Nephrol.* 1999;10(3):545–551.

[77] Suzuki K, Han GD, Miyauchi N, Hashimoto T, Nakatsue T, Fujioka Y, Koike H, Shimizu F, Kawachi H. Angiotensin II type 1 and type 2 receptors play opposite roles in regulating the barrier function of kidney glomerular capillary wall. *Am. J. Pathol.* 2007;170(6):1841–53.

[78] Takamatsu M, Urushihara M, Kondo S, Shimizu M, Morioka T, Oite T, et al. Glomerular angiotensinogen protein is enhanced in pediatric IgA nephropathy. *Pediatr Nephrol.* 2008;23(8):1257–1267.

[79] Singh R, Singh AK, Leehey DJ. A novel mechanism for angiotensin II formation in streptozotocin-diabetic rat glomeruli. *Am. J. Physiol. Ren. Physiol.* 2005;288(6):F1183–90.

[80] Arai M, Wada A, Isaka Y, Akagi Y, Sugiura T, Miyazaki M, et al. In vivo transfection of genes for renin and angiotensinogen into the glomerular cells induced phenotypic change of the mesangial cells and glomerular sclerosis. *Biochem. Biophys. Res. Commun.* 1995; 206(2):525–32.

[81] Shi L, Nikolic D, Liu S, Lu H, Wang S. Activation of renal renin-angiotensin system in upstream stimulatory factor 2 transgenic mice. *Am. J. Physiol. Ren. Physiol.* 2009;296(2):F257–65.

[82] Whaley-Connell A, Habibi J, Nistala R, Cooper SA, Karuparthi PR, Hayden MR, Rehmer N, DeMarco VG, Andresen BT, Wei Y, Ferrario C, Sowers JR. Attenuation of

NADPH oxidase activation and glomerular filtration barrier remodeling with statin treatment. *Hypertension.* 2008 51(2):474-80.

[83] Whaley-Connell A, Nistala R, Habibi J, Hayden MR, Schneider RI, Johnson MS, Tilmon R, Rehmer N, Ferrario CM, Sowers JR. Comparative effect of direct renin inhibition and AT1R blockade on glomerular filtration barrier injury in the transgenic Ren2 rat. *Am. J. Physiol. Renal. Physiol.* 2010 298(3):F655-61.

[84] Rakusan D, Kujal P, Kramer HJ, Husková Z, Vanourková Z, Vernerová Z, Mrázová I, Thumová M, Cervenka L, Vanecková I. Persistent antihypertensive effect of aliskiren is accompanied by reduced proteinuria and normalization of glomerular area in Ren-2 transgenic rats. *Am. J. Physiol. Renal. Physiol.* 2010 299(4):F758-66.

[85] Lee LK, Meyer TW, Pollock AS, Lovett DH. Endothelial cell injury initiates glomerular sclerosis in the rat remnant kidney. *J. Clin. Invest.* 1995;96(2):953–64.

[86] Nakamura T, Kataoka K, Tokutomi Y, Nako H, Toyama K, Dong YF, Koibuchi N, Yamamoto E, Yasuda O, Ogawa H, Kim-Mitsuyama S. Novel mechanism of salt-induced glomerular injury: critical role of eNOS and angiotensin II. *J. Hypertens.* 2011;29(8):1528–35.

[87] Oudit GY, Herzenberg AM, Kassiri Z, Wong D, Reich H, Khokha R, Crackower MA, Backx PH, Penninger JM, Scholey JW. Loss of angiotensin-converting enzyme-2 leads to the late development of angiotensin II-dependent glomerulosclerosis. *Am. J. Pathol.* 2006; 168(6):1808–20.

[88] Reich HN, Oudit GY, Penninger JM, Scholey JW, Herzenberg AM. Decreased glomerular and tubular expression of ACE2 in patients with type 2 diabetes and kidney disease. *Kidney Int.* 2008;74(12):1610–16.

[89] Mizuiri S, Hemmi H, Arita M, Aoki T, Ohashi Y, Miyagi M, Sakai K, Shibuya K, Hase H, Aikawa A. Increased ACE and decreased ACE2 expression in kidneys from patients with IgA nephropathy. *Nephron Clin. Pract.* 2011;117(1):c57-66.

[90] Oudit GY, Liu GC, Zhong J, Basu R, Chow FL, Zhou J, Loibner H, Janzek E, Schuster M, Penninger JM, Herzenberg AM, Kassiri Z, Scholey JW. Human recombinant ACE2 reduces the progression of diabetic nephropathy. *Diabetes.* 2010 59(2):529-38.

[91] Liu CX, Hu Q, Wang Y, Zhang W, Ma ZY, Feng JB, Wang R, Wang XP, Dong B, Gao F, Zhang MX, Zhang Y. Angiotensin-converting enzyme (ACE) 2 overexpression ameliorates glomerular injury in a rat model of diabetic nephropathy: a comparison with ACE inhibition. *Mol. Med.* 2011 17(1-2):59-69.

[92] Nadarajah R, Milagres R, Dilauro M, Gutsol A, Xiao F, Zimpelmann J, Kennedy C, Wysocki J, Batlle D, Burns KD. Podocyte-specific overexpression of human angiotensin-converting enzyme 2 attenuates diabetic nephropathy in mice. *Kidney Int.* 2012 82(3):292-303.

[93] Sachse A, Wolf G. Angiotensin II-induced reactive oxygen species and the kidney. *J. Am. Soc. Nephrol.* 2007 18(9):2439-46.

[94] Montezano AC, Burger D, Ceravolo GS, Yusuf H, Montero M, Touyz RM. Novel Nox homologues in the vasculature: focusing on Nox4 and Nox5. *Clin. Sci.* (Lond). 2011 120(4):131-41.

[95] Briones AM, Tabet F, Callera GE, Montezano AC, Yogi A, He Y, Quinn MT, Salaices M, Touyz RM. Differential regulation of Nox1, Nox2 and Nox4 in vascular smooth muscle cells from WKY and SHR. *J. Am. Soc. Hypertens.* 2011 5(3):137-53.

[96] Barnes JL, Gorin Y. Myofibroblast differentiation during fibrosis: role of NAD(P)H oxidases. *Kidney Int.* 2011 79(9):944-56.

[97] Satoh M, Fujimoto S, Arakawa S, Yada T, Namikoshi T, Haruna Y, Horike H, Sasaki T, Kashihara N. Angiotensin II type 1 receptor blocker ameliorates uncoupled endothelial nitric oxide synthase in rats with experimental diabetic nephropathy. *Nephrol. Dial Transplant.* 2008 23(12):3806-13.

[98] Bondi CD, Manickam N, Lee DY, Block K, Gorin Y, Abboud HE, Barnes JL. NAD(P)H oxidase mediates TGF-beta1-induced activation of kidney myofibroblasts. *J. Am. Soc. Nephrol.* 2010 21(1):93-102.

[99] Brezniceanu ML, Wei CC, Zhang SL, Hsieh TJ, Guo DF, Hébert MJ, Ingelfinger JR, Filep JG, Chan JS. Transforming growth factor-beta 1 stimulates angiotensinogen gene expression in kidney proximal tubular cells. *Kidney Int.* 2006 69(11):1977-85.

[100] Hsieh TJ, Zhang SL, Filep JG, Tang SS, Ingelfinger JR, Chan JS. High glucose stimulates angiotensinogen gene expression via reactive oxygen species generation in rat kidney proximal tubular cells. *Endocrinology.* 2002 143(8):2975-85.

[101] Kondo S, Shimizu M, Urushihara M, Tsuchiya K, Yoshizumi M, Tamaki T, Nishiyama A, Kawachi H, Shimizu F, Quinn MT, Lambeth DJ, Kagami S. Addition of the antioxidant probucol to angiotensin II type I receptor antagonist arrests progressive mesangioproliferative glomerulonephritis in the rat. *J. Am. Soc. Nephrol.* 2006 17(3):783-94.

[102] Nagai Y, Yao L, Kobori H, Miyata K, Ozawa Y, Miyatake A, Yukimura T, Shokoji T, Kimura S, Kiyomoto H, Kohno M, Abe Y, Nishiyama A. Temporary angiotensin II blockade at the prediabetic stage attenuates the development of renal injury in type 2 diabetic rats. *J. Am. Soc. Nephrol.* 2005 16(3):703-11.

[103] Maeda Y, Inoguchi T, Takei R, Sawada F, Sasaki S, Fujii M, Kobayashi K, Urata H, Nishiyama A, Takayanagi R. Inhibition of chymase protects against diabetes-induced oxidative stress and renal dysfunction in hamsters. *Am. J. Physiol. Renal. Physiol.* 2010 299(6):F1328-38.

In: Renin-Angiotensin System
Editors: Ayako Himura and Takeshi Sato

ISBN: 978-1-62417-788-0

Chapter VII

The Role of Vitamin D in the Renin Angiotensin System

Khanh vinh quốc Lương* and Lan Thi Hoàng Nguyễn
Vietnamese American Medical Research Foundation
Westminster, California, US

Abstract

The primary function of the renin-angiotensin system (RAS) is to maintain fluid homeostasis and regulate blood pressure. It has been noted that vitamin D and RAS share many of the same risk factors, including both indirect - environment (seasonal and air pollution) and direct - genetics risk factors (human leukocyte antigen, vitamin D receptor, angiotensin-converting enzyme variants, microRNA, and apolipoprotein E).

Vitamin D has been known as a regulator of bone and mineral metabolism by regulating of calcium absorption in the gut and reabsorption by the kidney. The vitamin D receptor (VDR) is present in many tissues. Vitamin D and VDR may effect on the endothelial cells, blood pressure, cardiopathy, renal functions, and keratinocytes via modulating RAS. The combination of vitamin D and RAS blockade has been proved to be effective synergistically in medicine.

Keywords: Vitamin D, renin angiotensin system, calcitriol, RAS

INTRODUCTION

The renin angiotensin system (RAS) plays an essential role in blood pressure regulation by affecting cardiac contractility, vascular resistance, and blood volume. RAS hyper-activation is a major pathogenic factor in hypertension. This process is mediated primarily

* Corresponding author: Khanh v.q. Lương, M.D., FACP, FACE, FACN, FASN, FCCP, and FACAAI (SC), 14971 Brookhurst St., Westminster, CA.92683, US, Telephone: 714 839 5898, Fax: 714 839 5989, E-mail: Lng2687765@aol.com.

through the activation of the angiotensin II (Angio II) type 1 receptor (AT_1R) by Angio II, which activates of several pro-hypertrophic signaling cascades (Paul et al., 2006). Over-stimulation of the RAS leads to hypertension, cardiac hypertrophy, and impaired cardiac activity (Ichihara et al., 2001). It is well known that vitamin D is an important factor in normal calcium and phosphate homeostasis and for promoting bone mineralization. Recent experimental animal and human studies have suggested that vitamin D may also have a role in regulating blood pressure, cardiac function, and kidney injury. Serum levels of calcitriol are inversely associated with blood pressure in normotensive and hypertensive subjects (Kristal-Boneh et al., 1997; Lind et al., 1995). It has been shown that vitamin D treatments reduced the blood pressure levels of hypertensive and elderly patients (Lind et al., 1989; Pfeifer et al., 2001; Judd et al., 2010). In a meta-analysis, high 25-hydrovitamin D_3 (25OHD) levels were associated with significantly improved survival rates in patients with chronic kidney disease (CKD) (Pilz et al., 2011). In CKD patients, paricalcitol significantly reduced albuminuria independently of its effect on hemodynamics or parathyroid hormone (PTH) suppression (Alborzi et al., 2008; Fishbane et al., 2009). In a model of 1α-hydroxylase knockout mice, the mice developed skeletal abnormalities that were characteristic of rickets and exhibited a phenotype of enhanced RAS activity, hypertension, and cardiac hypertrophy, treatment with calcitriol or RAS antagonists attenuated these symptoms (Zhou et al., 2008). In normal mice, vitamin D deficiency stimulates renin expression, whereas calcitriol reduces renin synthesis. Calcitriol directly suppresses renin gene transcription in cell cultures through a vitamin D receptor-dependent mechanism (Li et al., 2004). In addition, vitamin D analogs inhibit renin biosynthesis and suppress renin-angiotensin gene expression in the kidney (Qiao et al., 2005; Freundlich et al., 2008). These findings suggest that vitamin D plays a role in RAS activation.

1. Factors in the Development of Vitamin D Deficiency and Renin Angiotensin System Activation

It has been noted that vitamin D deficiency and the activation of the RAS share similar risk factors, including air pollution and seasonal variation.

1.1. Air Pollution

Exposure to ambient air pollution is associated with blood pressure increases (Delfino et al., 2005; Linn et al., 1999). Particulate matter (PM) exposure potentiates Angio II-induced hypertension, cardiac hypertrophy, and collagen deposition (Ying et al., 2009). In an Angio II-induced hypertensive Sprague-Dawley rat model, PM exposure for 10 weeks induced prolonged blood pressure recovery, compared with the filtered air-exposed group (Sun et al., 2008). PM exposure also produced vasoconstriction and enhanced the mitogen-activated protein kinase (MAPK) signaling pathway via the AT_1R and the local RAS (Li et al., 2005). There is a relationship between close (<50 m compared to >150 m) residential proximity to major roadways and elevated left ventricular mass (LVM) (Van Hee et al., 2009). In addition, an AT_1R variant is associated with residential proximity to major roadways and LVM (Van Hee et al., 2010). Similarly, it has been suggested that atmospheric pollution is a cause of reduced vitamin D synthesis in the skin. In Australia, one study demonstrated a large difference in the vitamin D synthesis in an urban canyon (an urbanized environment with tall building) and a typical suburban area (~2.5 km away from an urban area) (McKinley et al., 2011). Increased atmospheric pollution may be related to the haze from industrial and vehicle sources and may lead to a decrease ultraviolet-B (UVB) photons absorption, thereby reducing cutaneous vitamin D synthesis (Mims, 1996; Hollick, 1995). Another study reported that higher atmospheric pollution resulted in lower amounts of UVB light reaching ground level (Agarwal et al., 2002). This study also showed that children living in areas of high atmospheric pollution were at risk of developing vitamin D-deficient rickets. A Belgian study, in which postmenopausal women participated in outdoor activities during the summer, demonstrated that urban inhabitants had an increased prevalence of vitamin D deficiency compared with rural inhabitants (Manicourt and Devogelear, 2008). In a cross-sectional study, living in a polluted area was found to play a significant independent role in vitamin D deficiency (Hosseinpanah et al., 2010).

1.2. Seasonal Variation

After acute heat exposure, the plasma renin activity (PRA) and aldosterone levels increased more in the winter months than at the end of summer in residents living in a semi-desert zone (Finberg et al., 1974; Finberg and Berlyne, 1977). Plasma aldosterone also significantly increased 59% from summer to winter, whereas the PRA increased 17% from summer to winter (Radke and Izzo, 2010).

In addition, the plasma Angio II levels positively correlated to the outside temperature, which was lowest in January and highest in August (Kruse et al., 2002). Seasonal variations in the 25OHD levels were reported at both southern and northern latitudes (Oliveri et al., 1993; Stryd et al., 1979). Another study confirmed and quantified the relatively large seasonal fluctuations in the circulating 25OHD levels that were associated with the summer sun exposure among outdoor workers.

The workers' median serum 25OHD levels decreased from 122 nmol/l in late summer to 74 nmol/l in late winter (Barger-Lux and Heany, 2002).

2. The Genomic Factors Associated with Vitamin D and the Renin Angiotensin System

Genetic studies provide an excellent opportunity to link molecular variations with epidemiological data. DNA sequences variations, such as polymorphisms, have modest and subtle biological effects. Receptors play a crucial role in regulating cellular function, and small changes in their structure can influence the intracellular signal transduction pathways.

2.1. Human Leukocyte Antigen (HLA)

Studies have suggested that HLA genes are located in the major histocompatibility complex (MHC) class II region. Lower activity of angiotensin-converting enzyme (ACE) activity was associated with a favorable prognosis in Scandinavian HLA-DR-17 sarcoidosis patients (Planck et al., 2001). There was an increased prevalence of HLA-DR2 antigen reported in a Chinese hypertensive population (Tao et al., 1995). Hypertensive patients who have the ACE *DD* genotype have an increased prevalence of HLA-DR6 (Diamantopoulos et al., 2000). The genetic control of RAS activity correlates with the production of anti-HLA antibodies (Akçay et al., 2004). Angiotensin-(1-7), an Ang II metabolite, reportedly stimulates the hematopoietic progenitor cells *in vitro* and *in vivo*. Angio-(1-7) significantly increased the number of HLA-DR^+ cells in human bone marrow and the human spleen at a dose-dependent rate (Heringer-Walther et al., 2009). In addition, the *HLA-DRB1*04* allele increases the risk for autoantibodies against angiotensin AT_1 receptor production (Zhu et al., 2011). However, calcitriol is known to stimulate phagocytosis but suppress MHC class II antigen expression in human mononuclear phagocytes (Tokuda and Levy, 1995; Tokuda et al., 1992). Calcitriol also decreases interferon-gamma-induced HLA-DR antigen expression in normal and transformed human keratinocytes (Tamaki et al., 1990-1991; Tone et al., 1993).

2.2. Vitamin D Receptors (VDRs)

VDRs have been shown to affect RAS activation. The activation of VDRs was associated with the down-regulation of the RAS and attenuated the morphine-induced T-cell apoptosis; this activation is blocked by losartan, an AT_1R blocker (Chandel et al., 2012). The over-expression of VDRs in murine juxtaglomerular cells suppressed renin expression independently of the parathyroid hormone and calcium (Kong et al., 2008). The genetic disruption of VDRs resulted in over-stimulation of the RAS, leading to high blood pressure and cardiac hypertrophy (Xiang et al., 2005). VDRs attenuate obstructive renal injury, partly by suppressing the RAS. Compared with wild-type mice, VDR-null mice developed more severe renal damage in the obstructed kidney with the induction of extracellular matrix proteins, pro-fibrogenic factors, and pro-inflammatory factors. Treatment with losartan eliminated the difference in obstruction-induced interstitial fibrosis between the wild-type and VDR-null mice (Zhang et al., 2010). The RAS was also reported to promote atherosclerosis in the absence of VDRs in mice (Szeto et al., 2012). Furthermore, when combine with 25OHD levels, the *VDR FokI* polymorphism is associated with the risk of developing essential hypertension in Asian Indian population and low PRA levels in Caucasian hypertensive patients (Swapna et al., 2011; Vaidya et al., 2011a).

2.3. Angiotensin-Converting Enzyme (ACE) Variants

The VDR *BsmI* polymorphism was associated with greater quadriceps strength compared with normal controls, but the effect of *BsmI* on quadriceps strength was least apparent in patients who had the *ACE II* genotype (Hopkinson et al., 2008). The *ACE* and AT_1R *A1166C* polymorphisms were associated with incident hypertension in post-menopausal women who had inadequate calcium and vitamin D intakes (Forman et al., 2008). The use of ACE inhibitors in combination with the presence of the *DD* genotype decreased calcitriol levels (Pérez-Castrillón et al., 2006). The presence of the *D* allele was linked to a higher LVM index in the Turkish hypertensive population and negatively correlated with serum 25OHD levels (Kulah et al., 2007). In patients on hemodialysis, those with the *DD* allele had significantly higher serum PTH levels and received higher doses of vitamin D supplements than those without the *DD* allele (Kulah et al., 2006).

2.4. *MicroRNAs* (miRNAs)

miRNAs are small, non-coding, single-stranded RNA molecules that exist in cells and body fluids (Gilad et al., 2008) and play important roles in the pathogenesis of various diseases (Pauley et al., 2009; Lu and Liston, 2009). The miRNA-155 specifically interacts with the binding site harbored in the 3'-untranslated region (3'-UTR) of the human AT_1R mRNA and decreases the AT_1R expression by inhibiting the mRNA translation. The transfection of anti-miRNA-155 increases AT_1R expression and enhances Ang II-induced signaling (Martin et al., 2006 and 2007) In aerobic exercise training, the increased miRNA-27 expression inhibits the ACE levels (Fernandes et al., 2011a). In maternal protein restriction during pregnancy, fetal brains show increased mRNA expression of angiotensinogen and ACE-1, decreased mRNA levels of AT_1R, and up-regulation of miRNA-27a and 27b (Goyal et al., 2010). In antenatal maternal hypoxic stress, the angiotensinogen protein is detectable and increases significantly in association with decreased miRNA-27a, which results in increased ACE-1 translation (Goyal et al., 2011). A polymorphic miRNA-155 binding site in the AT_1R is associated with cardiac hypertrophy in Friedreich's ataxia (Kelly et al., 2011). In one study, the levels of miRNA-146 were significantly higher in the coronary artery disease (CAD) group than in the non-CAD group, and these levels decreased markedly after treatment with an AT_1R blocker or ACE inhibitor compared with the controls (Takahashi et al., 2010). MiRNA-125 is up-regulated in pathological cardiac hypertrophy (Fernandes et al., 2011b). Disturbed RAS activity has been reported in the systemic lupus erythematous disease (SLE) (Luong and Nguyen, 2012). The serum levels of miRNA-146a inversely correlate with the proteinuria and SLE activity index scores. Following calcitriol treatment, the serum miRNA-146a levels of SLE patients significantly increased (Wang et al., 2011). In another study, the levels of urinary miRNA-146a in patients with SLE were significantly higher than those of the healthy controls. Calcitriol generally reduces the levels of urinary miRNA-146a, which significantly correlate with the estimated glomerular filtration rate in SLE patients (Wang et al., 2012a). Serum miRNA-155 levels have also been shown to be lower in SLE patients than in the controls (Wang et al., 2011a), although urinary levels are significantly higher in the SLE patients than the healthy controls. Calcitriol also reduces the levels of urinary miRNA-155, which significantly correlate with proteinuria and the SLE disease activity index (Wang et al., 2012b).

Furthermore, many additional studies have documented the relationship between vitamin D and miRNAs. Plasma miRNA-146 levels significantly changed after supplementation with high doses of vitamin D (Jorde et al., 2012). Moreover, two miRNAs have been shown to down-regulate VDR expressions, as confirmed by immunoblots and qPCR analyses (Pan et al., 2009). Calcitriol reduces miRNA-27b expression in melanoma cell lines (Essa et al.,

2012). Human vitamin D_3 hydroxylase (CYP24), which catalyzes the inactivation of calcitriol, is post-transcriptionally regulated by miRNA-125b (Komagata et al., 2009). A potential miRNA-125b recognition element was identified in the 3'-UTR of human VDR mRNA (Mohri et al., 2009). Fifteen miRNAs are known to be differentially regulated by calcitriol in prostate cancer cells (Wang et al., 2011b), and the endogenous level of VDR mRNA is inversely correlated with the expression of miRNA-125b in melanoma cell lines (Essa et al., 2010).

2.5. Apolipoprotein E (ApoE)

ApoE has important functions in systemic and local lipid transport. Several studies have suggested a relationship between RAS and ApoE. In mice, the infusion of Angio II significantly reduced the ApoE expression in adipocytes (Rao et al., 2007). The ACE polymorphism is associated with dementia risk in carriers of the *ApoE ε 4* allele (Gustafson et al., 2010). There is an interaction between the *ACE* and *ApoE* genotypes; the combined carrier state for the *D ACE* and *ApoE* alleles substantially increases restenosis after coronary angioplasty (van Bockxmeer et al., 1995). In addition, *ApoE* and *Angiotensinogen* gene polymorphisms have a synergistic effect on the risk for early myocardial infarction (Batalla et al., 2000). In ApoE-deficient mice, severe hyperlipidemia impairs the RAS function (Mazzolai et al., 2006) and chronic angiotensin IV treatment reverses the endothelial dysfunction (Vinh et al., 2008). ACE and AT_1R inhibitors prevented the acceleration of atherosclerosis in ApoE-deficient mice (Candido et al., 2002; Bro et al., 2007; Blessing et al., 2008; Cheng et al., 2011). However, the *ApoE4* allele is reported to be associated with lower bone mass in post-menopausal Japanese women (Shiraki et al., 1997). Common *ApoE* polymorphisms had a complex effect on the bone metabolism of peri-menopausal Danish women; women who have the *ApoE2* polymorphism have reduced bone mineral loss in the femoral neck and hip region than other women, whereas women who have the *ApoE4* polymorphism gain more bone mineral than other women (Gerdes et al., 2001). *ApoE ε4*, however, is associated with higher serum levels of 25OHD (Huebbe et al., 2011). Calcitriol has been known to induce macrophages to exhibit specific saturable receptors for low-density lipoprotein (LDL) and acetyl-LDL; the LDL receptor of calcitriol-induced macrophages was found to exhibit specificity for ApoB- and E-containing lipoproteins (Jouni et al., 1991). In ApoE knockout mice with dyslipidemia, high oxidative stress, and pronounced atherosclerosis after uninephrectomy, the animals developed less plaque growth and calcification after vitamin D analog treatment (paricalcitol) compared with the control groups (Husain et al., 2010; Becker et al., 2011)

3. The Non-Genomic Role of Vitamin D in the Renin Angiotensin System

Vitamin D and VDRs may affect the endothelial cells, blood pressure, cardiac and kidney functions, and keratinocytes via RAS modulation.

3.1. Endothelial Dysfunction

Endothelial dysfunction, resulting from an imbalance between the release of endothelium-derived relaxing and contacting factors, is a predictor of impaired cardiovascular function. *In vivo* and *in vitro* studies have shown that calcitriol improves endothelial function in hypertension by normalizing the expressions of AT_1Rs and radical-generating and scavenging enzymes and thus preventing the over-production of reactive oxygen species (Dong et al., 2012). In vitamin D treated subculture endothelial cells, the ACE activity of the morphologically changed cells decreased to approximately one-third, and the plasminogen activator release increased approximately 12 times compared with the control cells (Hagiwara et al., 1988). Furthermore, a combination therapy of RAS blockade and calcitriol is associated with a 60% lower risk of deep-vein thrombosis in renal transplant recipients compared with the controls (Moscarelli et al., 2011). (Ravenell et al., 2012) demonstrated that premature atherosclerosis is associated with hypovitaminosis D and ACE inhibitor non-use in lupus patients. Treatment with paricalcitol alone or in combination with enalapril protected the inflammatory and oxidative endothelial injury of the aorta in atherosclerotic mice (Husain et al., 2010).

3.2. Hypertension

Plasma 25OHD levels were inversely associated with the risk of incident hypertension, which was independent of age, body mass index (BMI), physical activity, race, and menopausal status (Forman et al., 20070. Plasma calcitriol and PTH levels were higher in hypertensive patients with low PRA than in other hypertensive patients and the controls (Resnick et al., 1986). In subjects with high-renin hypertension, an increase in dietary sodium intakes resulted in the increased excretion of urinary calcium and increased serum calcitriol levels, which may mediate the response of high-renin hypertension to increased sodium intake (Burgess et al., 1990). (Tomaschitz et al. 2010) demonstrated an inverse relationship between plasma renin concentrations and both plasma 25OHD and calcitriol levels.

In a cross-sectional study, the plasma 25OHD levels were inversely associated with PRA in both high- and low-sodium diet and were positively associated with the salt sensitivity of blood pressure in low-renin hypertension subjects (Vaidya et al., 2011b). There is a positive association between the plasma 25OHD levels and vascular sensitivity to Ang II in obese hypertensive patients; vascular RAS activity may progressively increase when plasma 25OHD deficiency occurs in obesity (Vaidya et al., 2011c). In these obese hypertensive patients, vitamin D administration modified the renal plasma flow, the mean arterial pressure, and tissue sensitivity to Ang II, similar to an ACE inhibitor (Vaidya et al., 2012).

3.3. Cardiopathy

Low plasma calcitriol levels have been associated with RAS activation, increased pro-inflammatory cytokines, and an increase in plasma PTH levels, all of which may increase the risk for chronic heart failure (CHF) (Schleithoff et al., 2006). In children with CHF, vitamin D supplementations significantly improve their heart failure scores, increased serum anti-inflammatory cytokines IL-10 levels, significantly decreased serum pro-inflammatory cytokines TNF-α and IL-6 levels, decreased PTH levels, and improved the myocardial performance index with markedly increased serum 25OHD (Shedeed, 2012). Vitamin D analogs, such as paricalcitol and doxercalciferol, reduce cardiac hypertrophy in spontaneously hypertensive rats via the suppression of RAS activity. The combination of a vitamin D analog and losartan nearly prevented of this LVM (Kong et al., 2010).

3.4. Renal Function

VDRs are identified in various cells of the mouse kidney, such as the distal and proximal tubules, the macula densa of the juxtaglomerular apparatus, glomerular parietal cells, and podocytes (Wang et al., 2012b). Calcitriol suppresses high glucose-induced angiotensinogen expression in kidney cells by blocking the NF-κB pathway (Deb et al., 2009). Paricalcitol changes the peritoneal membrane permeability and proteinuria in patients on peritoneal dialysis (Coronel et al., 2012). Mouse models of diabetes develop proteinuria and renal injury with elevated intra-renal RAS activity. The administration of either calcitriol or paricalcitol decreases the RAS activity in these mice and attenuates the proteinuria and kidney injury. AT_1R blockers produce the same effects, but the synergistic effect is more prominent when using a combination of these drugs (Deb et al., 2010; Zhang et al., 2008; Ohara et al., 2011).

The addition of vitamin D to RAS inhibitor decreased albuminuria in type 2 diabetic nephropathy (Zhang et al., 2009; Lambers Heerspink et al., 2009; de Zeeuw et al., 2010; Kim et al., 2011). The combination therapy of an AT_1R blocker and a vitamin D analog markedly ameliorates diabetic nephropathy by suppressing the induction of fibronectin, the transforming growth factor-β1 (TGF-β1), and the monocyte chemoattractant protein-1 (MCP-1) (Zhang et al., 2008).

The combined therapy of ACE inhibitor and a vitamin D analog also suppresses the progression of renal insufficiency in uremic rats via TGF-β signaling pathway (Mizobuchi et al., 2007) and reduces renal fibrosis in obstructive nephropathy (Tan et al., 2009).

3.5. Keratinocytes

Captopril is an angiotensin-converting enzyme inhibitor that has sulfhydryl groups in its chemical structure. The capacity of captopril and pemphigus serum to induce acantholysis, *in vivo* or in *vitro*, has been demonstrated experimentally (Baroni et al., 2004). Vitamin D protects keratinocytes from captopril-induced cell detachment and apoptosis (Zeeli et al., 2011).

Conclusion

The relationship between vitamin D and the RAS is reviewed in the present paper. Vitamin D deficiency and RAS activation share some common risk factors. Genetic studies have provided opportunities to determine which proteins link vitamin D to the RAS pathology. Vitamin D acts to control the cardiovascular system and renal function partly via modulation of the RAS.

Acknowledgment

Conflict of interest statement: The authors, Dr. Khanh Luong and Dr. Lan Nguyen, report no competing interests.

Ethical approval: Not required

Funding: The authors, Dr. Khanh Luong and Dr. Lan Nguyen, received no funding for this study.

References

Agarwal, K. S., Mughal, M. Z., Upadhyay, P., Berry, J. L., Mawer, E. B., Puliyel, J. M. 2002. The impact of atmostpheric pollution on vitamin D status of infants and toddlers in Delhi, India. *Arch. Dis. Child.* 87:111-113.

Akçay, A., Ozdemir, F. N., Ataç, F. B., Sezer, S., Verdi, H., et al. 2004. Angiotensin-converting enzyme genotype is a predictive factor in the peak panel-reactive antibody response. *Transplant. Proc.* 36:35-37.

Alborzi, P., Patel, N. A., Peterson, C., Bills, J. E., Bekele, D. M., et al. 2008. Paricalcitol reduces albuminuria and inflammation in chronic kidney disease: a randomized double-blind pilot trial. *Hypertension.* 52:249-255.

Barger-Lux, M. J., Heany, R. P. 2002. Effects of above average summer sun exposure on serum 25-hydroxyvitamin D and calcium absorption. *J. Clin. Endocrinol. Metab.* 87:4952-4956.

Baroni, A., Buommino, E., Paoletti, I., Orlando, M., Ruocco, E., Ruocco, V. 2004. Pemphigus serum and captopril induce heat shock protein 70 and inducible nitric oxide synthase overexpression, triggering apoptosis in human keratinocytes. *Br. J. Dermatol.* 150:1070-1080.

Batalla, A., Alvarez, R., Reguero, J. R., Hevia, S., Iglesias-Cubero, G., et al. 2000. Synergistic effect between apolipoprotein E and angiotensinogen gene polymorphisms in the risk for early myocardial infarction. *Clin. Chem.* 46:1910-1915.

Becker, L. E., Koleganova, N., Piecha, G., Noronha, I. L., Zeier, M., et al. 2011. Effects of paricalcitol and calcitriol on aortic wall remodeling in uninephrectomized ApoE knockout mice. *Am. J. Physiol. Renal. Physiol.* 300:F772–F782.

Blessing, E., Preusch, M., Kranzhöfer, R., Kinscherf, R., Marx, N., et al. 2008. Anti-atherosclerotic properties of telmisartan in advanced atherosclerotic lesions in apolipoprotein E deficient mice. *Atherosclerosis.* 199:295-303.

Bro, S., Binder, C. J., Witztum, J. L., Olgaard, K., Nielsen, L. B. 2007. Inhibition of the renin-angiotensin system abolishes the proatherogenic effect of uremia in apolipoprotein E-deficient mice. *Arterioscler. Thromb. Vasc. Biol.* 27:1080-1086.

Burgess, E. D., Hawkins, R. G., Watanabe, M. 1990. Interaction of 1,25-dihydroxyvitamin D and plasma renin activity in high renin essential hypertension. *Am. J. Hypertens.* 3:903-905.

Candido, R., Jandeleit-Dahm, K. A., Cao, Z., Nesteroff, S. P., Burns, W. C., et al. 2002. Prevention of accelerated atherosclerosis by angiotensin-converting enzyme inhibition in diabetic apolipoprotein E-deficient mice. *Circulation.* 106:246-253.

Chandel, N., Sharma, B., Salhan, D., Husain, M., Malhotra, A., Buch, S., Singhal, P. C. 2012. Vitamin D Receptor Activation (VDR) and Down regulation of Renin Angiotensin System Attenuate Morphine-induced T Cell Apoptosis. *Endocrinol. Nutr.* 2012 Jul. 2. [Epub. ahead of print]

Cheng, X. W., Song, H., Sasaki, T., Hu, L., Inoue, A., et al. 2011._Angiotensin type 1 receptor blocker reduces intimal neovascularization and plaque growth in apolipoprotein E-deficient mice. *Hypertension.* 57:981-989.

Coronel, F., Cigarran, S., Gomis, A., Rodríguez-Cubillo, B., Herrero, J. A., et al. 2012. Changes in peritoneal membrane permeability and proteinuria in patients on peritoneal dialysis after treatment with paricalcitol: a preliminary study. *Clin. Nephrol.* 78:93-99.

De Zeeuw, D., Agarwal, R., Amdahl, M., Audhya, P., Coyne, D., et al. 2010. Selective vitamin D receptor activation with paricalcitol for reduction of albuminuria in patients with type 2 diabetes (VITAL study): a randomised controlled trial. *Lancet.* 376:1543-1551.

Deb, D. K., Chen, Y., Zhang, Z., Zhang, Y., Szeto, F. L., et al. 2009. 1,25-Dihydroxy-vitamin D_3 suppresses high glucose-induced angiotensinogen expression in kidney cells by blocking the NF-{kappa}B pathway. *Am. J. Physiol. Renal. Physiol.* 296:F1212-1218

Deb, D. K., Sun, T., Wong, K. E., Zhang, Z., Ning, G., et al. 2010. Combined vitamin D analog and AT1 receptor antagonist synergistically block the development of kidney disease in a model of type 2 diabetes. *Kidney Int.* 77:1000-1009.

Delfino, R. J., Sioutas, C., Malik, S. 2005. Potential role of ultrafine particles in associations between airborne particle mass and cardiovascular health. *Environ. Health Perspect.* 113:934-946.

Diamantopoulos, E. J., Andreadis, E. A., Vassilopoulos, C. V., Tabacila-Kakou, M. G., Sfakianakis, M. E., et al. 2000. Distribution of different HLA antigens in Greek hypertensives according to the angiotensin-converting enzyme genotype. *Am. J. Hypertens.* 13:438-441.

Dong, J., Wong, S. L., Lau, C. W., Lee, H. K., Ng, C. F., et al. 2012. Calcitriol protects renovascular function in hypertension by down-regulating angiotensin II type 1 receptors and reducing oxidative stress. *Eur. Heart J.* 2012 Jan. 19. [Epub. ahead of print]

Essa, S., Denzer, N., Mahlknecht, U., Klein, R., Collnot, E. M., et al. 2010. VDR microRNA expression and epigenetic silencing of vitamin D signaling in melanoma cells. *J. Steroid Biochem. Mol. Biol.* 121:110-113.

Essa, S., Reichrath, S., Mahlknecht, U., Montenarh, M., Vogt, T., Reichrath, J. 2012. Signature of VDR miRNAs and epigenetic modulation of vitamin D signaling in melanoma cell lines. *Anticancer Res.* 32:383-389.

Fernandes, T., Hashimoto, N. Y., Magalhães, F. C., Fernandes, F. B., Casarini, D. E., et al. 2011. Aerobic exercise training-induced left ventricular hypertrophy involves regulatory MicroRNAs, decreased angiotensin-converting enzyme-angiotensin ii, and synergistic regulation of angiotensin-converting enzyme 2-angiotensin (1-7). *Hypertension*. 58:182-189.

Fernandes, T., Soci, U. P., Oliveira, E. M. 2011. Eccentric and concentric cardiac hypertrophy induced by exercise training: microRNAs and molecular determinants. *Braz. J. Med. Biol. Res*. 44:836-847.

Finberg, J. P., Katz, M., Gazit, H., Berlyne, G. M. 1974. Plasma renin activity after acute heat exposure in nonacclimatized and naturally acclimatized man. *J. Appl. Physiol.* 36:519-523.

Finberg, J. P., Berlyne, G. M. 1977. Modification of renin and aldosterone response to heat by acclimatization in man. *J. Appl. Physiol*. 42:554-558.

Fishbane, S., Chittineni, H., Packman, M., Dutka, P., Ali, N., Durie, N. 2009. Oral paricalcitol in the treatment of patients. *Am. J. Kidney Dis*. 54:647-652

Forman, J. P., Giovannucci, E., Holmes, M. D., Bischoff-Ferrari, H. A., Tworoger, S. S., et al. 2007. Plasma 25-hydroxyvitamin D levels and risk of incident hypertension. *Hypertension*. 49:1063-1069.

Forman, J. P., Fisher, N. D., Pollak, M. R., Cox, D. G., Tonna, S., Curhan, G. C. 2008. Renin-angiotensin system polymorphisms and risk of hypertension: influence of environmental factors. *J. Clin. Hypertens*. (Greenwich). 10:459-466.

Freundlich, M., Quiroz, Y., Zhang, Z., Zhang, Y., Bravo, Y., et al. 2008. Suppression of renin-angiotensin gene expression in the kidney by paricalcitol. *Kidney Int.* 74:1394-1402.

Gerdes, L. U., Vestergaard, P., Hermann, A. P., Mosekilde, L. 2001. Regional and hormone-depenpent effects of Apolipoprotein E genotype on changes in bone mineral in perimenopausal women. *J. Bone Miner Res*. 16:1906-1916.

Gilad, S., Meiri, E., Yogev, Y., Benjamin, S., Lebanony, D., et al. 2008. Serum microRNAs are promising novel biomarkers. *PLoS One*. 3:e3148.

Goyal, R., Goyal, D., Leitzke, A., Gheorghe, C. P., Longo, L. D. 2010. Brain renin-angiotensin system: fetal epigenetic programming by maternal protein restriction during pregnancy. *Reprod. Sci*. 17:227-238.

Goyal, R., Lister, R., Leitzke, A., Goyal, D., Gheorghe, C. P., Longo, L. D. 2011. Antenatal maternal hypoxic stress: adaptations of the placental renin-angiotensin system in the mouse. *Placenta*. 32:134-139.

Gustafson, D. R., Melchior, L., Eriksson, E., Sundh, V., Blennow, K., Skoog, I. 2010. The ACE Insertion Deletion polymorphism relates to dementia by metabolic phenotype, APOEε 4, and age of dementia onset. *Neurobiol. Aging*. 31:910-916.

Hagiwara, H., Furuhashi, H., Nakaya, K., Nakamura, Y. 1988. Effects of vitamin D_3 and related compounds on angiotensin converting enzyme activity of endothelial cells and on release of plasminogen activator from them. *Chem. Pharm. Bull.* (Tokyo). 36:4858-4864

Heringer-Walther, S., Eckert, K., Schumacher, S. M., Uharek, L., Wulf-Goldenberg, A., et al. 2009. Angiotensin-(1-7) stimulates hematopoietic progenitor cells in vitro and in vivo. *Haematologica*. 94:857-860.

Hollick, M. F. 1995. Environmental factors that influence the cutaneous production of vitamin D. *Am. J. Clin. Nutr*. 61:638S-645S.

Hopkinson, N. S., Li, K. W., Kehoe, A., Humphries, S. E., Roughton, M., et al. 2008. Vitamin D receptor genotypes influence quadriceps strength in chronic obstructive pulmonary disease. *Am. J. Clin. Nutr.* 87:385-390.

Hosseinpanah, F., Pour, S. H., Heibatollahi, M., Moghbel, N., Asefzade, S., Azizi, F. 2010. The effects of air pollution on vitamin D status in healthy women: A cross section study. *BMC Pub. Health*. 10:519.

Huebbe, P., Nebel, A., Siegert, S., Moehring, J., Boesch-Saadatmandi, C., et al. 2011. APOE ε4 is associated with higher vitamin D levels in targeted replacement mice and humans. *FASEB J.* 25:3262-3270.

Husain, K., Suarez, E., Isidro, A., Ferder, L. 2010. Effects of paricalcitol and analapril on atherosclerotic injury in mouse aortas. *Am. J. Nephrol.* 32:296–304.

Ichihara, S., Senbonmatsu, T., Price, E. Jr, Ichiki, T., Gaffney, F. A., Inagami, T. 2001. Angiotensin II type 2 receptor is essential for left ventricular hypertrophy and cardiac fibrosis in chronic angiotensin II-induced hypertension. *Circulation*. 104:346-351.

Jorde, R., Svartberg, J., Joakimsen, R. M., Coucheron, D. H. 2012. Plasma profile of microRNA after supplementation with high doses of vitamin D_3 for 12 months. *BMC Res. Notes*. 5:245.

Jouni, Z. E., McNamara, D. J. Lipoprotein receptors of HL-60 macrophages. 1991. Effect of differentiation with tetramyristic phorbol acetate and 1,25-didroxyvitamin D_3. *Arterioscler. Thromb.* 11:995–1006.

Judd, S. E., Raiser, S. N., Kumari, M., Tangpricha, V. 2010. 1,25-dihydroxyvitamin D_3 reduces systolic blood pressure in hypertensive adults: a pilot feasibility study. *J. Steroid Biochem. Mol. Biol.* 121:445-447.

Kelly, M., Bagnall, R. D., Peverill, R. E., Donelan, L., Corben, L., et al. 2011. A polymorphic miR-155 binding site in AGTR1 is associated with cardiac hypertrophy in Friedreich ataxia. *J. Mol. Cell Cardiol.* 51:848-854.

Kim, M. J., Frankel, A. H., Donaldson, M., Darch, S. J., Pusey, C. D., et al. 2011. Oral cholecalciferol decreases albuminuria and urinary TGF-β1 in patients with type 2 diabetic nephropathy on established renin-angiotensin-aldosterone system inhibition. *Kidney Int.*;80:851-860.

Komagata, S., Nakajima, M., Takagi, S., Mohri, T., Taniya, T., Yokoi, T. 2009. Human CYP24 catalyzing the inactivation of calcitriol is post-transcriptionally regulated by miR-125b. *Mol. Pharmacol.* 76:702-709.

Kong, J., Qiao, G., Zhang, Z., Liu, S. Q., Li, Y. C. 2008. Targeted vitamin D receptor expression in juxtaglomerular cells suppresses renin expression independent of parathyroid hormone and calcium. *Kidney Int.* 74:1577-1581.

Kong, J., Kim, G. H., Wei, M., Sun, T., Li, G., et al. 2010. Therapeutic effects of vitamin D analogs on cardiac hypertrophy in spontaneously hypertensive rats. *Am. J. Pathol.* 177:622-631.

Kristal-Boneh, E., Froom, P., Harari, G., Ribak, J. 1997. Association of calcitriol and blood pressure in normotensive men. *Hypertension*. 30:289-1294.

Kruse, H. J., Wieczorek, I., Hecker, H., Creutzig, A., Schellong, S. M. 2002. Seasonal variation of endothelin-1, angiotensin II, and plasma catecholamines and their relation to outside temperature. *J. Lab. Clin. Med.* 140:236-241.

Kulah, E., Sezer, S., Uyar, M., Arat, Z., Ozdemir, F. N. 2006. Effects of ACE gene polymorphism on vitamin D therapy according to parathyroid hormone level in patients on hemodialysis. *Adv. Ther.* 23:778-786.

Kulah, E., Dursun, A., Aktunc, E., Acikgoz, S., Aydin, M., et al. 2007. Effects of angiotensin-converting enzyme gene polymorphism and serum vitamin D levels on ambulatory blood pressure measurement and left ventricular mass in Turkish hypertensive population. *Blood Press Monit.* 2:207-213.

Manicourt, D. H., Devogelaer, J. P. 2008. Urban tropospheric ozone increases the prevalence of vitamin D deficiency among Belgian postmenopausal women with outdoor activities during summer. *J. Clin. Endocrinol. Metab.* 93:3893-3899.

Martin, M. M., Lee, E. J., Buckenberger, J. A., Schmittgen, T. D., Elton, T. S. 2006. MicroRNA-155 regulates human angiotensin II type 1 receptor expression in fibroblasts. *J. Biol. Chem.* 281:18277-18284.

Martin, M. M., Buckenberger, J. A., Jiang, J., Malana, G. E., Nuovo, G. J., et al. 2007. The human angiotensin II type 1 receptor +1166 A/C polymorphism attenuates microrna-155 binding. *J. Biol. Chem.* 282:24262-24269.

Mazzolai, L., Korber, M., Bouzourene, K., Aubert, J. F., Nussberger, J., et al. 2006. Severe hyperlipidemia causes impaired renin-angiotensin system function in apolipoprotein E deficient mice. *Atherosclerosis.* 186:86-91.

McKinley, A., Janda, M., Auster, J., Kimlin, M. 2011. In vitro model of vitamin D synthesis by UV radiation in an Australian urban environment. Photochem Photobiol. *Photochem. Photobiol.* 87:447-451.

Mims, F. M. 3rd. 1996. Significant reduction of UVB caused by smoke from biomass burning in Brazil. *Photochem. Photobiol.* 64:814-816.

Mizobuchi, M., Morrissey, J., Finch, J. L., Martin, D. R., Liapis, H., et al. 2007. Combination therapy with an angiotensin-converting enzyme inhibitor and a vitamin D analog suppresses the progression of renal insufficiency in uremic rats. *J. Am. Soc. Nephrol.* 18:1796-1806.

Mohri, T., Nakajima, M., Takagi, S., Komagata, S., Yokoi, T. 2009. MicroRNA regulates human vitamin D receptor. *Int. J. Cancer.* 125:1328-1333.

Moscarelli, L., Zanazzi, M., Bertoni, E., Caroti, L., Rosso, G., et al. 2011. Renin angiotensin system blockade and activated vitamin D as a means of preventing deep vein thrombosis in renal transplant recipients. *Clin. Nephrol.* 75:440-450.

Lambers Heerspink, H. J., Agarwal, R., Coyne, D. W., Parving, H. H., Ritz, E., et al. 2009. The selective vitamin D receptor activator for albuminuria lowering (VITAL) study: study design and baseline characteristics. *Am. J. Nephrol.* 30:280-286.

Li, Y. C., Qiao, G., Uskokovic, M., Xiang, W., Zheng, W., Kong, J. 2004. Vitamin D: a negative endocrine regulator of the renin-angiotensin system and blood pressure. *J. Steroid Biochem. Mol. Biol.* 89-90:387-392.

Li, Z., Carter, J. D., Dailey, L. A., Huang, Y. C. 2005. Pollutant particles produce vasoconstriction and enhance MAPK signaling via angiotensin type I receptor. *Environ. Health Perspect.* 113:1009-1014.

Lind, L., Wengle, B., Wide, L., Ljunghall, S. 1989. Reduction of blood pressure during long-term treatment with active vitamin D (alphacalcidol) is dependent on plasma renin activity and calcium status. A double-blind, placebo-controlled study. *Am. J. Hypertens.* 2:20-25.

Lind, L., Hänni, A., Lithell, H., Hvarfner, A., Sörensen, O. H., Ljunghall, S. 1995. Vitamin D is related to blood pressure and other cardiovascular risk factors in middle-aged men. *Am. J. Hypertens*. 8:894-901.

Linn, W. S., Gong, H. Jr, Clark, K. W., Anderson, K. R. 1999. Day-to-day particulate exposures and health changes in Los Angeles area residents with severe lung disease. *J. Air Waste Manag. Assoc*. 49:108-115.

Lu, L. F., Liston, A. 2009. MicroRNA in the immune system, microRNA as an immune system. *Immunology*. 127:291-298.

Luong, V. Q. K., Nguyen, L. T. H. 2012. The beneficial role of vitamin D in systemic lupus erythematosus (SLE). *Clin. Rheumatol*. 2012 Jul. 17. [Epub. ahead of print].

Ohara, I., Tanimoto, M., Gohda, T., Yamazaki, T., Hagiwara, S., et al. 2011. Effect of combination therapy with angiotensin receptor blocker and 1,25-dihydroxyvitamin D_3 in type 2 diabetic nephropathy in KK-A(y)/Ta mice. *Nephron. Exp. Nephrol*. 117:e124-132.

Oliveri, M. B., Ladizesky, M., Mautalen, C. A., Alonso, A., Martinez, L. 1993. Seasonal variations of 25-hydroxyvitamin D and parathyroid hormone in Ushuala (Argentina), the southernmost city of the world. *Bone Miner*. 20:99-108.

Pan, Y. Z., Gao, W., Yu, A. M. 2009. MicroRNAs regulate CYP3A4 expression via direct and indirect targeting. *Drug Metab. Dispos*. 37:2112-2117.

Pauley, K. M., Cha, S., Chan, E. K. 2009. MicroRNA in autoimmunity and autoimmune diseases. *J. Autoimmun*. 32:189-194.

Pérez-Castrillón, J. L., Justo, I., Sanz, A., De Luis, D., Dueñas, A. 2006. Effect of angiotensin converting enzyme inhibitors on 1.25-$(OH)_2$ D levels of hypertensive patients. Relationship with ACE polymorphisms. *Horm. Metab. Res*. 38:812-816.

Pfeifer, M., Begerow, B., Minne, H. W., Nachtigall, D., Hansen, C. 2001. Effects of a short-term vitamin D_3 and calcium supplementation on blood pressure and parathyroid hormone levels in elderly women. *J. Clin. Endocrinol. Metab*. 86:1633-1637.

Pilz, S., Iodice, S., Zittermann, A., Grant, W. B., Gandini, S. 2011. Vitamin D status and mortality risk in CKD: a meta-analysis of prospective studies. *Am J. Kidney Dis*. 58:374-382,

Planck, A., Eklund, A., Grunewald, J. 2001. Inflammatory BAL-fluid and serum parameters in HLA DR17 positive vs. DR17 negative patients with pulmonary sarcoidosis. *Sarcoidosis Vasc. Diffuse Lung Dis*. 18:64-69.

Qiao, G., Kong, J., Uskokovic, M., Li, Y. C. 2005. Analogs of 1alpha,25-dihydroxyvitamin D_3 as novel inhibitors of renin biosynthesis. *J. Steroid Biochem. Mol. Biol*. 96:59-66.

Radke, K. J., Izzo, J. L. Jr. 2010. Seasonal variation in haemodynamics and blood pressure-regulating hormones. *J. Hum. Hypertens*. 24:410-416.

Rao, P., Huang, Z. H., Mazzone, T. 2007. Angiotensin II regulates adipocyte apolipoprotein E expression. *J. Clin. Endocrinol. Metab*. 92:4366-4372.

Ravenell, R. L., Kamen, D. L., Spence, J. D., Hollis, B. W., Fleury, T. J., et al. 2012. Premature Atherosclerosis Is Associated With Hypovitaminosis D and Angiotensin-Converting Enzyme Inhibitor Non-use in Lupus Patients. *Am. J. Med. Sci*. 2012 Jan. 4. [Epub. ahead of print]

Resnick, L. M., Müller, F. B., Laragh, J. H. 1986. Calcium-regulating hormones in essential hypertension. Relation to plasma renin activity and sodium metabolism. *Ann. Intern. Med.* 105:649-654.

Schleithoff, S. S., Zittermann, A., Tenderich, G., Berthold, H. K., Stehle, P., et al. Vitamin D supplementation improves cytokine profiles in patients with congestive heart failure: a double-blind, randomized, placebo-controlled trial. *Am. J. Clin. Nutr.* 83:754-759.

Shedeed, S. A. 2012. Vitamin D supplementation in infants with chronic congestive heart failure. *Pediatr. Cardiol.* 33:713-719.

Shiraki, M., Shiraki, Y., Aoki, C., Hosoi, T., Inoue, S., et al. 1997. Association of bone mineral density with Apolipoprotein E phenotype. *J. Bone Miner Res.* 12:1438-1445.

Stryd, R. P., Gilbertson, T. J., Bruden, M. N. 1979. A seasonal variation study of 25-hydroxyvitamin D_3 serum levels in normal human. *J. Clin. Endocrinol. Metab.* 48:771-775.

Sun, Q., Yue, P., Ying, Z., Cardounel, A. J., Brook, R. D., et al. 2008. Air pollution exposure potentiates hypertension through reactive oxygen species-mediated activation of Rho/ROCK. *Arterioscler. Thromb. Vasc. Biol.* 28:1760-1766.

Swapna, N., Vamsi, U. M., Usha, G., Padma, T. 2011. Risk conferred by FokI polymorphism of vitamin D receptor (VDR) gene for essential hypertension. *Indian. J. Hum. Genet.* 17:201-206.

Szeto, F. L., Reardon, C. A., Yoon, D., Wang, Y., Wong, K. E., et al. 2012. Vitamin d receptor signaling inhibits atherosclerosis in mice. *Mol. Endocrinol.* 26:1091-1101.

Takahashi, Y., Satoh, M., Minami, Y., Tabuchi, T., Itoh, T., Nakamura, M. 2010. Expression of miR-146a/b is associated with the Toll-like receptor 4 signal in coronary artery disease: effect of renin-angiotensin system blockade and statins on miRNA-146a/b and Toll-like receptor 4 levels. *Clin. Sci.* (Lond.). 119:395-405.

Tamaki, K., Saitoh, A., Kubota, Y. 1990-1991. 1,25-hydroxyvitamin D_3 decreases the interferon-gamma (IFN-gamma) induced HLA-DR expression but not intercellular adhesion molecule 1 (ICAM-1) on human keratinocytes. *Reg. Immunol.* 3:223-227.

Tan, X., He, W., Liu, Y. 2009. Combination therapy with paricalcitol and trandolapril reduces renal fibrosis in obstructive nephropathy. *Kidney Int.* 76:1248-1257.

Tokuda, N., Levy, R. B. 1996. 1,25-hydroxyvitamin D_3 stimulates phagocytosis but suppresses HLA-DR and CD13 antigen expression in human mononuclear phagocytes. *Proc. Soc. Exp. Biol. Med.* 211:244-250.

Tokuda, N., Mizuki, N., Kasahara, M., Levy, R. B. 1992. 1,25-hydroxyvitamin D_3 down-regulation of HLA-DR on human peripheral blood monocytes. *Immunol.* 75:349-354.

Tomaschitz, A., Pilz, S., Ritz, E., Grammer, T., Drechsler, C., et al. 2010. Independent association between 1,25-dihydroxyvitamin D, 25-hydroxyvitamin D and the renin-angiotensin system: The Ludwigshafen Risk and Cardiovascular Health (LURIC) study. *Clin. Chim. Acta.* 411:1354-1360.

Tone, T., Eto, H., Katou, T., Otani, F., Nishiyama, S. 1993. 1 alpha,25-dihydroxy vitamin D_3 modulation of HLA-DR mRNA induced by gamma-interferon in cultured epithelial tumor cell lines. *J. Dermatol.* 20:581-584.

Xiang, W., Kong, J., Chen, S., Cao, L. P., Qiao, G., et al. 2005. Cardiac hypertrophy in vitamin D receptor knockout mice: role of the systemic and cardiac renin-angiotensin systems. *Am. J. Physiol. Endocrinol. Metab*. 288:E125-132.

Ying, Z., Yue, P., Xu, X., Zhong, M., Sun, Q., et al. 2009. Air pollution and cardiac remodeling: a role for RhoA/Rho-kinase. *Am. J. Physiol. Heart Circ. Physiol.* 296:H1540-1550.

Vaidya, A., Sun, B., Forman, J. P., Hopkins, P. N., Brown, N. J., et al. 2011a. The Fok1 vitamin D receptor gene polymorphism is associated with plasma renin activity in Caucasians. *Clin. Endocrinol.* (Oxf.). 74:783-790.

Vaidya, A., Forman, J. P., Hopkins, P. N., Seely, E. W., Williams, J. S. 2011b. 25-Hydroxyvitamin D is associated with plasma renin activity and the pressor response to dietary sodium intake in Caucasians. *J. Renin. Angiotensin. Aldosterone Syst.* 12:311-319.

Vaidya, A., Forman, J. P., Williams, J. S. 2011c. Vitamin D and the vascular sensitivity to angiotensin II in obese Caucasians with hypertension. *J. Hum. Hypertens.* 25:672-678.

Vaidya, A., Sun, B., Larson, C., Forman, J. P., Williams, J. S. 2012. Vitamin D_3 Therapy Corrects the Tissue Sensitivity to Angiotensin II Akin to the Action of a Converting Enzyme Inhibitor in Obese Hypertensives: An Interventional Study. *J. Clin. Endocrinol. Metab*. 97:2456-2465.

Van Bockxmeer, F. M., Mamotte, C. D., Gibbons, F. A., Burke, V., Taylor, R. R. 1995. Angiotensin-converting enzyme and apolipoprotein E genotypes and restenosis after coronary angioplasty. *Circulation*. 92:2066-2071.

Van Hee, V. C., Adar, S. D., Szpiro, A. A., Barr, R. G., Bluemke, D. A., et al. 2009. Exposure to traffic and left ventricular mass and function: the Multi-Ethnic Study of Atherosclerosis. *Am. J. Respir. Crit. Care Med*. 179:827-834.

Van Hee, V. C., Adar, S. D., Szpiro, A. A., Barr, R. G., Diez Roux, A., et al. 2010. Common genetic variation, residential proximity to traffic exposure, and left ventricular mass: the multi-ethnic study of atherosclerosis. *Environ. Health Perspect*. 118:96296-9.

Vinh, A., Widdop, R. E., Drummond, G. R., Gaspari, T. A. 2008. Chronic angiotensin IV treatment reverses endothelial dysfunction in ApoE-deficient mice. *Cardiovasc. Res*. 77:178-187.

Wang, G., Tam, L. S., Li, E. K., Kwan, B. C., Chow, K. M., et al. 2011a. Serum and urinary free microRNA level in patients with systemic lupus erythematosus. *Lupus*. 20:493-500.

Wang, W. L., Chatterjee, N., Chittur, S. V., Welsh, J., Tenniswood, M. P. 2011b. Effects of 1α,25 dihydroxyvitamin D3 and testosterone on miRNA and mRNA expression in LNCaP cells. *Mol. Cancer*. 10:58.

Wang, G., Tam, L. S., Kwan, B. C., Li, E. K., Chow, K. M., et al. 2012a. Expression of miR-146a and miR-155 in the urinary sediment of systemic lupus erythematosus. *Clin. Rheumatol*. 31:435-440.

Wang, Y., Borchert, M. L., Deluca, H. F. 2012b. Identification of the vitamin D receptor in various cells of the mouse kidney. *Kidney Int*. 81:993-1001.

Zhang, Z., Zhang, Y., Ning, G., Deb, D. K., Kong, J., Li, Y. C. 2008. Combination therapy with AT1 blocker and vitamin D analog markedly ameliorates diabetic nephropathy: blockade of compensatory renin increase. *Proc. Natl. Acad. Sci. U S* 105:15896-15901

Zhang, Y., Deb, D. K., Kong, J., Ning, G., Wang, Y., et al. 2009. Long-term therapeutic effect of vitamin D analog doxercalciferol on diabetic nephropathy: strong synergism with AT1 receptor antagonist. *Am. J. Physiol. Renal. Physiol.* 297:F791-801.

Zhang, Y., Kong, J., Deb, D. K., Chang, A., Li, Y. C. 2010. Vitamin D receptor attenuates renal fibrosis by suppressing the renin-angiotensin system. *J. Am. Soc. Nephrol.* 21:966-973.

Zhou, C., Lu, F., Cao, K., Xu, D., Goltzman, D., Miao, D. 2008. Calcium-independent and 1,25$(OH)_2D_3$-dependent regulation of the renin-angiotensin system in 1alpha-hydroxylase knockout mice. 74:170-179.

Zhu, F., Sun, Y., Wang, M., Ma, S., Chen, X., et al. 2011. Correlation between HLA-DRB1, HLA-DQB1 polymorphism and autoantibodies against angiotensin AT_1 receptors in Chinese patients with essential hypertension. *Clin. Cardiol.* 34:302-308.

In: Renin-Angiotensin System
Editors: Ayako Himura and Takeshi Sato
ISBN: 978-1-62417-788-0

Chapter VIII

The Renin-Angiotensin System in the Pathogenesis of Intracranial Aneurysms and Its Complications

***Christoph J. Griessenauer*[1], *Joel Raborn*[1], *R. Shane Tubbs*[1], *Martim Mortazavi*[1] *and Mohammadali M. Shoja*[1,2*]**
[1]Pediatric Neurosurgery, Children's Hospital, Birmingham, AL and Division of Neurosurgery, University of Alabama at Birmingham, AL, USA
[2]Medical Philosophy and History Research Center, Tabriz University of Medical Sciences, Tabriz, Iran

Abstract

"In recent years, the pathophysiology of intracranial (cerebral) aneurysms has been explored by several studies and multiple factors involved in the formation and rupture of intracranial aneurysms have been identified. Currently, researches indicate that the renin-angiotensin system (RAS) is one of the many factors potentially involved in the pathogenesis of intracranial aneurysms. This chapter discusses the pathogenesis of intracranial aneurysms, the nature and pathophysiology of the RAS, and how the RAS, specifically the brain RAS, plays a role in the pathogenesis of intracranial aneurysms."

Introduction

In recent years, the pathophysiology of intracranial (cerebral) aneurysms (IAs) has been explored and multiple factors involved in the formation and rupture of IAs have been identified. Currently, research indicates that the Renin-Angiotensin System (RAS) is one of

* Correspondence: Mohammadali M. Shoja, MD 1600 7th Avenue South ACC 400 Birmingham, AL 35233 USA, E-mail: shoja.m@gmail.com, Phone: 001-2057670575 Fax: 001-2059399972.

the many factors potentially involved in the pathogenesis of IAs. [52] This chapter discusses the pathogenesis of IAs, the nature and pathophysiology of the RAS, and how the RAS, specifically the brain RAS, plays a role in the pathogenesis of IAs.

Pathophysiology of Intracranial Aneurysms

IAs are classified as saccular, commonly referred to as 'berry aneurysms', dissecting, and fusiform. They may be caused by inherited conditions, [36, 43] or other acquired factors including head trauma, infection[4] and head and neck tumors. [58] One of the most important risk factors for IAs appears to be hypertension, including factors contributing to hypertension such as atherosclerosis, cigarette smoking and drug or alcohol abuse. [8, 14, 43].

Several biological factors play a role in the pathogenesis of IAs. First, extracellular matrix (ECM) degradation may play an important role in the formation and progression of aneurysms. Matrix metalloproteinases (MMPs) attack elastic fibers in the arterial wall and are inhibited by tissue inhibitors of matrix metalloproteinases (TIMPs). [38] TIMP-1 and TIMP-2 in arterial walls are down-regulated early in the pathogenic process, while later stages show highly elevated levels of MMP activity.

When the balance between MMPs and TIMPs is changed, the arterial wall structure is altered, which may lead to the development of IA. [2] Next, tumor necrosis factor-alpha (TNFα) and the Fas death pathway were up-regulated in weakened cerebral arterial walls, though interleukin-10 (IL-10) was not, implying the involvement of apoptosis in the pathogenesis of IA. [27] Another factor in the pathogenesis of IA may include inflammation, especially the recruitment macrophages and neutrophils secreting endothelin and free radicals. NF-κB was found to be up-regulated in the cerebral artery walls early in pathogenesis, inducing the expression of genes involved in the recruitment and activation of macrophages. [3, 21].

Furthermore, sodium balance has been examined in the pathogenesis of IA. In spontaneously hypertensive stroke-prone rats, sodium loading increased the incidence of IA. [61] Finally, multiple genes have been associated in the predisposition to IA, although more research is necessary because genetic issues such as low penetrance, late onset, and uncertain modes of inheritance have inhibited efforts to determine susceptibility loci. Many of the genes currently implicated in the pathogenesis of IAs relate to genes involved in vascular development and repair, muscle activity, cell adhesion, inflammation, and components of the ECM. For instance, small nucleotide polymorphisms (SNPs) identified on chromosome 9p involve gene CDKN2A that is associated with various arterial diseases including IA, while SNPs on loci 8q probably act through SOX17 and play a role in development and repair of vasculature. [7].

Another study of global gene expression patterns of ruptured IA and unruptured IA compared to control arteries showed that muscle activity and cell adhesion were down-regulated while the inflammatory response was up-regulated, suggesting a role in the pathogenesis of IAs. [42] In a similar gene expression study of aneurysm walls compared to control temporal arteries, differential expression was found in focal adhesion, ECM receptor interactions, cell communication, the inflammatory response, and apoptosis. [51].

The Renin-Angiotensin System

With widespread effects on the cardiovascular system including the brain, the RAS is responsible for the intricate balance between vasoconstriction and vasorelaxation [10, 18] as well as maintaining the vascular wall. [39] The RAS has been associated with both systemic and local vascular diseases, including hypertension, atherosclerosis, and aneurysms, when not functioning properly. [10, 13, 17, 34]. In the kidney, the enzyme renin is produced by the juxtaglomerular cells in response to decreased sodium chloride delivery in the distal convoluted tubule and decreased intrarenal blood pressure. [24] This enzyme acts to cleave angiotensinogen, an α2 globulin zymogen constitutively produced by the liver. Angiotensinogen plasma levels are elevated by corticosteroids, thyroxin, estrogen, and angiotensin II (Ang II). [35].

Renin cleaves the N-terminus of angiotensinogen to form angiotensin I, [24] which is then cleaved again at the C-terminus by an isoform of angiotensin-converting enzyme (ACE) found primarily in the capillary endothelia of the lungs to produce Ang II. [12, 20]. Ang II acts on angiotensin receptor type 1 (AT1) and 2 (AT2) [20, 56] to regulate renal blood flow, glomerular filtration, and aldosterone secretion from the adrenal cortex. In addition, Ang II produces a vasoconstrictor action by binding to AT1 on vascular smooth muscle cells (VSMCs) [44] activating the G_q protein, and thus resulting in muscle contraction through the IP3 pathway. [50].

Along with calcium mobilization and influx via the IP3 pathway to produce muscle contraction, [9] activation of VSMC AT1 leads to VSMC proliferation and hypertrophy through increased DNA synthesis and gene expression of contractile proteins. [10, 23] Conversely, when Ang II activates AT1 on endothelial cells (EC), endothelial nitric oxide (NO) synthase (eNOS) is activated to produce NO and create a vasodilatory effect as well as inhibit proliferation in the neighboring VSMCs. [15, 45] Additionally, Ang II acts on AT2 to activate eNOS through the bradykinin-dependent pathway [60] and to induce prostaglandin production, [24] both causing vasodilation. Thus, Ang II is an important mediator in regulating vasodilation and vasoconstriction and vascular wall integrity, depending on the type of cells (VSMC or EC) acted upon. [49] In circulation, Ang II appears to have more interaction with ECs to promote vasodilation and inhibit VSMC proliferation, promoting vascular wall atrophy. In contrast, Ang II from the vascular wall stimulates VSMC proliferation and induces vasoconstriction. The RAS has been shown to have important properties in the brain. [22, 25] Ang II can be transported into or synthesized in the brain since angiotensinogen, renin, ACE, and other catalysts required to generate Ang II can all be synthesized in situ. [33] A receptor bound prorenin present in the brain cleaves angiotensinogen that is mainly produced by astrocytes, [33, 37] and even though ACE is found in small quantities on the cerebral capillary ECs, the quantity of ACE secretion is higher than in other parts of the vasculature. [5] Ang II receptors are located in circumventricular organs and cerebrovascular ECs that respond to tissue and circulating Ang II and inside the blood brain barrier that respond to Ang II both made in and transported into the brain. [47].

Thus, Ang II appears to be involved mostly via AT1 receptors in development including neuronal migration, sensory processing, other cognitive and emotional response functions, and cerebral blood flow. [47] In adults, AT2 receptors are mostly involved in sensory information processing, [47] while AT4 receptors in the brain function in memory. [33] Ang II may play a role in maintaining normal baroreflex control of vasopressin secretion in the hindbrain in conditions of sodium depletion, [11] yet excess Ang II inhibits this baroreceptor reflex and indirectly alters sympathetic tone to the kidneys. [30, 31, 57, 59] Consequently, asRAS plays an important role in the maintenance of the vascular wall, such as balance between vasoconstriction and vasodilation, and regulation of other factors related to blood pressure, that dysfunction in the RAS may be involved in the pathogenesis of hypertension, stroke/ischemia, and aneurysms, as previously mentioned.

The RAS Involvement in the Pathogenesis of Intracranial Aneurysms

The RAS plays a role in several of the many factors associated with IAs, including hypertension, vessel wall integrity, and ECM interactions and dynamics. First, a decrease in expression of AT1 and Ang II may cause a loss of EC and VSMC, weakening the vessel walls. In a study comparing patients with ruptured and unruptured cerebral aneurysms, AT1 and Ang II were down-regulated in both, while ruptured aneurysms showed a larger decrease. [39].

Next, research demonstrates that specific variation in the alleles of the ACE gene may be connected to IAs. In these studies, the I allele represents an insertion polymorphism while the D allele represents a deletion polymorphism. [53] Of the DD, DI, and II genotypes, the II genotype of the ACE gene tends to have the highest association with IAs and is associated with lower concentrations of serum ACE. [36, 118, 120, 121].

In three studies of Polish, [53] British, [36] and Japanese patients, [120] researchers found varying associations between the DI and II genotypes of the ACE gene and IAs. In the Polish study, [53] the II genotype was the independent risk factor for aneurysmal subarachnoid hemorrhage with an odds ratio of 4.57, perhaps due to increased bradykinin activity with this genotype. Nevertheless, a single I genotype did not represent an independent risk factor. [119] Interestingly, the British study of ruptured IAs showed that, although the II genotype represented the majority of IAs in the study, the single I allele may be linked to the incidence of IAs as well. [36] In the Japanese study of saccular IAs, [120] a low DD frequency was detected in patients with aneurysms (6% versus 15% in controls), similar to the Polish study. [28, 46, 53, 55] A similar study of the Caucasian population in the US failed to find any link between the various genotypes of the ACE gene and IAs. [40] Given that these studies were conducted in different parts of the world and included different race and ethnicities, a meta-analysis using the fixed-effect model of the data from these four studies showed an association between the ACE genotype II and subarachnoid hemorrhage or ruptured IAs with an odds ratio of 1.64. [41].

Another association between the RAS and IAs involves the effects of angiotensin receptor blockers, while ACE inhibitors may be associated with IAs but in a RAS independent manner.

The ACE inhibitor imidapril has been shown to reduce the size and medial thinning of induced cerebral aneurysms (CA) in rats. Interestingly, ACE expression and activity was not changed with administration of imidapril, suggesting that this drug's inhibitory effects were independent of the RAS. Furthermore, imidapril inhibited MMP-9 that is upregulated in CA walls, blocking extracellular matrix degradation. Thus, imidapril acts in an ACE independent and MMP-9 dependent manner to reduce the formation of CAs. [26] AT1 blockers, among other drugs that improve vascular wall integrity and prevent injury, may inhibit the formation of aneurysms. In a study of the development of IAs in rats, the effects of an AT1 blocker olmesartan and the statin pravastatin were studied. [29] The results showed that pravastatin reduced fully developed saccular aneurysms at stage III and stage II+III, while olmesartan reduced the fully developed saccular aneurysm at stage III. With these results and since olmesartan and pravastatin inhibit different molecules, these two drugs act on different stages of IA pathogenesis. [1] Although these studies were conducted in rats, a human study of the effects of olmesartan on cerebral hemodynamics in hypertensive patients after stroke showed that autoregulation of cerebral blood flow improved regardless of systemic blood pressure. [32].

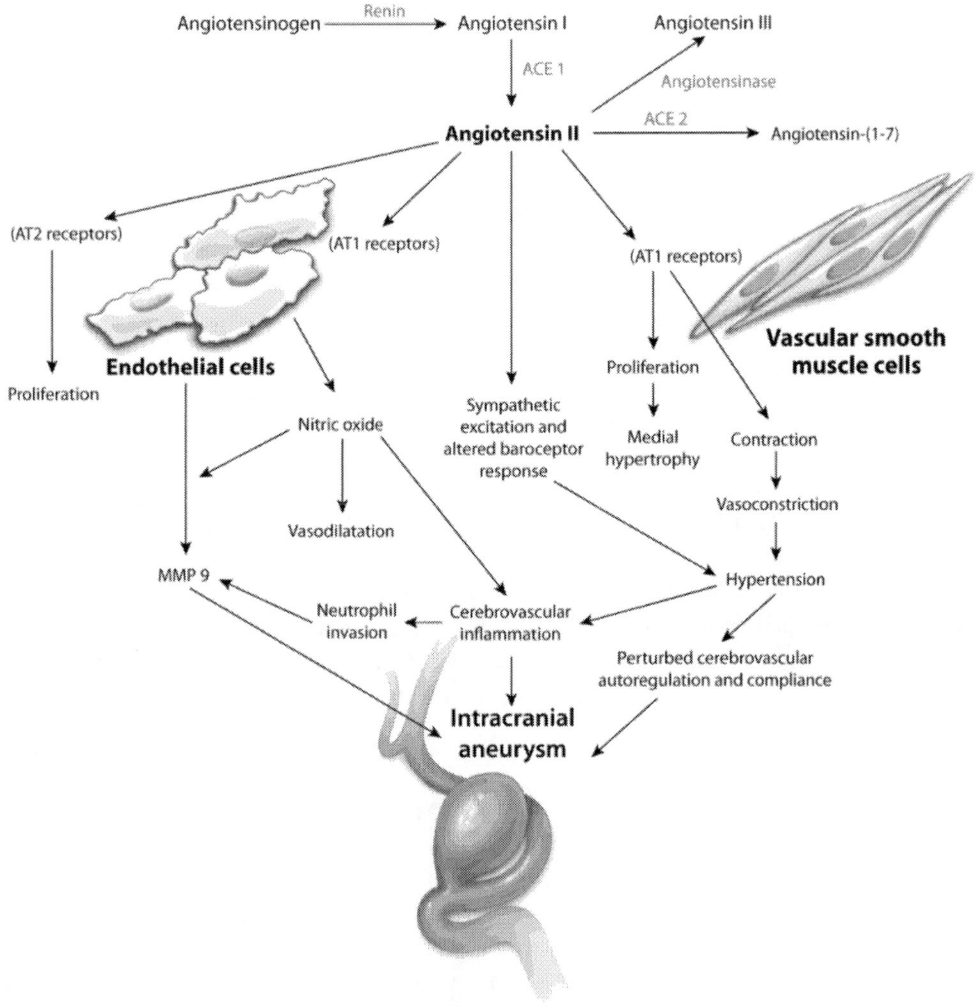

Figure 1. The role of the renin-angiotensin system in the pathogenesis of intracranial aneurysm formation (reproduced from Shoja et al., 2011 [54] ©Journal of the Renin-Angiotensin-Aldosterone System, Volume 12/Issue 3, September/2011, SAGE Publications Ltd./SAGE Publications, Inc).

The RAS is involved in the inflammatory cascade, [19] which is a factor in the pathogenesis of IAs. In the aorta, Ang II up-regulates local expression of vascular endothelial growth factor (VEGF) and its receptor, which have been associated with vascular inflammation. [62] In the adult rat brain, VEGF has been shown to increase vascular permeability, induce angiogenesis, and promote further inflammation. [16] AT1 blockers have anti-inflammatory effects in the brain, [6] and although aneurysms in cerebral and systemic arteries most likely undergo different pathological mechanisms, [4] RAS blockers and other anti-inflammatory medications may be effective against IAs. Finally, aldosterone may play a role in IAs. Aldosterone is a mineralocorticoid that is released from the adrenal cortex in response to Ang II, as well as other signals. In a study conducted with the mineralocorticoid receptor blocker eplerenone in rats, the incidence of IA was lowered when eplerenone was administered. [54] Ang II and nitrotyrosine, as well as the mRNA levels of pro-inflammatory molecules such as ACE 1, NADPH oxidase subunits, and monocyte chemoattractant protein 1, were elevated at the site of the aneurysm compared to surrounding vascular tissue.

Eplerenone reduced the expression of these molecules and inhibited the oxidative stress, inflammation, and RAS. Thus, aldosterone and its receptor may promote the pathogenesis of IAs. Additionally, primary aldosteronism, a condition in which the adrenal glands produce too much aldosterone, may be a risk factor for IAs. [48].

Conclusion

With so many factors playing a role in the pathogenesis of IAs and given the complex intertwine of hormones, enzymes, and other molecules in the RAS, studies associating RAS and IAs should account for these multiple interactions in the RAS and other factors that play a role in the development and progression of IA.

Given current research, there does appear to be an association between the RAS and IAs; however, further investigation is warranted to strengthen this relationship and answer many of the questions that remain elusive.

For instance, the synthesis and distribution of Ang II in the brain and the relationship between AT1 receptor stimulation and inflammation are unknown. With further research, a clearer understanding of the RAS and IAs will become more apparent paving the way for more effective treatment options to prevent or reduce the incidence of IAs.

Acknowledgments

This chapter is an update on the previous publication of the authors (MM Shoja and RS Tubbs) (Journal of the Renin-Angiotensin-Aldosterone System; Year 2011; Volume 12/Issue 3; pp. 262-273). The authors are authorized to use any part of the previous publication for this chapter. The authors would like to thank Dr. Paul S. Agutter and Drs TD Payner, K Ghabili, AA Cohen-Gadol for their assistance and advices.

References

[1] Agata J, Ura N, Yoshida H, Shinshi Y, Sasaki H, Hyakkoku M, Taniguchi S, Shimamoto K (2006) Olmesartan is an angiotensin II receptor blocker with an inhibitory effect on angiotensin-converting enzyme. *Hypertension Research* 29: 865-874.

[2] Aoki T, Kataoka H, Moriwaki T, Nozaki K, Hashimoto N (2007) Role of TIMP-1 and TIMP-2 in the progression of cerebral aneurysms. *Stroke* 38: 2337-2345.

[3] Aoki T, Kataoka H, Shimamura M, Nakagami H, Moriwaki T, Ishibashi R, Nozaki K, Morishita R, Hashimoto N (2007) NF-kappaB is a key mediator of cerebral aneurysm formation. *Circulation* 116: 2830-2840.

[4] Aoki T, Nishimura M, Kataoka H, Ishibashi R, Miyake T, Takagi Y, Morishita R, Hashimoto N (2009) Role of angiotensin II type 1 receptor in cerebral aneurysm formation in rats. *International Journal of Molecular Medicine* 24: 353-359.

[5] Baudin B, Berard M, Carrier J, Legrand Y, Drouet L (1997) Vascular origin determines angiotensin I-converting enzyme expression in endothelial cells. *Endothelium* 5: 73-84.

[6] Benicky J, Sánchez-Lemus E, Pavel J, Saavedra J (2009) Anti-inflammatory effects of angiotensin receptor blockers in the brain and the periphery. *Cellular and Molecular Neurobiology* 29: 781-792.

[7] Bilguvar K, Yasuno K, Niemelä M, Ruigrok Y, von Und Zu Fraunberg M, van Duijn C, van den Berg L, Mane S, Mason C, Choi M, Gaál E, Bayri Y, Kolb L, Arlier Z, Ravuri S, Ronkainen A, Tajima A, Laakso A, Hata A, Kasuya H, Koivisto T, Rinne J, Ohman J, Breteler M, Wijmenga C, State M, Rinkel G, Hernesniemi J, Jääskeläinen J, Palotie A, Inoue I, Lifton R, Günel M (2008) Susceptibility loci for intracranial aneurysm in European and Japanese populations. *Nature Genetics* 40: 1472-1477.

[8] Brisman J, Song J, Newell D (2006) Cerebral aneurysms. *New England Journal of Medicine* 355: 928-939.

[9] Brock T, Alexander R, Ekstein L, Atkinson W, Gimbrone MJ (1985) Angiotensin increases cytosolic free calcium in cultured vascular smooth muscle cells. *Hypertension* 7: I105-109.

[10] Brooks D, Ruffolo R (1994) Functions mediated by peripheral angiotensin II receptors. In: Ruffolo R (ed) Angiotensin II Receptors, Vol 1: Molecular Biology, Biochemistry, Pharmacology and Clinical Perspectives. CRC Press, Boca Raton, Fla, pp 71-102.

[11] Brooks V, Keil L, Reid I (1986) Role of the renin-angiotensin system in the control of vasopressin secretion in conscious dogs. *Circulation Research* 58: 829-838.

[12] Campbell D (1987) Circulating and tissue angiotensin systems. *Journal of Clinical Investigation* 79: 1-6.

[13] Cassis L, Helton M, Howatt D, King V, Daugherty A (2005) Aldosterone does not mediate angiotensin II-induced atherosclerosis and abdominal aortic aneurysms. *British Journal of Pharmocology* 144: 443-448.

[14] Clarke M (2008) Systematic review of reviews of risk factors for intracranial aneurysms. *Neuroradiology* 50: 653-664.

[15] Cornwell T, Arnold E, Boerth N, Lincoln T (1994) Inhibition of smooth muscle cell growth by nitric oxide and activation of cAMP-dependent protein kinase by cGMP. *American Journal of Physiology* 267: C1405-1413.

[16] Croll S, Ransohoff R, Cai N, Zhang Q, Martin F, Wei T, Kasselman L, Kintner J, Murphy A, Yancopoulos G, Wiegand S (2004) VEGF-mediated inflammation precedes angiogenesis in adult brain. *Experimental Neurology* 187: 388-402.

[17] Daugherty A, Cassis L (2004) Angiotensin II and abdominal aortic aneurysms. *Current Hypertension Reports* 6: 442-446.

[18] Drenjancevic-Peric I, Phillips S, Falck J, Lombard J (2005) Restoration of normal vascular relaxation mechanisms in cerebral arteries by chromosomal substitution in consomic SS.13BN rats. *American Journal of Physiology Heart and Circulatory Physiology* 289: H188-195.

[19] Emsley H, Tyrrell P (2002) Inflammation and infection in clinical stroke. *Journal of Cerebral Blood Flow and Metabolism* 22: 1399-1419.

[20] Fyhrquist F, Saijonmaa O (2008) Renin-angiotensin system revisited. *Journal of Internal Medicine* 264: 224-236.

[21] Gallo G, Tamargo R (2006) Leukocyte-endothelial cell interactions in chronic vasospasm after subarachnoid hemorrhage. *Neurological Research* 28: 750-758.

[22] Ganten D, Hermann K, Unger T, Lang R (1983) The tissue renin-angiotensin systems: focus on brain angiotensin, adrenal gland and arterial wall. *Clinical and Experimental Hypertension A* 5: 1099-1118.

[23] Geisterfer A, Peach M, Owens G (1988) Angiotensin II induces hypertrophy, not hyperplasia, of cultured rat aortic smooth muscle cells. *Circulation Research* 62: 749-756.

[24] Haber E, Burton J (1979) Inhibitors of renin and their utility in physiologic studies. *Federation Proceedings* 38: 2768-2773.

[25] Haberl R, Decker-Hermann P, Hermann K (1996) Effect of renin on brain arterioles and cerebral blood flow in rabbits. *Journal of Cerebral Blood Flow and Metabolism* 16: 714-719.

[26] Ishibashi R, Aoki T, Nishimura M, Miyamoto S (2012) Imidapril inhibits cerebral aneurysm formation in an angiotensin-converting enzyme-independent and matrix metalloproteinase-9-dependent manner. *Neurosurgery* 70: 722-730.

[27] Jayaraman T, Berenstein V, Li X, Mayer J, Silane M, Shin Y, Niimi Y, Kiliç T, Günel M, Berenstein A (2005) Tumor necrosis factor alpha is a key modulator of inflammation in cerebral aneurysms. *Neurosurgery* 57: 558-564.

[28] Keramatipour M, McConnell R, Kirkpatrick P, Tebbs S, Furlong R, Rubinsztein D (2000) The ACE I allele is associated with increased risk for ruptured intracranial aneurysms. *Journal of Medical Genetics* 37: 498-500.

[29] Kimura N, Shimizu H, Eldawoody H, Nakayama T, Saito A, Tominaga T, Takahashi A (2010) Effect of olmesartan and pravastatin on experimental cerebral aneurysms in rats. *Brain Research* 1322: 144-152.

[30] Lochard N, Silversides D, van Kats J, Mercure C, Reudelhuber T (2003) Brain-specific restoration of angiotensin II corrects renal defects seen in angiotensinogen-deficient mice. *Journal of Biological Chemistry* 278: 2184-2189.

[31] Mathias C (1987) Role of the central nervous system in human secondary hypertension. . *Journal of Cardiovascular Pharmocology* 10: S93-99.

[32] Matsumoto S, Shimodozono M, Miyata R, Kawahira K (2009) Benefits of the angiotensin II receptor antagonist olmesartan in controlling hypertension and cerebral hemodynamics after stroke. *Hypertension Research* 32: 1015-1021.

[33] McKinley M, Albiston A, Allen A, Mathai M, May C, McAllen R, Oldfield B, Mendelsoh F, Chai S (2003) The brain renin-angiotensin system: location and physiological roles. *International Journal of Biochemistry and Cell Biology* 35: 901-918.

[34] Mehta P, Griendling K (2007) Angiotensin II cell signaling: physiological and pathological effects in the cardiovascular system. *American Journal of Physiology Cell Physiology* 292: C82-97.

[35] Ménard J, Bouhnik J, Clauser E, Richoux J, Corvol P (1983) Biochemistry and regulation of angiotensinogen. *Clinical and Experimental Hypertension A* 5: 1005-1019.

[36] Nekrysh S (2000) Association between heritable connective tissue disorders and intracranial aneurysms. *Surgical Neurology* 54: 77-78.

[37] Nguyen G, Burckle C, Sraer J (2003) The renin receptor: the facts, the promise and the hope. *Current Opinion in Nephrology and Hypertension* 12: 51-55.

[38] Nuki Y, Tsou T, Kurihara C, Kanematsu M, Kanematsu Y, Hashimoto T (2009) Elastase-induced intracranial aneurysms in hypertensive mice. *Hypertension* 54: 1337-1344.

[39] Ohkuma H, Suzuki S, Fujita S, Nakamura W (2003) Role of a decreased expression of the local renin-angiotensin system in the etiology of cerebral aneurysms. *Circulation* 108: 785-787.

[40] Pannu H, Tran-Fadulu V, Milewicz D (2005) Genetic basis of thoracic aortic aneurysms and aortic dissections. *American Journal of Medical Genetics Part C Seminars in Medical Genetics* 139C: 10-16.

[41] Peck G, Smeeth L, Whittaker J, Casas J, Hingorani A, Sharma P (2008) The genetics of primary haemorrhagic stroke, subarachnoid haemorrhage and ruptured intracranial aneurysms in adults. *PLoS One* 3: e3691.

[42] Pera J, Korostynski M, Krzyszkowski T, Czopek J, Slowik A, Dziedzic T, Piechota M, Stachura K, Moskala M, Przewlocki R, Szczudlik A (2010) Gene expression profiles in human ruptured and unruptured intracranial aneurysms: what is the role of inflammation? *Stroke* 41: 224-231.

[43] Pfohman M, Criddle L (2001) Epidemiology of intracranial aneurysm and subarachnoid hemorrhage. *Journal of Neuroscience Nursing* 33: 39-41.

[44] Pueyo M, Michel J (1997) Angiotensin II receptors in endothelial cells. *General Pharmacology* 29: 691-696.

[45] Pueyo M, Arnal J, Rami J, Michel J (1998) Angiotensin II stimulates the production of NO and peroxynitrite in endothelial cells. *American Journal of Physiology* 274: C214-220.

[46] Rigat B, Hubert C, Alhenc-Gelas F, Cambien F, Corvol P, Soubrier F (1990) An insertion/deletion polymorphism in the angiotensin I-converting enzyme gene accounting for half the variance of serum enzyme levels. *Journal of Clinical Investigation* 86: 1343-1346.

[47] Saavedra J (2005) Brain angiotensin II: new developments, unanswered questions and therapeutic opportunities. *Cellular and Molecular Neurobiology* 25: 485-512.

[48] Sawada K, Maehara T, Inaji M, Toriyama H, Okada T, Nariai T, Aoyagi M, Doi M, Ohno K (2010) Case of ruptured multiple cerebral aneurysms associated with primary aldosteronism. *No Shinkei Geka* 38: 347-351.

[49] Schulman I, Raij L (2008) The angiotensin II type 2 receptor: what is its clinical significance. *Current Hypertension Reports* 10: 188-193.

[50] Shelat S, Flanagan-Cato L, Fluharty S (1999) Glucocorticoid and mineralocorticoid regulation of angiotensin II type 1 receptor binding and inositol triphosphate formation in WB cells. *Journal of Endocrinology* 162: 381-391.

[51] Shi C, Awad I, Jafari N, Lin S, Du P, Hage Z, Shenkar R, Getch C, Bredel M, Batjer H, Bendok B (2009) Genomics of human intracranial aneurysm wall. *Stroke* 40: 1252-1261.

[52] Shoja M, Agutter P, Tubbs R, Payner T, Ghabili K, Cohen-Gadol A (2011) The role of the renin--angiotensin system in the pathogenesis of intracranial aneurysms. *Journal of the Renin Angiotensin Aldosterone System* 12: 262-273.

[53] Slowik A, Borratynska A, Pera J, Betlej M, Dziedzic T, Krzyszkowski T, Czepko R, Figlewicz D, Szczudlik A (2004) II genotype of the angiotensin-converting enzyme gene increases the risk for subarachnoid hemorrhage from ruptured aneurysm. *Stroke* 35: 1594-1597.

[54] Tada Y, Kitazato K, Tamura T, Yagi K, Shimada K, Kinouchi T, Satomi J, Nagahiro S (2009) Role of mineralocorticoid receptor on experimental cerebral aneurysms in rats. *Hypertension* 54: 552-557.

[55] Takenaka K, Yamakawa H, Sakai H, Yoshimura S, Murase S, Okumura A, Nakatani K, Kimura T, Nishimura Y, Yoshimi N, Sakai N (1998) Angiotensin I-converting enzyme gene polymorphism in intracranial saccular aneurysm individuals. *Neurological Research* 20: 607-611.

[56] Tirapelli C, Fukada S, de Godoy M, de Oliveira A (2006) Analysis of the mechanisms underlying the vasorelaxant action of angiotensin II in the isolated rat carotid. *Life Sciences* 78: 2676-2682.

[57] Wei S, Felder R (2002) Forebrain renin-angiotensin system has a tonic excitatory influence on renal sympathetic nerve activity. *American Journal of Physiology Heart and Circulatory Physiology* 282: H890-895.

[58] Wong G, Knuckey N, Gubbay S (1983) Subarachnoid haemorrhage in children caused by cerebral tumour. *Psychiatry* 46: 449-450.

[59] Yamamoto K, Ueno Y, Arita M, Suruda H, Hano T, Masuyama Y (1988) Contributions of the sympathetic nervous system, vasopressin and baroreceptor function in brain angiotensin II excess-induced hypertension in the dog. *Clinical and Experimental Hypertension A* 10: 309-316.

[60] Yayama K, Okamoto H (2008) Angiotensin II-induced vasodilation via type 2 receptor: role of bradykinin and nitric oxide. *International Immunopharmocology* 8: 312-318.

[61] Zhang W, Liu A, Yi-Ming W, Liu J, Shen F, Su D (2008) Pressor and non-pressor effects of sodium loading on stroke in stroke-prone spontaneously hypertensive rats. *Clinical and Experimental Pharmocology and Physiology* 35: 83-88.

[62] Zhao Q, Ishibashi M, Hiasa K, Tan C, Takeshita A, Egashira K (2004) Essential role of vascular endothelial growth factor in angiotensin II-induced vascular inflammation and remodeling. *Hypertension* 44: 264-270.

In: Renin-Angiotensin System
Editors: Ayako Himura and Takeshi Sato
ISBN: 978-1-62417-788-0

Chapter IX

The Discrepancy of Angiotensin-Converting Enzyme Inhibitor for Contrast-Induced Nephropathy Prophylaxis

Hongliang Cong, Ximing Li and Tingting Li
Department of Cardiology, Tianjin Chest Hospital, Tianjin, China

Abstract

Contrast-induced nephropathy (CIN) is reported to be the third leading cause of acute renal failure.The role of angiotensin-converting enzyme (ACE) inhibitors in CIN is controversial. Some studies pointed out that it was effective in the prevention of CIN, while some concluded that it was a risk for CIN, especially for patients with pre-existing renal impairment. Nevertheless, it is a common practice in many centers to prescribe ACE inhibitors before coronary angiography. The most likely mechanisms leading to CIN are medullary hypoxia due to decreased renal blood flow (RBF) secondary to renal artery vasoconstriction and direct tubular toxicity by contrast media. Furthermore, experimental data suggest that an activated renin-angiotensin-aldosterone system, increased endothelin-1, and reactive oxygen species play a role in the pathogenesis of CIN and these can be inhibited by using ACE inhibitors.

In this context, we review the medical literatures and discuss the pathogenesis, the role of renin-angiotensin-aldosterone system on the development of CIN and ACEI's effect on CIN.

Introduction and Background

With the increasing use of contrast media (CM) for diagnostic and interventional procedures, nephropathy induced by CM has become the third leading cause of hospital-acquired acute renal failure, accounting for 12% of cases [1]. Although there is no universally accepted definition, CIN refers to the development of acute renal impairment following the intravascular administration of radiocontrast in the absence of other identifiable causes of renal failure. Most studies have used a 25% elevation in serum creatinine (SCr) or an absolute increase of 0.5 mg/dL (44 μmol/L) 2 to 3 days following CM administration [2].

The incidence of CIN is usually <2% in patients who do not have any risk factor for CIN, but it can rise up to 50% or more in patients with multiple risk factors [3]. CIN most commonly occurs in patients with pre-existing renal impairment, diabetes mellitus, congestive heart failure, hypovolemia, increased volume of CM, advanced age, and concurrent intake of potentially nephrotoxic drugs [4-7]. The incidence of CIN is over 20% in patients with renal insufficiency and over 10% in elderly [4, 7].

Patients experiencing CIN have a much worse outcome than patients without CIN following coronary angiography [8], associated with significant consequences, including prolonged hospitalization, the requirement for dialysis, and an increased risk of death [9]. Dangas et al. [10] showed that in-hospital outcome rates, such as of death (6.3% vs. 0.8%), cardiac death (4.0% vs. 0.5%), coronary artery bypass grafting (5.8% vs. 0.5%), major adverse cardiac events (9.3% vs. 1.1%), packed red cell transfusions (28% vs. 6%), and postprocedure length of stay (6.8±7.1 days vs. 2.3±2.5 days), were significantly higher in patients who developed CIN as compared with control patients ($p<0.0001$).Clinical outcomes associated with acute renal failure following cardiac catheterization can be catastrophic, with an in-hospital mortality rate of 20% in unselected patients and a 1-year mortality rate of up to 66% in patients with acute myocardial infarction and pre-existing renal dysfunction [11, 12].

Mechanism Developing CIN

The mechanism by which CM induces nephropathy is complex and not very clear. The proposed mechanisms are medullary hypoxia due to decreased renal blood flow (RBF) secondary to renal artery vasoconstriction and direct tubular toxicity by CM [13, 14]. The viscosity of the CM may play an additional role in contributing to the fall in glomerular filtration rate (GFR) and renal medullary blood flow.

The injection of CM induces early, rapid renal vasodilatation followed by prolonged vasoconstriction, with an increase in intrarenal vascular resistances, a reduction of total RBF and a decrease in GFR. Conversely, the effect on the extrarenal vasculature is transient vasoconstriction that precedes a stable decrease in vascular peripheral resistances [15]. The reduction in renal plasmatic flow is not uniform and occurs especially in the medulla, since medullar perfusion and partial O2 pressure (PO2) are much lower than in the cortex [16].

Direct tubular toxicity has also been proposed, with proximal tubular vacuolar changes and simplification of brush border considered as a characteristic CM-induced tubular injury pattern [17]. Pathological changes induced by contrast medium (e.g. epithelial cell vacuolization, interstitial inflammation and cellular necrosis) suggest a direct toxic effect of contrast media on renal tubular epithelial cells [18, 19]. Apoptosis is also involved as a result of cellular injury [18]. Contrast media have been found to reduce antioxidant enzyme activity in the rat kidney, and direct cytotoxic effects mediated by oxygen free radicals have been found in canine and rat models of contrast-medium nephropathy [18-20]. According to a study conducted on pig's renal cells, lesions on the proximal tubule could be related to CM-induced inhibition of mitochondrial enzymatic activity [21], which is supported by the observed increase in adenosine concentration and evidence of altered metabolism of ATP. In fact, the adenosine itself could be responsible for contrast-induced tubule toxicity.

Other factors that may decrease renal blood flow include increased viscosity of contrast media and increased erythrocyte aggregation induced by contrast media, which results in diminished oxygen delivery [22].

Experimental studies performed on rats who have undergone CM administration have shown decreases in capillary blood flow in the renal papilla, reductions in erythrocyte velocity and O2 tension and increases in erythrocyte aggregation [23]. The hypertonic effect of high osmolality CM reduces the volume and deformability of the erythrocyte membrane, contributing to an increase in haematic viscosity and to the worsening of selective medullar hypoperfusion: in fact, the plasma hyperviscosity can alter RBF particularly in the inner medulla, where the haemoconcentration is usually increased. It has been suggested that the higher viscosity of iodixanol may cause a reduced transit time of these agents in the renal tubules and subsequent increased tubular pressures, which in turn can cause a decrease in glomerular filtration rate [18].

Therefore, most authors agree that the peculiar viscosity of some CM can play a role in the pathogenesis of CIN, at least in animal studies [23].

Renin-Angiotensin-Aldosterone System Activated during Administratin of CM

Experimental data suggest that an activated renin-angiotensin-aldosterone system, increased endothelin-1, and reactive oxygen species play a role in the pathogenesis of CIN [22, 24]. Endothelin-1, renin, and angiotensin II are some of the potential mediators leading to intrarenal vasoconstriction in experimental models of CIN [15, 22].

A few studies on the action of angiotensin II have been done on sodium-depleted dogs, in which this depletion accentuates both the magnitude and duration of the vasoconstrictive phase of the RBF response to injection of CM, and the blockade of the intrarenal renin–angiotensin system shortens the duration of this response [25]. Animal models of acute renal failure have been induced by administration of a CM bolus, following activation of the renin–angiotensin system by sodium restriction and PG synthesis inhibition with indomethacin [26]. Activation of the renin–angiotensin system could cause vasoconstriction of the efferent glomerular arteriole while at the same time increasing the ex novo synthesis of vasodilator prostaglandins resulting in almost stable or slightly increased intrarenal resistance.

From above all, renin–angiotensin system contribute to the development of CIN [31]. Theoretically, RAS as potential mediators can be inhibited by ACE inhibitors [28-32]. Inhibition of angiotensin II prevents vasoconstriction and generation of reactive oxygen species and increases the synthesis and bioactivity of nitric oxide [29, 31, 32]. However, The available data on the use of angiotensin converting enzyme inhibitors with its associated risks for CIN are sparse and conflicting [27, 33].

Paradoxical Literatures for ACE Inhibitor's Effect on CIN

Some reports have implicated ACEI as nephrotoxic and exacerbating renal failure with CIN, especially for patients with pre-existing renal impairment [34] and the olderly [35]. ACEIs can often cause a decrease in GFR and can increase serum creatinine, which may predispose to the development of CIN in patients taking ACEIs.

Toprak O [36] performed a randomized controlled study in 80 patients with serum creatinine below 2 mg/dL, who were assigned to captopril group (n=48) and control group(n=32). 5 patients (10.4%) in the captopril group developed CIN, compared with only one patient (3.1%) in the control group (p = 0.02). Krusová D et al. [37] showed combination of ACEI and furosemide is risky medication which resulted in a significant statistical decline in GFR and a rise in proteinuria in the sub-group.ACEI is harmful for renal function when coronary angiography [38]. Some published reviews on the subject have suggested to hold these drugs for 24 hours prior to an angiogram [24, 39].

Other reports have pointed out the use of ACEI to protect the kidneys from the effects of CIN and under normal conditions, ACEI are not nephrotoxic [29]. It has been speculated that ACEIs may confer protection against CIN by counteracting afferent arteriolar vasoconstriction and subsequent medullary ischemia caused by angiotensin II activation after CM administration.A study by Gupta et al. [28] in India randomized patients to captopril 25 mg TID for three days (starting one hour prior to contrast administration) and found a 79 percent risk reduction in developing CIN compared to controls who received no therapy.Patients with moderate renal impairment treated with ACEIs were ever reported to have no significant change in their serum creatinine 48 hours after procedure compared with patients not receiving ACEIs [40]. Using a large prospectively collected database of 7,230 patients undergoing a coronary intervention, ACEIs were found retrospectively to decrease the risk of CIN by 39% in patients with GFR<60 ml/min [5]. It signified that ACEI has a potentially protective effect on the renal function of patients undergoing coronary angioplasty.

Caldicott et al. showed that renal vasoconstriction occurs after CM administration, and the renin–angiotensin system is responsible for this vasoconstriction [41]. ACEIs preferentially dilate the efferent arteriole, and therefore increase the renal medullary plasma flow by diminishing the filtration fraction. It is conceivable that ACEIs could mitigate a decrease in the reduction of medullary blood flow induced by the contrast agent.Inhibition of angiotensin II prevents vasoconstriction and generation of reactive oxygen species and increases the synthesis and bioactivity of nitric oxide [29]. Moreover, angiotensin II injection aggravates CIN in rats [42]. Conversely, in the presence of acute contrast-induced reduction of renal blood flow, blunting the vasoconstriction of efferent arteries by angiotensin II may have a deleterious effect on GFR by reducing the intraglomerular pressure. These opposite effects explain probably why the studies to date have been controversial on this issue.

As the role of ACE inhibitors in CIN is paradoxical and under the condition that it is widely used in clinical practices before CM administration, larger randomized controlled trials are urgently required to furtherly and deeply investigate the role of ACE inhibitors in the development of CIN.

References

[1] Nash, K., Hafeez, A., Hou, S. Hospital-acquired renal insufficiency. *Am. J. Kidney Dis.* 2002;39:930-936.

[2] McCullough, P. A.Contrast-induced acute kidney injury. *J. Am. Coll. Cardiol.*, 2008,51(15):1419-1428.

[3] Omer Toprak, Mustafa Cirit. Risk Factors for Contrast-Induced Nephropathy. *Kidney Blood Press. Res.* 2006;29:84–93.

[4] McCullough, P. A., Soman, S. S. Contrast-induced nephropathy. *Crit. Care Clin.* 2005; 21: 261–280.

[5] Toprak, O., Cirit, M., Bayata, S., Yesil, M. Review of the radiocontrast nephropathy risk profi les and risk stratifi cation. *Anadolu Kardiyol. Derg.* 2004; 4: 331–335.

[6] Mehran, R., Aymong, E. D., Nikolsky, E., et al. A simple risk score for prediction of contrast-induced nephropathy after percutaneous coronary intervention: development and initial validation. *J. Am. Coll. Cardiol.* 2004; 44: 1393–1399.

[7] Kohli, H. S., Bhaskaran, M. C., Muthukumar, T., et al. Treatment-related acute renal failure in the elderly: a hospital-based prospective study. *Nephrol Dial. Transplant.* 2000; 15: 212–217.

[8] Gruberg, L., Mintz, G. S., Mehran, R., et al. The prognostic implications of further renal function deterioration within 48 h of interventional coronary procedures in patients with pre-existent chronic renal insufficiency. *J. Am. Coll. Cardiol.* 2000;36: 1542–1548.

[9] Rihal, C. S., Textor, S. C., Grill, D. E., et al. Incidence and prognostic importance of acute renal failure after percutaneous coronary intervention. *Circulation.* 2002; 105: 2259–2264.

[10] Dangas, G., Iakovou, I., Nikolsky, E., et al. Contrast-induced nephropathy after percutaneous coronary interventions in relation to chronic kidney disease and hemodynamic variables. *Am. J. Cardiol.* 2005; 95(1): 13–19.

[11] Liss, P., Carlsson, P. O., Palm, F., Hansell, P. Adenosine A1 receptors in contrast-media induced renal dysfunction in the normal rat. *Eur. Radiol.* 2004; 14: 1297–1302

[12] Best, P. J., Lennon, R., Ting, H. H., et al. The impact of renal insufficiency on clinical outcomes in patients undergoing percutaneous coronary interventions. *J. Am. Coll. Cardiol.* 2002;39:1113-1119.

[13] McCullough, P. A., Stacul, F., Becker, C. R., et al., for the Contrast-Induced Nephropathy Consensus Working Panel.Executive summary. *Rev. Cardiovasc. Med.* 2006;7(4):177–197.

[14] Tumlin, J., Stacul, F., Adam, A., et al. on behalf of the CIN Consensus Working Panel. Pathophysiology of contrast-induced nephropathy. *Am. J. Cardiol.* 2006;98 (Suppl.):14K–20K

[15] Detrenis, S., Meschi, M., Musini, S., Savazzi, G. Lights and shadows on the pathogenesis of contrast-induced nephropathy: state of the art. *Nephrol. Dial. Transplant.* 2005; 20: 1542–1550.

[16] Heyman, S. N., Rosen, S., Brezis, M. Radiocontrast nephropathy: a paradigm for the synergism between toxic and hypoxic insults in the kidney. *Exp. Nephrol.* 1994;2:153–157.

[17] Aspelin, P., Aubry, P., Fransson, S. G., et a1. Nephortoxic effects in high-risk patients undergoing angeography. *N Engl. J. Med.* 2003; 348(6): 491-499.

[18] Ueda, J., Nygren, A., Hansell, P., Ulfendahl, H. R. Effect of intravenous contrast media on proximal and distal tubular hydrostatic pressure in the rat kidney. *Acta Radiologica.* 1993;34:83-87.

[19] Battenfeld, R., Khater, A. el-R, Drommer, W., Guenzel, P., Kaup, F. J. Ioxaglate-induced light and electron microscopic alterations in the renal proximal tubular epithelium of rats. *Invest. Radiol.* 1991;26:35-39.

[20] Hizoh, I., Haller, C. Radiocontrast-induced renal tubular cell apoptosis: hypertonic versus oxidative stress. *Invest. Radiol.* 2002;37:428-434.

[21] Hardiek, K., Katholi, R. E., Ramkumar, V., Deitrick, C. Proximal tubule cell response to radiographic contrast media. *Am. J. Physiol. Renal. Physiol.* 2001; 280: 61–70

[22] Persson, P. B., Hansell, P., Liss, P. Pathophysiology of contrast medium-induced nephropathy. *Kidney Int.* 2005; 68: 14–22.

[23] Lancelot, E., Idee, J. M., Couturier, V., et al. Influence of the viscosity of iodixanol on medullary and cortical blood flow in the rat kidney: a potential cause of nephrotoxicity. *J. Appl. Toxicol.* 1999; 19: 341–346

[24] Gami, A. S., Garovic, V. D. Contrast nephropathy after coronary angiography. *Mayo. Clin. Proc.* 2004; 79: 211–219.

[25] Larson, T. S., Hudson, K., Mertz, J. I., et al. Renal vasoconstrictive response to contrast media. The role of sodium balance and the renin-angiotensin system. *J. Lab. Clin. Med.* 1983; 101: 385–391.

[26] Heyman, S. N., Brezis, M., Reubinoff, C. A., et al. Acute renal failure with selective medullary injury in the rat. *J. Clin. Invest.* 1988; 82:401–412.

[27] Toprak, O., Bayata, S., Tanrısev, M. Can we use the ACE inhibitors on prevention of radiocontrast nephropathy? *Turkiye Klinikleri J. Cardiol.* 2004; 17: 375–381.

[28] Gupta, R. K., Kapoor, A., Tewari, S., Sinha, N., Sharma, R. K. Captopril for preventing of contrastinduced nephropathy in diabetic patients: a randomized study. *Indian Heart J.* 1999; 51: 521–526.

[29] Brewster, U. C., Perazella, M. A. The renin-angiotensin- aldosterone system and the kidney: effects on kidney disease. *Am. J. Med.* 2004; 116 (4): 263–272.

[30] Gibbons, G. H. Vasculoprotective and cardioprotective mechanisms of angiotensin-converting enzyme inhibition: the homeostatic balance between angiotensin II and nitric oxide. *Clin. Cardiol.* 1997; 20 (suppl. 2):18–25.

[31] Fleming, I., Kohlstedt, K., Busse, R.: New fACEs to the Renin-Angiotensin System. *J. Appl. Physiol.* 2005; 20: 91–95.

[32] Munzel, T., Keaney, J. F. Jr. Are ACE inhibitors a'magic bullet' against oxidative stress? *Circulation.* 2001; 104: 1571–1574.

[33] Toprak, O., Cirit, M., Bayata, S., et al.The effect of pre-procedural captopril on contrast media induced nephropathy who underwent coronary angiography. *Anadolu Kardiyol. Derg.* 2003;3(2):98-103.

[34] Cirit, M., Toprak, O., Yesil, M., et al. Angiotensin-converting enzyme inhibitors as a risk factor for contrast-induced nephropathy. *Nephron. Clin. Pract.* 2006; 104(1): c20-c27.

[35] Mahajan, S., Tiwari, S., Bhowmik, D., Agarwal, S. K., Tiwari, S. C., Dash, S. C. Factors affecting the outcome of acute renal failure among the elderly population in India: a hospital based study. *Int. Urol. Nephrol.* 2006; 38: 391-396.

[36] Omer Toprak .Letter to the editor:Angiotensin Converting Enzyme Inhibitors and Contrast-Induced Nephropathy. *Renal. Failure.* 2006;28(1): 99 – 100.

[37] Krusová, D., Sevela, K., Králová, D.,et al. Risky medication and contrast media-induced nephropathy in patients with diabetes and hypertension. *Vnitr Lek.* 2006;52(11):1014-1020.

[38] Huber, W., Schipek, C., Ilgmann, K., et al. Effectiveness of theophylline prophylaxis of renal impairment after coronary angiography in patients with chronic renal insufficiency. *Am. J. Cardiol.* 2003;91(10):1157– 1162.

[39] Maeder, M., Klein, M., Fehr, T., Rickli, H.. Contrast nephropathy: review focusing on prevention. *J. Am. Coll Cardiol.* 2004;44(9):1763-1771.

[40] El-Harakeeh, M. A., Kleiner, M., Ahern, K., Saggi, S. Effects of chronic angiotensin receptor blockers and ACE inhibitors use on the incidence of contrast induces nephropathy in patients with chronic renal insufficiency. *J. Am. Soc. Nephrol.* 2004;15:347A, SA-PO214.

[41] Caldicott, W. J., Hollenberg, N. K., Abrams, H. L. Characteristics of response of renal vascular bed to contrast media. Evidence for vasoconstriction induced by renin-angiotensin system. *Invest. Radiol.* 1970;5(6):539–547.

[42] Brezis, M., Greenfeld, Z., Shina, A., Rosen, S. Angiotensin II augments medullary hypoxia and predisposes to acute renal failure. *Eur. J. Clin. Invest.* 1990;20(2):199-207.

Index

A

B

C

D

E

F

G

H

I

J

K

L

M

N

O

P

Q

R

S

T

U

V